Assistive Technology Intervention in Healthcare

Assistive Technology Intervention in Healthcare

Edited by Shruti Jain and Sudip Paul

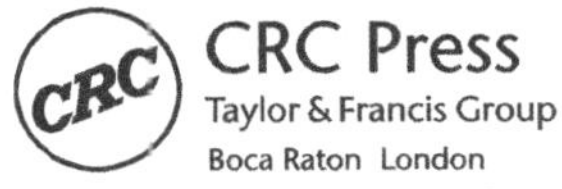

CRC Press is an imprint of the
Taylor & Francis Group, an **informa** business

First edition published 2022
by CRC Press
6000 Broken Sound Parkway NW, Suite 300, Boca Raton, FL 33487–2742

and by CRC Press
2 Park Square, Milton Park, Abingdon, Oxon, OX14 4RN

CRC Press is an imprint of Taylor & Francis Group, LLC

Library of Congress Cataloging-in-Publication Data
Names: Jain, Shruti, editor. | Paul, Sudip, 1984– editor.
Title: Assistive technology intervention in healthcare / edited by Shruti Jain and Sudip Paul.
Description: First edition. | Boca Raton : CRC Press, 2022. | Includes bibliographical references and index.
Identifiers: LCCN 2021032813 | ISBN 9781032075976 (hardback) | ISBN 9781032075983 (paperback) | ISBN 9781003207856 (ebook)
Subjects: LCSH: Medical technology. | Robotics in medicine. | Medical care—Data processing.
Classification: LCC R855.3 .A87 2022 | DDC 610.285—dc23
LC record available at https://lccn.loc.gov/2021032813

ISBN: 978-1-032-07597-6 (hbk)
ISBN: 978-1-032-07598-3 (pbk)
ISBN: 978-1-003-20785-6 (ebk)

DOI: 10.1201/9781003207856

Typeset in Times
by Apex CoVantage, LLC

Contents

Preface

Assistive technology (AT) in healthcare and rehabilitation has had consistent applications in the treatment of and intervention in several conditions. AT is nothing but a type of product, system or equipment used to improve the functional capabilities of different-aged people, from children to older people. It may improve the quality of life and ease dependence on family members or caregivers for the person with disabilities. Nowadays, many types of AT are commercially available on the market, such as hearing aids, wheelchairs, augmented communication, and so on. Internet of Things (IoT)-enabled devices have made remote monitoring possible in the healthcare sector by unleashing the potential to keep patients safe and healthy and enabling medical professionals to provide superlative care.

Adolescent idiopathic scoliosis, commonly known as AIS, is a major severe orthopedic anomaly observed in a significant part of the human population. The disease arises during adolescence and may become fatal if untreated. Detection of the region of interest (RoI) based on histogram analysis, localization of vertebrae segments and edges with the help of advanced image processing methods and deep-learning algorithms has the potential for better treatment strategies. The IoT has revealed a paradigm shift in health, introducing benefits like availability, accessibility and cost-effective delivery of individualized care. Enabling such a shift requires that hardware and software work together to enable widespread technical innovations. Electronic health records (EHRs) are becoming popular among radiologists, clinicians, pharmacists, healthcare providers and researchers for effective treatment and diagnosis, as they contain confidential and critical information about patients.

Reversible logic (RL) has received immense consideration in recent years due to its ability to lower power dissipation. There are six different types of reversible gates, based on simulation and evaluation of different parameters using Verilog and SPICE; the Toffoli gate shows remarkable results. Using a Toffoli gate, different combinational and sequential circuits are designed and simulated using both reversible and irreversible logic. It has been observed that results using reversible logic are exceptional.

COVID-19 has bought about disruptive and transformative digital automation in the health sector worldwide with multifold investments in upgrades. The situation has led to many developing cost-effective digital health technologies by using existing smartphones and integrating smart watches. Epilepsy disease management systems can also be made affordable. Among these, the technique known as segmented microaneurysm using the measures of entropy, skewness and kurtosis gives high performance regardless of image contrast. Augmented continuous particle swarm optimization successfully detects microaneurysms and helps to diagnose diabetic retinopathy in the early stages in an efficient way. In the same way, another technique known as computational fluid dynamics (CFD) has been an effective tool for obtaining insight into the circulatory system's physical functioning. Similarly, gait analysis has become a significant way to gauge movement debilities and provide therapeutic interventions in the early phases of neurological diseases.

Biosensors are analytical devices used for identifying alterations in biological processes or biological elements such as tissues, cells, acids, enzymes or microorganisms, converting them to electrical signals. A biosensor is a combination of transducer and biological sensing elements used for modifying data into electric signals. Autism spectrum disorder (ASD) is a neurodevelopmental disability that impairs the social interaction and communication skills of an individual and can include repetitive behavior. The behavioral features of ASD emerge during the later part of the first and second years of life. The early detection of abnormalities in an EEG may be used as a biomarker for developmental cognitive disorders and is emphasized in this book.

Acknowledgments

We want to extend our gratitude to all the chapter authors for their sincere and timely support to make this book a grand success. We are equally thankful to all Taylor & Francis/CRC Press executive board members for their kind approval and granting permission for us as editors of this book. We want to extend our sincere thanks to *Dr. Gagandeep Singh* and other members of Taylor & Francis/CRC Press for their valuable suggestions and encouragement throughout the project.

It is with immense pleasure that we express thankfulness to our colleagues for their support, love and motivation in all our efforts during this project. We are grateful to all the reviewers for their timely reviews and consent, which helped us improve the quality of the book.

We may have inadvertently left out many others, and we sincerely thank all of them for their help.

Dr. Shruti Jain
Dr. Sudip Paul

Editors

Dr. Shruti Jain is an associate professor in the Department of Electronics and Communication Engineering at Jaypee University of Information Technology, Waknaghat, H.P., India, and received her doctor of science (DSc) in electronics and communication engineering. She has around 16 years of teaching experience. She has filed five patents, of which one has been granted and four are published. She has published more than 21 book chapters and 125 research papers in reputed indexed journals and at international conferences. She has also published 12 books. She has completed two government-sponsored projects. She has guided six PhD students and now has four registered students; and has also guided 11 MTech scholars and more than 90 BTech undergraduates. Her research interests are image and signal processing, soft computing, bio-inspired computing and computer-aided design of FPGA and VLSI circuits. She is a senior member of IEEE, life member and editor in chief of the Biomedical Engineering Society of India and a member of IAENG. She is a member of the editorial board of many reputed journals. She is also a reviewer of many journals and a member of TPCs of different conferences. She was awarded the Nation Builder Award in 2018–19.

Dr. Sudip Paul is currently an assistant professor and teacher in-charge in the Department of Biomedical Engineering, School of Technology, North-Eastern Hill University (NEHU), Shillong, India. He completed his postdoctoral research at the School of Computer Science and Software Engineering, University of Western Australia, Perth. He was an awardee of one of the most prestigious fellowships (Biotechnology Overseas Associateship for the Scientists Working in the North Eastern States of India: 2017–18 supported by the Department of Biotechnology, Government of India). He received his PhD from the Indian Institute of Technology (Banaras Hindu University), Varanasi, with a specialization in electrophysiology and brain signal analysis. He has also organized many workshops and conferences; the most significant are the IEEE Conference on Computational Performance Evaluation 2020, IRBO/APRC Associate School 2017 and 29th Annual Meeting of the Society for Neurochemistry, India, 2015. Dr. Sudip has published more than 40 international journal papers and more than 35 conference papers on different international/national platforms. He has filed eight patents, out of which one has been granted. He completed more than ten book projects for Springer Nature, Elsevier, IGI Global, and so on. Dr. Sudip is a member of different societies and professional bodies, including APSN, ISN, IBRO, SNCI, SfN, IEEE and IAS. He has received many awards, including the World Federation of Neurology (WFN) traveling fellowship, Young Investigator Award, IBRO Travel Award and ISN Travel Award. Dr. Sudip has also contributed his knowledge to different international journals as an editorial board member and reviewer. He has presented his research accomplishments in many countries including the United States, Greece, France, South Africa and Australia.

Contributors

N. Madhu Baala is a senior physiotherapist at Gleneagles Global Health City, Chennai, India. She is a qualified postgraduate in physiotherapy with 12+ years' experience specializing in clinical knowledge and competencies in assessment, examination, diagnosis, treatment and rehabilitation in recent trends. She holds experience in teaching international students at the International Human Resource Development Centre and is also experienced in conducting ergonomic sessions in the IT and BPO sectors. She is certified in reiki, an alternative healing therapy. She holds lifetime membership in the Indian Association of Physiotherapists and is also a member of the Singapore Physiotherapy Association.

Hritam Basak is a senior undergraduate student pursuing a BE in electrical engineering at Jadavpur University, India, and will be graduating in 2021. His research interests lie in the domain of deep learning and computer vision, and he has vast experience in the domain, having authored several papers.

C. Chandralekha completed a PhD at Anna University, Chennai. She is currently serving as the Head of IT Wing, Unnadha Ulagam, Coimbatore, Tamilnadu, India. She has many publication credits, including Annexure–II, Web of Science, Springer Lecture Series, UGC Care Groups and many international journals. She has organized and conducted several international, national and state-level webinars, seminars, guest lectures, awareness programs, webinar series and faculty development programs.

Pradeep Kumar Chaudhary received a BE in electrical and electronics engineering from Rajiv Gandhi Technological University, Bhopal, India, in 2016 and an MTech in electrical engineering from the National Institute of Technology Hamirpur, India, in 2018. Currently, he is pursuing a PhD in electrical engineering from the Indian Institute of Technology, Indore, India. His current research interests include medical signal processing, image processing and machine learning. He has published several research papers for reputed international journals and conference papers. He served as a reviewer for *Biomedical Signal Processing and Control* and the *IEEE Sensor Journal*.

K.K. Deepak is currently serving as head of the Department of Physiology at AIIMS, New Delhi, India. He initiated the Autonomic Function Lab in the department in 1989. It was the first lab of its kind in the country. It has been providing patient care services and a platform for research in clinical physiology. To date, over 16,000 human subjects have been investigated in this lab. He has a deep interest in biomedical engineering. He developed a blood pressure simulation model. He was involved in harnessing EEG and EOG signals for the purpose of moving prostheses. He developed the techniques of EMG biofeedback for patients of hand dystonia. He also set up a technique for recording gastric motility from the surface called electrogastrography (EGG) for the first time in India. He has also been interested in designing and developing software for analysis of physiological signals. His team has indigenously developed software for quantification of autonomic tone. He has more than 90 full-length refereed research papers published in indexed journals and has written 13 chapters in various books. He has co-authored three books. His work has been abstracted in more than 260 scientific communications.

Santosha K. Dwivedy received a PhD in mechanical engineering from the Indian Institute of Technology Kharagpu (IIT Kharagpur), India, in 2000. He is currently professor in the Department of Mechanical Engineering at the Indian Institute of Technology Guwahati (IIT Guwahati). He was also a visiting professor at the Institute of Engineering and Computational Mechanics, University of Stuttgart, Germany, under the DAAD-IIT Faculty Exchange Scheme. He has over 180 journal and conference publications, with a focus on integrating robotics and dynamics in various fields. His research interests include both industrial and medical robotics, biomechanics, nonlinear vibration and control, along with applications.

Renuka Garg completed her graduation and masters in chemical engineering. She is pursuing her PhD in the field of nanotechnology. She has published research papers in reputed journals. She has also filed two patents. One is under evaluation, and the second is published.

Vandana Guleria completed her PhD under the mentorship of Dr. Varun Jaiswal, assistant professor at Shoolini University Himachal Pradesh. She has been awarded for her doctoral studies at Shoolini University Himachal Pradesh and her thesis entitled "Comparative Transcriptome Analysis of Different Stages of Plasmodium Falciparum for Discovery of Vaccine and Drug Candidates." Most of her work involves computational study. Her doctoral research work has been published in the *Genomics Journal* and *International Journal of Plant Research*. She has published a good range of research articles in reputed journals and book chapters at publishing houses like NOVA Publications and Springer. She was actively involved in computational work in NGS analysis. During her academic career, she secured 82% in master of philosophy (biotechnology) as well as the first division in her postgraduate degree in bioinformatics.

N. Hemapriya is an aspiring web developer and a machine-learning enthusiast currently pursuing her undergraduate in information technology from St Joseph's College of Engineering at Anna University. She has crafted a role as a "change leader" at the World Youth Council, a part of Google's Women Tech Makers (WTM), and is a member of the Computer Society of India (CSI). She is an active volunteer at the NGO "Asha for Education"–Chennai chapter, mentoring in the education of underprivileged children. She has served as a project intern at Grroom, a tech-based fashion start-up, and was a part of the TakenMind Global internship program recognized by the United Nations SDGs. Her current research interests include medical image analysis, blockchain technology, GANs and NLP. She is deeply interested in crafting and implementing research papers, ML frameworks and libraries. She is a recipient of the AICTE-sponsored Lilavati Award 2020 and runner-up at the GovTechThon for a project on blockchain-based seed certification.

Varun Jaiswal is a researcher of Indian origin working in the area of bioinformatics, which spans medical informatics to artificial intelligence and genomics of hosts and pathogens. He is presently working as assistant professor at Gachon University South Korea. He is an alumnus of JNU, New Delhi, and served as assistant director in the National Centre of Disease Control (NCDC), New Delhi. During the COVID-19 pandemic, he played a key role in the development of the initial testing, training and genome-sequencing facility to combat COVID-19 in India at the NCDC with high-end machines such as COBAS 6800 and Illumina NextSeq. He has expertise in dry- and wet-lab experiments and administration. He has applied machine-learning methods in diverse fields which include biology, chemistry, medicine, computer science and social science. He has authored dozens of research papers in reputed top-tier journals of diverse fields. Several students have completed their PhD and master's degrees under his able guidance. He prefers to work with new and emerging technology to answer different challenging problems of the nation and the world. He strongly believes that artificial intelligence powered by machine learning will change the global scenario in favor of humanity in almost all fields.

A.K. Jayanthy is a professor in the Department of Biomedical Engineering. She received her PhD and MTech from the Indian Institute of Technology, Madras, in the field of biomedical optics and biomedical engineering. Her articles have appeared in *Optics and Lasers in Engineering*; the *International Journal of Biomedical and Biological Engineering*; *Biomedical Engineering: Applications, Basis and Communications*; the *Journal of Supercomputing*; and others. She has around 23 years of teaching experience, 4.5 years of research experience and 2 years of industrial experience. She is a fellow member of the Institute of Biomedical Engineers (India), fellow member of the Institute of Engineers (India), life member of the Indian Society for Technical Education and also a life member of the Biomedical Engineering Society of India. Her fields of interest are biomedical optics, biomedical sensors, EEG signal analysis and wearable devices.

Shashi Kala is a young bioinformatician who is a postgraduate in bioinformatics at Guru Nanak Dev University, Amritsar. She is a bronze medal holder in master's. She did research work on "Computational Analysis of Textile Dyes Decolorizing Plant Peroxidase Found in Industrial Waste Water" during her master's. Her areas of interest are system biology and meta-analysis. She also taught for two years as a lecturer in the Department of Bioinformatics at the reputed college of Jalandhar, Punjab, India. Now she is working on some minor projects and wants to continue her journey in bioinformatics to enhance her skills.

S. Karunakaran has 25 years of overall experience and is currently working as an associate professor of spine surgery. He pioneered percutaneous endoscopic lumbar discectomy under local anesthesia for disc prolapse. He was the first in South India to use an INSPACE-interspinous implant for lumbar canal stenosis-keyhole spine surgery under local anesthesia. He has performed more than 1000 spine surgeries for scoliosis, cervical spine pathologies, thoracotomies, laparotomies and disc replacement surgeries. He has presented various papers. He is also an esteemed member of the Tamil Nadu Orthopedic Association, Association of South Indian States, Association of Spine Surgeons of India and Asian Academy of Minimally Invasive Spinal Surgery.

Kunal Kundu is currently a final-year undergraduate student, pursuing a bachelor's of technology (BTech) in the Department of Mechanical Engineering, Indian Institute of Technology, Guwahati. His research interests are in the domains of machine learning, artificial intelligence and robotics.

Rohit Kundu is a junior undergraduate student pursuing a BE in electrical engineering at Jadavpur University, India, and will be graduating in 2022. His research interests lie in the domains of deep learning, computer vision, image and video processing and evolutionary optimization. He has significant experience in working with deep learning for biomedical image diagnosis, having authored several papers in notable peer-reviewed journals and conferences.

G.S. Anandha Mala received a BE from Bharathidhasan University in 1992, an ME from the University of Madras in 2001 and a PhD from Anna University in 2007. Currently she is working as professor at Easwari Engineering College, Chennai, India. She has published more than 100 technical papers in various international journals/conferences. She has 26 years of teaching experience at both the graduate and postgraduate level. She is a recognized supervisor of Anna University, Sathyabama University and Jawaharlal Technological University. She has guided 12 PhD students from Anna University and Jawaharlal Nehru Technological University. She has received a research grant of 20 lakhs from DST under a device development program. She has received the IET CLN Exemplary Teacher Award from IET and Distinguished Women Administrator Award from VIWA. Her areas of interest include natural language processing and image processing.

Qaysar Mohi Ud Din is a research scholar at the SRM Institute of Science and Technology. He has completed his MTech and BTech in biomedical engineering from the Bharath Institute of Science and Technology.

V. Muthulakshmi is currently working as associate professor in the Department of Information Technology, St. Joseph's College of Engineering, Chennai, India. She has a total of 26 years of experience in teaching and research. She received her PhD in philosophy from Anna University, Chennai, India. She holds a bachelor of engineering (BE) in electronics and telecommunication engineering and a master's in computer science and engineering. Her interests include artificial intelligence, machine learning and cloud computing. She has published several papers in national and international refereed journals and conferences. She is a member of various professional organizations such as the Computer Society of India (CSI) and Indian Society for Technical Education (ISTE).

Jyotindra Narayan received his master of engineering (ME) from Thapar University, Patiala, in 2017 with the specialization of CAD/CAM and robotics, where he worked on patient-side medical manipulators. He is currently a PhD student in the Mechanical Engineering Department at the Indian Institute of Technology Guwahati (IIT Guwahati), India. His focused research interests are medical assisted robotics, rehabilitation devices for motion assistance and adaptive as well as intelligent control designs in robotics. Moreover, he employs intelligent and soft computing algorithms in his research. He has substantial experience in kinematics, dynamics and control of robotic devices for medical applications. He has published several in journals, book chapters and conference papers on the broad topic of medical and rehabilitation devices.

Ram Bilas Pachori received a BE with honors in electronics and communication engineering from Rajiv Gandhi Technological University, Bhopal, India, in 2001, and his MTech and PhD in electrical engineering from the Indian Institute of Technology (IIT), Kanpur, India, in 2003 and 2008, respectively. He worked as a postdoctoral fellow at Charles Delaunay Institute, University of Technology of Troyes, France, during 2007–2008. He has been working as a professor in the Department of Electrical Engineering at IIT Indore since 2017. He is also associated faculty with the Department of Biosciences & Biomedical Engineering and Center for Advanced Electronics at IIT Indore. He is an associate editor of *Electronics Letters, Biomedical Signal Processing and Control* and an editor of *IETE Technical Review*. He is a senior member of IEEE and a fellow of IETE and IET. He has 218 publications, which include journal papers, conference papers, books and book chapters. His publications have around 7900 citations with an h index of 47 (Google Scholar, April 2021). His research interests are in the areas of signal and image processing, biomedical signal processing, non-stationary signal processing, speech signal processing, brain-computer interfacing, machine learning and artificial intelligence in healthcare.

Vaidehi Patil is a graduate mechanical engineer from Sardar Patel College of Engineering, Mumbai (2020). She is the creator of TechTackled, a platform to discuss, develop and design technology related to robotics and automation. Her research interests include machine design and robotics, specifically robot manipulation, legged robotics and robot learning.

Pinki Paul is a research scholar in the Department of Management, Banasthali Vidyapith. She completed her MBA from Sikkim Manipal University and has published two international journal papers and three chapters in international books.

S. Poonguzhali is an associate professor in the Department of ECE, CEG, Anna University, Chennai, India, and is also associated with the Centre for Medical Electronics. With about 20 years' experience in the field of biomedical engineering, her research interests include biomedical instrumentation, biomedical image processing and developing low-cost rehabilitation aids, to name a few. She also holds life membership in the Biomedical Society of India. She has published several research papers in this field and has also successfully completed a couple of Government of India-funded projects.

J. Antony Prince is an information technology undergraduate at St. Joseph's College of Engineering, Chennai, with great interest in the field of blockchain. He has six months of experience as a research intern for a US-based start-up in the domains of blockchain and data science. He is functioning as the Microsoft Learn Student Ambassador for his college and is an active member of the Computer Society of India (CSI). He is a Certified Google Python Automation professional. He won the runner-up position under the Blockchain 'Seed-Certification' category in Gov-TechThon 2020, a virtual hackathon organized by IEEE in collaboration with the National Informatics Centre, MeitY, GoI and Oracle. He reached the grand finale of the COVID-19 National Bio-Informatics Hackathon organized by Anna University and endorsed by AICTE. He was selected for the Google FooBar challenge and has contributed open-source code to the Github Arctic Code Vault. He has assisted research work on prediction of CPU job waiting time using regression analysis and also on using generative adversarial networks for super-resolution imaging. He has worked on proofs of concept using blockchain for the digital transformation of the supply chain. Currently, he is researching the potential use cases of decentralized artificial intelligence to combine blockchain with AI.

Geetanjali Rathee received her PhD in computer science engineering from Jaypee University of Information Technology (JUIT), Waknaghat, Himachal Pradesh, India, in 2017. She is currently working as an assistant professor in the Department of Computer Science Engineering and Information Technology at JUIT. Her research interests include handoff security, cognitive networks, blockchain technology, resilience in wireless mesh networking, routing protocols and networking and Industry 4.0. To date, she has approximately 25 publications in peer-reviewed journals and more than 15 publications in international and national conferences. She is also a reviewer for various journals, such as *IEEE Transactions on Vehicular Technology*, *Wireless Networks*, *Cluster Computing*, *Ambience Computing*, *Transactions on Emerging Telecommunications Engineering* and the *International Journal of Communication Systems*.

Rehab A. Rayan is a PhD scholar in public with an epidemiology major and an epidemiologist in the response monitoring and evaluation team of the HIM/WHE where she prepares relevant reports about COVID-19; assists in the data management of COVID-19 and collects indicators relevant to COVID-19. She is also an assistant lecturer in the College of Pharmacy, AASTMT. She is an Erasmus+ Virtual Exchange Facilitator. Furthermore, she has taken part in several international conferences with research abstracts and scientific posters. She is a junior researcher at the UNESCO's Youth Against COVID-19 (YAR) initiative. In addition, she is a volunteer associate editor at *NovelMeds* where she proofreads submitted articles and used to be a peer reviewer at *URNCST Journal* where she reviewed submissions for publication in the journal. She has also worked for Caritas Egypt as Counselling and Health Promotion Associate in a UNHCR project that provides refugees with primary healthcare services.

R. Reena Roy received her BTech from Anna University in 2012 and ME from Anna University in 2014. Currently, she is working as assistant professor in the Department of Information Technology in Easwari Engineering College, Chennai, India. She has six years of teaching experience. She has published various research papers in various international journals/conferences. Her research area of interest are data mining, artificial intelligence and image processing.

Hemraj Saini is currently working as associate professor in the Department of Computer Science & Engineering, Jaypee University of Information Technology, Waknaghat. Prior to that, he worked in AIET, Alwar (2011–2012); OEC, Bhubaneswar (2008–2011); HIE, Baniwalid (Libya) (2007–2008); BITS, Pilani (2005–2007); IET, Alwar (2001–2005); REIL, Jaipur (2000–2001); and Dataman System, Delhi (1999–2000), for almost 20 years in academics, administration and industry. He obtained a PhD (computer science) from Utkal University, VaniVihar, Bhubaneswar; MTech (information technology) from Punjabi University, Patiala; and BTech (computer science and engineering) from Regional Engineering College, Hamirpur (H.P.), now NIT. Five PhDs have been awarded under his valuable guidance. He is an active member of various professional technical and scientific associations, such as IEEE, ACM, IAENG and others. Presently, he is providing his services in various modes like editor; member of editorial boards; member of different subject research committees; reviewer for international journals and conferences, including Springer, Science Direct, IEEE, Wiley, IGI Global, Bentham Science and others; and resource person for various workshops and conferences. He has published more than 140 research papers in international/national journals and conferences of repute.

S. Saranya has 10+ years' experience in teaching and research in the biomedical division of the Department of ECE, CEG, Anna University, Chennai. Her research interests include biosignal processing and biomechanics with expertise in human movement analysis and musculoskeletal modeling. Her research focuses on the realization of enabling technologies for personalized rehabilitative therapy. She has many refereed publications to her credit. She also holds a life membership in the Biomedical Society of India.

Vishwajeet Shankhwar received his BTech in electronics and communication engineering from IP University, Delhi, and his MTech in control and instrumentation from the National Institute of Technology, Jalandhar, India, in 2016 and is currently pursuing his PhD in the area of biomedical signal processing from the National Institute of Technology, Jalandhar, India. His research interests include biomedical signal processing, space physiology, microgravity countermeasures, computational fluid dynamics and cardiovascular. He holds a lifetime membership in the Association of Physiologists and Pharmacologists of India. He has patents filed on a microgravity countermeasure device.

Ajay Sharma is currently a PhD research scholar in the Department of Biotechnology and Bioinformatics at Jaypee University of Information Technology, Solan, Himachal Pradesh. Before joining JUIT, he obtained his master's degree in computer science and bachelor's degree in bioinformatics from Shoolini University. Mr. Ajay obtained his diploma in computer science from Lovely Professional University, Jalandhar, Punjab. During his bachelor's, he received the certificate of merit.

Ghanshyam Shivhare is currently a final-year undergraduate student, pursuing a bachelor of technology (BTech) in the Department of Mechanical Engineering, Indian Institute of Technology, Guwahati. He has a great interest in machine learning and robotics.

Balgopal Singh is currently an associate professor in the Faculty of Management Studies, WISDOM, Banasthali Vidyapith. He has published many international journal papers and book chapters and guided many PhD students.

D. Singh received his BE (Hons.) in electrical engineering from Punjab Engineering College, Chandigarh, in 1991; ME in control and guidance from the University of Roorkee in 1993; and PhD in engineering from the Indian Institute of Technology Roorkee in 2004. His PhD thesis was developed at the Instrumentation and Signal Processing Laboratory of the Electrical Engineering Department under the direction of Prof. Vinod Kumar, IIT Roorkee; Prof. S.C. Saxena, ex-director, IIT Roorkee; and Prof. K.K. Deepak, All India Institute of Medical Sciences, New Delhi, on "Analysis and Interpretation of Heart Rate and Blood Pressure Variability."

Rashi Singh is a pre-final year student pursuing her bachelor's in computer science and engineering from Jaypee University of Information Technology, Himachal Pradesh, India. Currently, she is working in data visualization for e-signing of loans. Her areas of interest include data visualization, natural language and processing, networks and security.

Christos Tsagkaris is a medical doctor from Greece. Christos has worked as a research or clinical intern in academic institutions in Lebanon, Brazil, Taiwan and

Mexico. In March 2020, he gave a talk at TEDx Larissa in Greece and in March 2019 he was selected to attend the Human Space Physiology training course of the European Space Agency. He has a keen interest in digital health and medical humanities. He has authored articles and book chapters in peer reviewed journals and books, has taken part in numerous conferences as a presenter or member of the organizing committee and has received awards for scientific projects, healthcare advocacy and literary writing.

Bhimavarapu Usharani's research areas are data mining, text mining, web mining, sentiment analysis, deep learning and image processing.

Apoorv Vats is a pre-final year student pursuing his bachelor's in computer science and engineering from Jaypee University of Information Technology, Himachal Pradesh, India. Currently, he is working in data visualization for e-signing of loans. His areas of interest include data visualization, computer vision, networks and security.

Kamleshwar Kumar Verma is a mechanical engineer who holds a master's degree in the relevant field with experience in AutoCAD, Creo and Ansys. He has publications in computational simulation work.

1 Detection of Scoliosis from Anteroposterior X-Ray Images

Hritam Basak and Rohit Kundu

CONTENTS

1.1 INTRODUCTION: BACKGROUND AND DRIVING FORCES

The human spinal cord consists of 33 vertebrae named cervical (7), thoracic (12), lumbar (5), sacral (5) and coccygeal (4). Among them, the upper 24 vertebrae are movable, while the lower 9 are fixed [15]. Scoliosis refers to a condition where the otherwise straight human spine has a lateral curvature, forming an angle, and the spine becomes "C"- or "S"-shaped.

This angle, called the "Cobb angle" [14], is the angle formed between the most tilted vertebrae above and below the apex of the curvature and is the measure of the severity of the disease. A Cobb angle in the range of 10 to 20 degrees is deemed mild scoliosis; it is moderate when the angle is between 20 and 40 degrees and severe when the angle is more than 40 degrees [7]. The diagnosis of scoliosis is done by determining the Cobb angle through the analysis of computed tomography (CT) scans, X-ray scans or magnetic resonance imaging (MRI).

The need for surgery can be avoided with early diagnosis of the disease. However, the detection of scoliosis from X-ray or MRI images sometimes turn out to be extremely difficult due to morphological differences between patients.

DOI: 10.1201/9781003207856-1

Also, there are limitations on the intensity of radioactive rays that can be used, which often results in underdeveloped radiograph images.

Deep learning is an essential component of artificial intelligence (AI), which gained popularity due to its ability to learn non-redundant, informative features on its own through back-propagation, unlike machine-learning techniques, where handcrafted features need to be extracted and selected manually [23, 12].

In the literature, there exist numerous computer-aided methods, but all of them have shortcomings. Mathematical filter-based segmentation methods like the active contour model [2] and charged-particle models [18] were proposed to segment the vertebrae before calculating the Cobb angle. These methods suffered from excess computational requirements and were susceptible to errors due to slight variations in images. Alharbi et al. [1] proposed a fuzzy spatial relation associated with deformable models to perform semi-supervised segmentation of the vertebrae. Recently convolutional neural network (CNN) and deep neural network models have been widely used for this purpose, with a significant improvement in the result [3]. Fu et al. [9] proposed a lightweight multitask network that primarily detects the corner points followed by accurate contour segmentation. In the literature, there exist other deep-learning based object-detection and segmentation methods [8, 6], but they suffer from the problem of extreme computation requirements.

In this chapter, we develop an automated method for the detection of vertebrae to measure the Cobb angle for scoliosis using deep learning and image processing. For this, first, the region of interest (RoI), that is, the vertebral column in this case, is extracted from the images using image processing. Then the vertebral column is segmented from the RoI by locating spine centers (SCs)

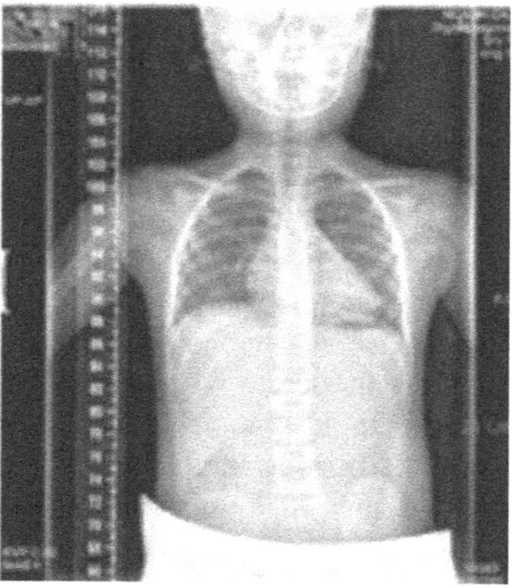

FIGURE 1.1 An example of the anteroposterior radiograph image from the dataset used in this research.

and the spine boundary. Next, deep learning is used to segment the vertebrae from the vertebral column and, finally, the Cobb angle is measured using a method known as minimum bounding rectangle (MBR). In this research, we use the VGG-19 [19] convolutional neural network as the backbone for U-Net [17] architecture to perform semantic segmentation of the vertebral column from X-ray images. Semantic segmentation refers to the pixel-level classification of each image; that is, each pixel is classified as belonging to an object class or background class.

1.2 MATERIALS AND METHODS

In this section, we describe in detail the proposed method for determining scoliosis by calculating the Cobb angle from anteroposterior (AP) X-ray images.

1.2.1 Dataset Descriptions

In this chapter, we use the publicly available dataset by Wu et al. [22] consisting of 609 X-ray anteroposterior images of the spine. Each image contains four landmarks for every vertebra for measurement of the Cobb angle.

1.2.2 Isolation of the Spine

The first step of the process is to select the spinal column from the entire radiograph image by cropping and resizing those images for the sake of ease of computation. In this case, the RoI is the spinal cord, specifically the zone between thoracic and lumbar (between L5 and T1).

It is clear from the X-ray image shown in Figure 1.1 that the pixel intensities have higher values along the center-line of the spine. Therefore, we plot the horizontal and vertical histogram projection of pixel intensity values of the images as shown in Figure 1.2. From the vertical distribution of the histogram, we select the mean

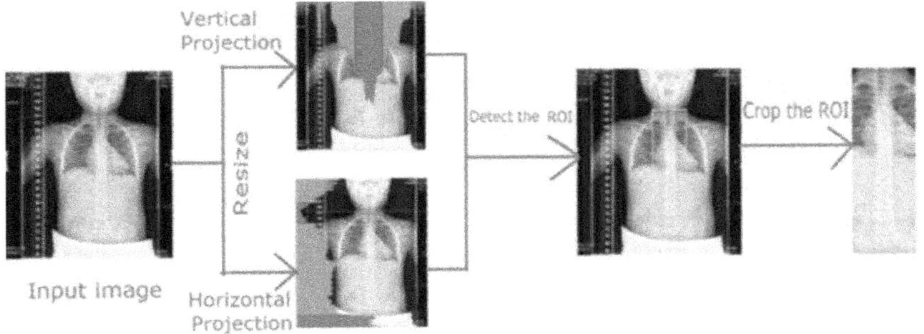

FIGURE 1.2 Isolating the RoI from the raw X-ray images.

intensity and some standard deviation (SD) value of intensity around it for the selection of vertical pixel columns in the RoI. Also, they have a comparatively lower-intensity distribution along the thoracic region, though it has higher-intensity values along the lumbar region of the spine. To resolve this, we plot the horizontal distribution of the pixel intensities as shown in Figure 1.2 and select the minimum intensity value as the upper limit of the RoI and the largest discontinuity of intensity as the lower limit of RoI. Thus, the complete RoI is selected and cropped accordingly.

1.2.3 Detection of Vertebrae

After selecting the RoI, our next task is to detect the vertebrae from the RoI. For this purpose, we distribute our job in three steps: (a) detection of the spine center-line, (b) detection of the spine border and (c) detection of the vertebra. From Figure 1.1, it is clear that the spine is characterized by higher pixel intensity values, so it is easier for us to detect the spine border using some basic mathematical operations based on the intensity and gradient distribution of the image.

For detecting the spine center-line, we assign a window of 50 × 13 pixels and move it along the RoI from left to right, calculating the sum of the pixel intensity values inside that window. The size of the window is set experimentally. Thus, we obtain a window with a maximum sum of pixel intensity value and mark its top-middle point as the first point of the SC. Then we move the window down by 12 pixels and continue the operation but this time not through the entire RoI but across the boundary of 10 pixels left and 10 pixels right of the previous SC point. Thus, we obtain the CS point along with the complete RoI and join the points using a polynomial fitting method using the best curve to join most of the points. Thus, after obtaining the center-line of the spine, we move on to the next step, detection of the spine boundary.

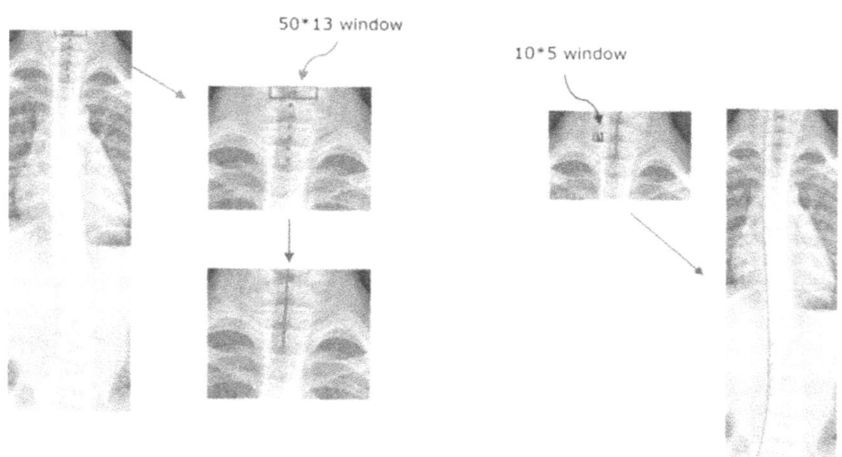

FIGURE 1.3 Detection of spine center-lines and boundaries.

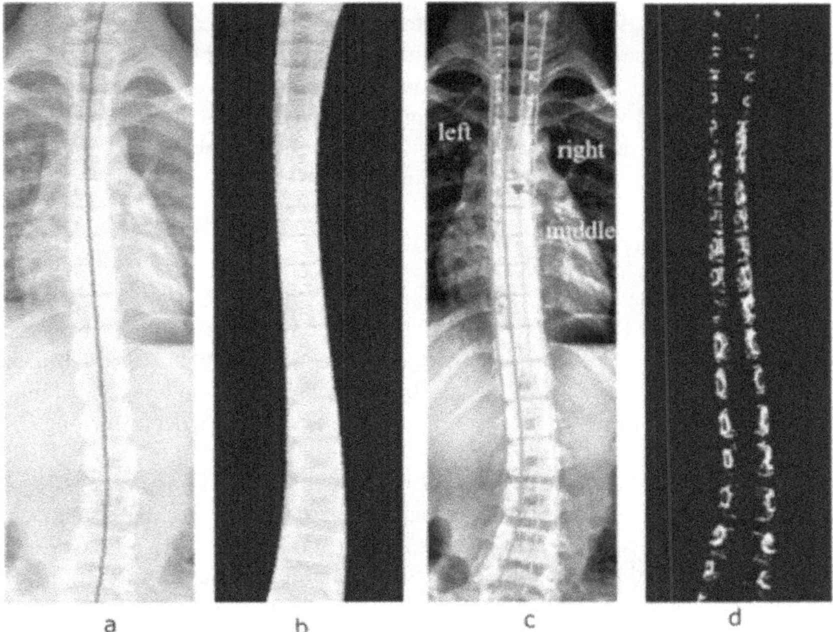

FIGURE 1.4 (a) Spine center-line; (b) threshold foreground of spine; (c) separating regions; (d) result of threshold.

To detect the boundary of the spine, we select two similar windows of size 10 × 5 pixels. We move these windows within the boundary of 40 pixels horizontally each at one side of the SC points that were previously obtained in the earlier steps. The one with the maximum intensity gradient is marked, and its top-middle point is allocated as the boundary point of the spine. Then the windows are brought down by 5 pixels, and the process continues throughout the complete RoI similar to the SC detection process. After obtaining the boundary points, we join them through curve fitting by choosing the best-fit polynomial curve. The window sizes and the pixel values of horizontal and vertical window-movement limits are obtained experimentally. The entire process of SC and boundary detection of the spine is described in Figure 1.3.

Further, the region between the two boundaries of the spine is separated into three regions; the two extreme regions are used for selecting the threshold image Ix with a value of $16x$, where x has integral values between 1 and 15 inclusive. The intensity of each image is projected vertically on the SC line, and a summation of histogram-projection is obtained. The new projection is assigned by Ax values given by Equation (1.1).

$$\begin{aligned} Ax &= 0, \text{ if } histogram - projection \geq 0 \\ &= 1, \text{ otherwise} \end{aligned} \tag{1.1}$$

The summation-histogram is calculated by $S = \sum_{n=1}^{15} Ax$, which is a voting mechanism. By analyzing the histogram of the RoI, it is observed that the vertebrae regions always have a value of 0 compared to the sub-vertebral region, which mostly assigns the value 1. By selecting the sharp changes in the histogram, we select the inter-vertebral spaces and thus segment the vertebra. This gives rise to 15 rectangular vertebral zones, shown in Figure 1.4.

1.2.4 Segmentation of Vertebrae

After detecting the vertebrae segments, our next task is to segment each of the vertebrae from the RoI. The radiograph images contain uneven intensity distributions, and normal image processing algorithms cannot detect the vertebrae segments from the spine images. Besides, there may be a different intensity of images due to the different morphology of the subjects. So, we use a deep learning-based method for this purpose.

In the literature, there exist several methods based on image processing [11, 13], clustering methods [12], deep learning-based methods [21] and machine learning [20]. Based on recent studies, U-Net models have greater accuracy in segmentation and detection tasks [10, 16]. Any model for feature extraction which is trained for classification can be used in the encoding phase of the U-Net. In this chapter, we use the VGG-19 model as the backbone of the U-Net in the encoding phase for feature extraction. After feature extraction, we perform semantic segmentation by aggregating those features using long skip connections along with the upsampled features in the decoding stage of the U-Net, similar to [5, 4].

1.2.5 Measurement of the Cobb Angle

Cobb's method is the most widely used technique for the measurement of spine curvature, where the angle between the upper border of the topmost vertebrae and the lower border of the bottommost vertebrae is measured as the Cobb angle. In the normal manual method, straight lines parallel to the borders are drawn, and the angle is measured between these two lines.

In our approach, we try an automated method, known as the minimum bounding rectangle method. In this approach, the smallest rectangle that fits the segmented vertebrae contour inside it is assigned, and the upper and lower sides of the rectangle are considered the upper and lower border of the vertebra. This MBR method is described in Figure 1.5.

After obtaining the borders, the Cobb angle (ϕ) is determined by Equation 1.2, where $(i, j) \in (u, v); (u, v) \in \mathbb{I}$, and $(v - u) \geq 2; v \leq N$. Here, u is the upper vertebrae and v is considered the lower vertebrae with at least one vertebra between them. Here θ_i and θ_j are considered the slopes of the upper border of upper vertebrae and lower border of lower vertebrae, respectively. N is the total number of vertebra segments.

$$\theta = \max \left| \tan^{-1} \left(\frac{\theta_i - \theta_j}{1 + \theta_i \theta_j} \right) \right| \tag{1.2}$$

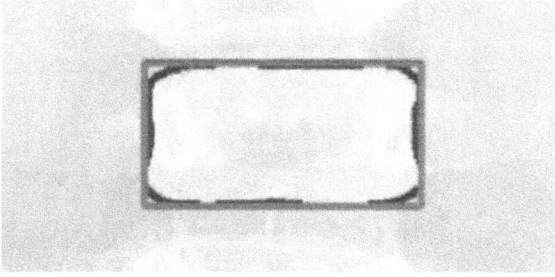

FIGURE 1.5 MBR method for selecting the upper and lower boundaries of vertebrae.

We calculate every possible angle and consider the maximum value among them Cobb's angle.

1.3 RESULTS AND DISCUSSION

In this section, we evaluate the proposed method on the publicly available dataset described and compare the model's performance with the results from two doctors – one novice and another expert.

1.3.1 Evaluation of Segmentation

The segmentation of vertebrae is performed using a convolution neural network based on a deep learning algorithm, as mentioned earlier. We trained the network based on the ground truth available of the vertebrae, and the relevant statistical results were obtained using the following equations:

$$Accuracy = \frac{TP + TN}{TP + FP + TN + FN} \tag{1.3}$$

$$Sensitivity = \frac{TP}{FN + TP} \tag{1.4}$$

$$Specificity = \frac{TN}{FP + TN} \tag{1.5}$$

where TP = true positive, TN = true negative, FP = false positive and FN = false negative. Our network gave a satisfactory result, with $Sensitivity \geq 0.98$ and $Specificity \geq 0.97$. The accuracy and loss plots are shown in Figure 1.6. Data augmentation is applied to enhance performance and to avoid overfitting. The detected vertebrae are shown in Figure 1.7, whereas the segmentation results exemplifying the efficacy of the proposed method are shown in Figure 1.8.

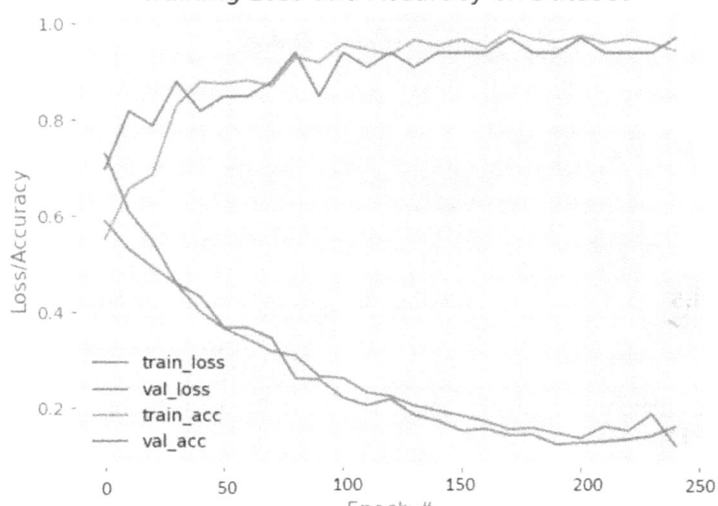

FIGURE 1.6 Plot of training and validation loss/accuracy.

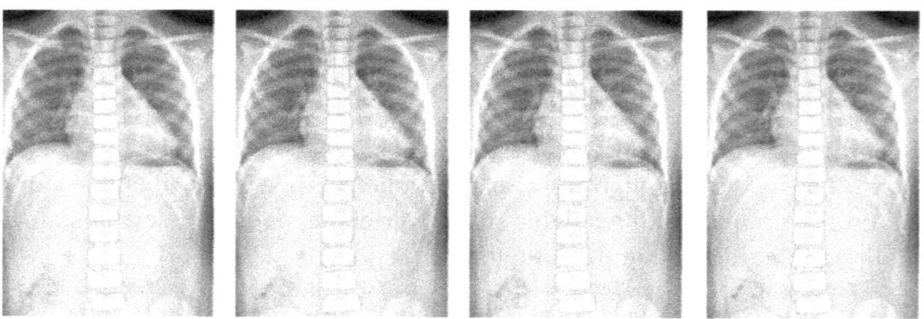

FIGURE 1.7 Detected vertebra by the proposed method.

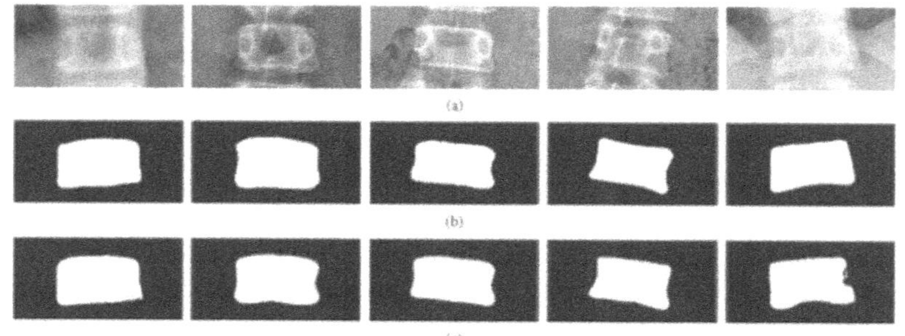

FIGURE 1.8 (a) Original input image; (b) ground truth; and (c) segmentation result.

1.3.2 Evaluation of Cobb Angle Measurement

We evaluate the Cobb angle using the proposed method and validate the results by comparing them to the results from two orthopedic doctors, of whom one was an expert in this field and the other was a novice doctor. The measured angle gave both positive and negative results, indicating the curvature of the spine on the left and right side, respectively. Each of the orthopedics measured the same radiograph images at two different times, and their measured angle was noted. These results are compared with the results achieved by the proposed model using the same images of spinal radiography shown in Table 1.1.

Next, we calculate the accuracy of our results by comparing and correlating these results with those obtained from the doctors. For this purpose, we use two methods: interclass correlation coefficient (ICC) and Pearson's correlation coefficient (PCC). Based on the results, the ICC is categorized in the following groups: (a) poor (≤ 0.39), (b) moderate (0.4 to 0.59), (c) good (0.60 to 0.74) and (d) excellent (0.75 to 1.0). The correlation result is described in Table 1.2.

TABLE 1.1
Comparison of Cobb Angle Measured by the Proposed Method with the Results Obtained by the Two Orthopedic Doctors

	First Observer (Expert)						Second Observer (Novice)						Proposed Method		
	Lower Vertebrae		Upper Vertebrae		Cobb Angle		Lower Vertebrae		Upper Vertebrae		Cobb Angle		Lower Vertebrae	Upper Vertebrae	Cobb Angle
Image Index	t1	t2	t1	t2	t1	t2	t1	t2	t1	t2	t1	t2			
1	L2	L2	T7	T7	14.6	13.5	L2	L3	T8	T6	14.2	12.2	L2	T8	10.2
2	L4	L4	T11	T11	8.3	7.9	L4	L4	T11	T10	6.3	6.7	L3	T10	3.6
3	L2	L3	T10	T10	−9.8	−8.5	L2	L3	T10	T6	−8.2	−7.9	L4	T8	−9.2
4	L4	L4	T8	T7	11.3	11.4	L4	L1	T6	T7	16.8	14.6	L2	T7	14.2
5	L4	L2	T8	T8	−4.5	−5.2	L2	L4	T6	T6	−6.8	−9.1	L1	T5	−8.5
6	L1	L2	T7	T8	−8.7	−9	L1	L1	T9	T7	−8.9	−9.9	L1	T9	−9
7	L3	L3	T9	T8	−17.8	−18.2	L1	L3	T10	T10	−14.3	−13.5	L4	T12	−13.2
8	L2	L2	T11	T11	11.4	11.7	L2	L2	T8	T7	10.2	12.6	L3	T9	12.4
9	L2	L3	T11	T11	2.6	6.8	L3	L4	T11	T9	3.2	3.2	L3	T6	2.5
10	L4	L4	T10	T10	17.6	12.7	L4	L4	T5	T6	16.6	14.7	L4	T8	14.7
11	L4	L4	T11	T11	16.5	15.9	L4	L4	T6	T6	19.2	20.3	L4	T6	18.6
12	L3	L3	T7	T7	−18.8	−17.8	L3	L3	T9	T8	−14.4	−13.9	L3	T8	−14.1
13	L3	L1	T8	T9	−5.6	−6.2	L1	L2	T7	T7	−3.6	−4.7	L4	T10	−4
14	NO SCOLIOSIS						T12	T11	T5	T5	2.6	1.3	L1	T6	3.1
15	L3	L3	T8	T8	−4.9	−3.9	L2	L4	T8	T4	−7.8	−9.7	L1	T5	−8
16	L1	L2	T9	T9	5.8	6	L4	L4	T4	T7	6.2	1.5	L3	T6	4.5
17	L2	L2	T11	T9	12.3	11.9	L2	L1	T5	T5	11.9	13.8	L2	T7	12
18	L3	L3	T11	T11	13.5	13.4	L1	L3	T8	T9	9.6	10.7	L3	T8	10.5
19	L4	L2	T5	T8	6.8	6.7	L1	L1	T5	T8	5.9	6.1	L1	T9	8.5
20	L2	L2	T8	T10	−14.8	−15.4	L2	L4	T6	T9	−13.6	−11.6	L2	T9	−12.6

TABLE 1.2
Correlation Results between the Expert and Novice Doctors and Our Proposed Method

Correlation	Expert to Novice	Expert to Our Result	Novice to Our Result
Interclass Correlation Coefficient	0.946	0.945	0.934
Pearson's Correlation Coefficient	0.954	0.949	0.94

1.4 CONCLUSION AND FUTURE WORK

In this chapter, we suggested an autonomous method for the detection of scoliosis by measuring the Cobb angle using computer vision and deep learning. The entire process consists of three different parts: Detection of spine center-line, segmentation of vertebrae using deep learning and finally measurement of the Cobb angle. The result obtained by this method closely matches with those obtained from clinical experts. The statistical evaluation also suggests very high correlation values using the Pearson correlation coefficient and interclass correlation coefficient. This method also suggests that U-Net provides mostly accurate results for segmentation for biomedical purposes.

Since this method produces significantly accurate results, it can be applied in the practical field, that is, for measuring the Cobb angle and determining the severity of scoliosis for clinical purposes. However, further development can be done by using a deeper network for training and by increasing the number of images for training as well as testing purposes. Further studies may be conducted regarding the severity of scoliosis using the length of the spine center-line and the three-dimensional reconstruction of the spine from the radiograph images of vertebrae AP view. Though our method only focuses on the determination of scoliosis, many further studies may prove more accurate and exacting regarding the assessment of scoliosis, and our work serves as a baseline for such studies.

REFERENCES

[1] Alharbi, R. H., Alshaye, M. B., Alkanhal, M. M., Alharbi, N. M., Alzahrani, M. A., & Alrehaili, O. A. (2020). Deep learning based algorithm for automatic scoliosis angle measurement. In *2020 3rd International Conference on Computer Applications & Information Security (ICCAIS)* (pp. 1–5). IEEE.

[2] Anitha, H., & Prabhu, G. (2012). Automatic quantification of spinal curvature in scoliotic radiograph using image processing. *Journal of Medical Systems*, *36*, 1943–1951.

[3] Banerjee, S., Ling, S. H., Lyu, J., Su, S., & Zheng, Y.-P. (2020). Automatic segmentation of 3D ultrasound spine curvature using convolutional neural network. In *2020 42nd Annual International Conference of the IEEE Engineering in Medicine & Biology Society (EMBC)* (pp. 2039–2042). IEEE.

[4] Basak, H., Ghosal, S., Sarkar, M., Das, M., & Chattopadhyay, S. (2020). Monocular depth estimation using encoder-decoder architecture and transfer learning from single RGB image. In *2020 IEEE 7th Uttar Pradesh Section International Conference on Electrical, Electronics and Computer Engineering (UPCON)* (pp. 1–6). IEEE.

[5] Basak, H., & Kundu, R. (2020). Comparative study of maturation profiles of neural cells in different species with the help of computer vision and deep learning. In *International Symposium on Signal Processing and Intelligent Recognition Systems* (pp. 352–366). Springer.

[6] Basak, H., Kundu, R., Agarwal, A., & Giri, S. (2020). Single image super-resolution using residual channel attention network. In *2020 IEEE 15th International Conference on Industrial and Information Systems (ICIIS)* (pp. 219–224). IEEE.

[7] Chan, E. W., Gannon, S. R., Shannon, C. N., Martus, J. E., Mencio, G. A., & Bonfield, C. M. (2017). The impact of curve severity on obstetric complications and regional anesthesia utilization in pregnant patients with adolescent idiopathic scoliosis: a preliminary analysis. *Neurosurgical Focus*, *43*, E4.

[8] Chattopadhyay, S., & Basak, H. (2020). Multi-scale attention U-Net (MsAUNet): A modified U-Net architecture for scene segmentation. *arXiv preprint arXiv: 2009.06911*.

[9] Fu, X., Yang, G., Zhang, K., Xu, N., & Wu, J. (2020). An automated estimator for Cobb angle measurement using multi-task networks. *Neural Computing and Applications*, 1–7.

[10] Huang, C., Tang, H., Fan, W., Cheung, K., To, M., Qian, Z., Terzopoulos, D. et al. (2020). Fully-automated analysis of scoliosis from spinal X-ray images. In *2020 IEEE 33rd International Symposium on Computer-Based Medical Systems (CBMS)* (pp. 114–119). IEEE.

[11] Kim, H. S., Ishikawa, S., Ohtsuka, Y., Shimizu, H., Shinomiya, T., & Viergever, M. A. (2001). Automatic scoliosis detection based on local centroids evaluation on moiré topographic images of human backs. *IEEE Transactions on Medical Imaging*, *20*, 1314–1320.

[12] Kusuma, B. A. (2017). Determination of spinal curvature from scoliosis X-ray images using k-means and curve fitting for early detection of scoliosis disease. In *2017 2nd International conferences on Information Technology, Information Systems and Electrical Engineering (ICITISEE)* (pp. 159–164). IEEE.

[13] Lu, J., Xin, L., Qian, Z., & Ye, K. (2019). Rapid detection of scoliosis based on digital image processing. *Zhongguo yi Liao qi xie za zhi = Chinese Journal of Medical Instrumentation*, *43*, 259–262.

[14] Morrissy, R., Goldsmith, G., Hall, E., Kehl, D., & Cowie, G. (1990). Measurement of the Cobb angle on radiographs of patients who have scoliosis. Evaluation of intrinsic error. *Journal of Bone and Joint Surgery. American Volume*, *72*, 320–327.

[15] Panjabi, M. M., Takata, K., Goel, V., Federico, D., Oxland, T., Duranceau, J., & Krag, M. (1991). Thoracic human vertebrae. Quantitative three-dimensional anatomy. *Spine*, *16*, 888–901.

[16] Pisov, M., Kondratenko, V., Zakharov, A., Petraikin, A., Gombolevskiy, V., Morozov, S., & Belyaev, M. (2020). Keypoints localization for joint vertebra detection and fracture severity quantification. In *International Conference on Medical Image Computing and Computer-Assisted Intervention* (pp. 723–732). Springer.

[17] Ronneberger, O., Fischer, P., & Brox, T. (2015). U-Net: Convolutional networks for biomedical image segmentation. In *International Conference on Medical image computing and computer-assisted intervention* (pp. 234–241). Springer.

[18] Sardjono, T. A., Wilkinson, M. H., Veldhuizen, A. G., van Ooijen, P. M., Purnama, K. E., & Verkerke, G. J. (2013). Automatic Cobb angle determination from radiographic images. *Spine*, *38*, E1256–E1262.

[19] Simonyan, K., & Zisserman, A. (2014). Very deep convolutional networks for large-scale image recognition. *arXiv preprint arXiv:1409.1556*.

[20] Tajdari, M., Pawar, A., Li, H., Tajdari, F., Maqsood, A., Cleary, E., Saha, S., Zhang, Y. J., Sarwark, J. F., & Liu, W. K. (2021). Imagebased modelling for adolescent idiopathic scoliosis: Mechanistic machine learning analysis and prediction. *Computer Methods in Applied Mechanics and Engineering*, *374*, 113590.

[21] Vergari, C., Skalli, W., & Gajny, L. (2020). A convolutional neural network to detect scoliosis treatment in radiographs. *International Journal of Computer Assisted Radiology and Surgery*, *15*, 1069–1074.

[22] Wu, H., Bailey, C., Rasoulinejad, P., & Li, S. (2017). Automatic landmark estimation for adolescent idiopathic scoliosis assessment using BoostNet. In *International Conference on Medical Image Computing and Computer-Assisted Intervention* (pp. 127–135). Springer.

[23] Yi, J., Wu, P., Huang, Q., Qu, H., & Metaxas, D. N. (2020). Vertebrafocused landmark detection for scoliosis assessment. In *2020 IEEE 17th International Symposium on Biomedical Imaging (ISBI)* (pp. 736–740). IEEE.

2 Review of Healthcare Management

Pinki Paul and Balgopal Singh

CONTENTS

2.1 INTRODUCTION

Globally, healthcare systems are progressing tremendously these days. Healthcare is undergoing significant changes. To provide more comprehensive and holistic care to an ever-increasing global population, advanced practice is required to improve the quality of services provided and ultimately patient care and assessment. In healthcare, technology is increasingly gaining a position in nearly all processes, from patient registration to record tracking, from lab assessments to self-care tools. Devices like smartphones are beginning to update traditional tracking and recording systems, and people are currently given the choice of a complete consultation in the privacy of their own homes. Technological improvements in healthcare have contributed to offerings being taken out of the confines of health facilities and integrated with user-friendly, convenient devices.

DOI: 10.1201/9781003207856-2

2.1.1 Past, Present, and Future Prospects

The entire healthcare industry evolved to become what it is today. Before World War II, healthcare was very like a cottage industry. Physicians typically ran independent practices, and non-profits and religious-affiliated businesses ran hospitals and clinics. Over time, coverage grew to include more of healthcare. Only in healthcare can medical health insurance expand to cover more of our everyday, predictable fitness problems and costs. Insurance has become like pay-as-you-go medical to take care of any services, and it has become a luxury product typically accessed through employers or the authorities in many cases, as with the arrival of Medicare and Medicaid [1].

Healthcare in India is in a very early stage and is undergoing a massive shift from static to dynamic status. The growth trend in this industry is impressive. Figure 2.1 shows statistics on the growth of healthcare in India.

In 2008, it was $45 billion growth in India. The healthcare enterprise has grown to $110 billion in 2016 and is anticipated to reach $280 billion by 2020. The marketplace recorded an increase of 16.5 GR and is anticipated to reach 23% in 2020. India's quality of medicine is the equal of that of any Western country, but it's significantly less expensive. Hence, many foreign patients go to India for their care. Most of the superior techniques and technology utilized in advanced nations can also now be found in India. Medical tourism is anticipated to develop from the present $3 billion to $8 billion by 2020. Due to the recognition of many

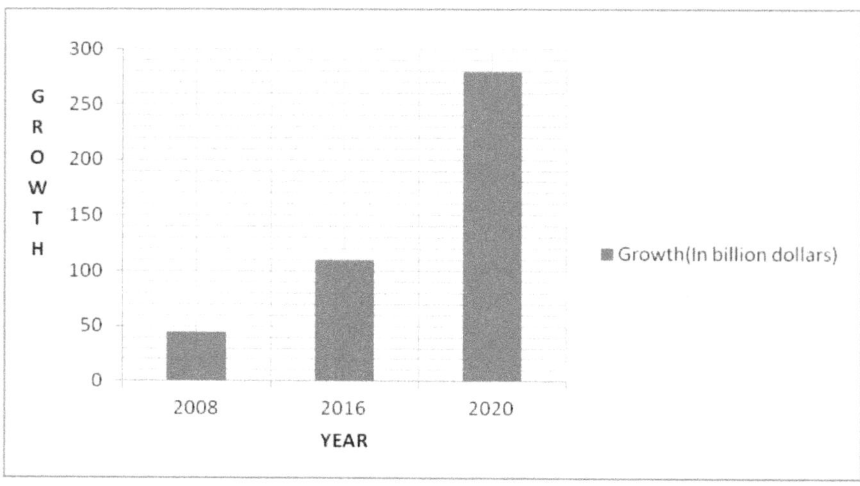

FIGURE 2.1 Healthcare growth in India [2].

leaders in India, many hospitals are choosing accreditation. Healthcare industries contribute the following to the growth healthcare in India:

- Raising income
- Affordability for the population
- Insurance penetration
- Improved average lifespan of the population
- Encouraging clinical tourism flow
- Wide knowledge of disorders

Due to improvements in technology, the average lifespan improved from 62 years to 67 years for adult males and 63.9 years to 69.6 years for women from 2005 to 2015. This means a developing older population. Better immunization and nutrition, mixed with the prevention and remedy of infectious disease, have contributed to this. Presently, India is dealing with a sizable undertaking with a wide range of disorders present. Earlier communicable diseases like malaria and tuberculosis had been widespread in the healthcare sector. People are threatened at the moment by non-communicable diseases like blood pressure, diabetes, and heart attacks [2].

Some of the technological advancements in healthcare in the last ten years are as follows [3]:

1. Electronic health records
2. Telemedicine and m-health services
3. Self-service systems
4. Wearable tracking devices
5. Genome sequencing or pharmacogenomics

Some of the future concerns for the healthcare sector are as follows [4]:

1. AI to drive sector growth
2. Big data to result in preventive care
3. Blockchain to bring about healthcare efficiency
4. Cloud technology to change healthcare scenarios
5. Innovative insurance models for preventive healthcare

2.2 HEALTHCARE SYSTEMS

When a system organizes and finances healthcare and provides this facility to people, it is called the healthcare system. A healthcare system always tries to fulfill the requirements of the targeted population. The basic need for a healthcare system is to maintain public health most efficiently with society's available resources. The healthcare system consists of four main components: (1) individual patients; (2) a professional care-providing team, which includes clinicians, pharmacists, family members of the patient, and so on; (3) the organization that

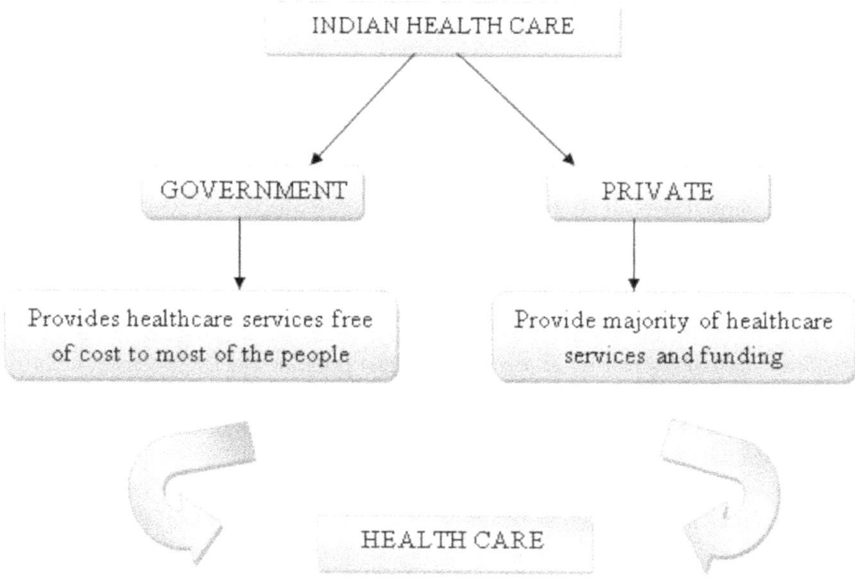

FIGURE 2.2 Structure of the Indian healthcare system.

provides a proper work environment and infrastructure to the working team; and (4) political and economic environments like regulatory, financial, and payment regimes and markets that provide feasible working conditions and environments for the organization, care-providing team, and service providers. There are different kinds of healthcare systems around the world. Management procedures within the healthcare system can be different depending on the country. A few countries distribute their healthcare system among various vendors in the market, whereas in some countries, the system is managed by the government, trade unions, charities, religious organizations, or others. There are two types of Indian healthcare systems as shown in Figure 2.2.

2.2.1 Public Healthcare

Public healthcare is mainly for people below the poverty line. They are provided with free and subsidized healthcare facilities. The Indian public health sector makes up 18% of total outpatient care and 44% of total inpatient care. Public health systems are commonly defined as "all public, private, and voluntary entities that contribute to the delivery of essential public health services within a jurisdiction." This concept ensures that all entities' contributions to community or state health and well-being are recognized in assessing public health services [5].

The public health system includes:

- Public health agencies at state and local levels
- Healthcare providers
- Public safety agencies
- Human service and charity organizations
- Education and youth development organizations
- Recreation and arts-related organizations
- Economic and philanthropic organizations
- Environmental agencies and organizations

Figure 2.3 shows a structural representation of a public healthcare system. The dark lines represent that all individual entities have a direct relationship with the public healthcare agency – or we can say they are all part of the healthcare agency. The light lines represent the relationship between two individual entities. They are also dependent upon each other or share information and help each other provide better service in the public healthcare agency [6].

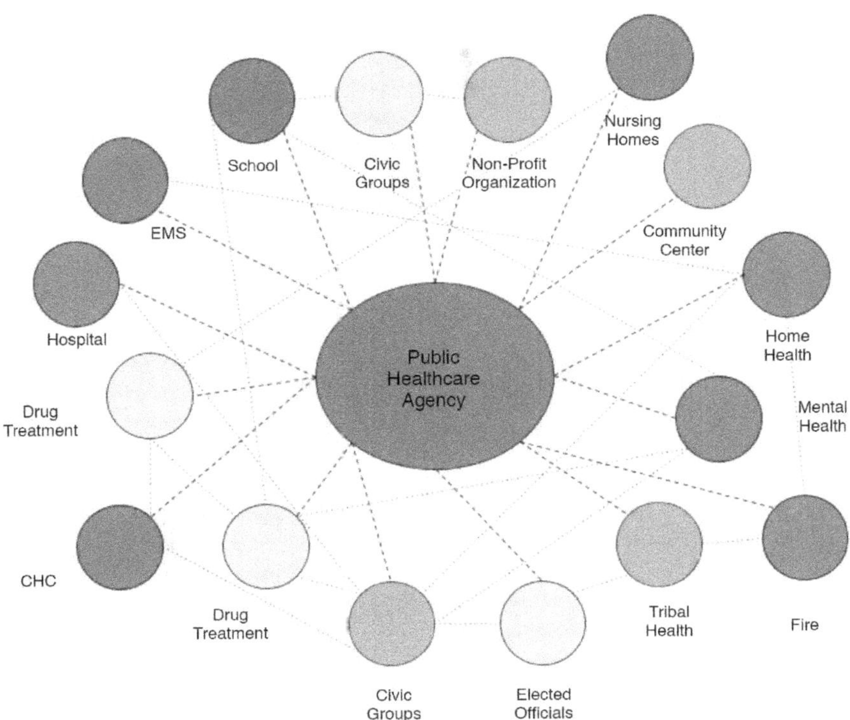

FIGURE 2.3 Public healthcare system.

2.2.2 Private Healthcare

Currently in Indian society, the private healthcare sector has become a strong force, gaining an immense national and international reputation. Starting from high-end technologies, superior devices, and advanced surgical procedures, the private healthcare sector is gaining greater preference by Indians for their health-related needs. According to reports, it is estimated that Indians spend nearly eight times more on private hospitals than on public ones, contributing to the greater flow of revenue and resources to the private healthcare sector. On the other hand, there is less public spending, constituting only 29% of the total expenditure. This means that the private healthcare sector has increased tremendously. Moreover, the gross inefficiency, dysfunction, and shortage of healthcare delivery systems in the public sector makes them insufficient to match the population's growing needs [7].

2.2.3 Capacity Healthcare Devices

Primary care is the main pillar of realistic, quality healthcare. Primary care clinicians have accelerated care through diverse vendors and control of extra patients with complicated conditions. Enabling technology can expand top care

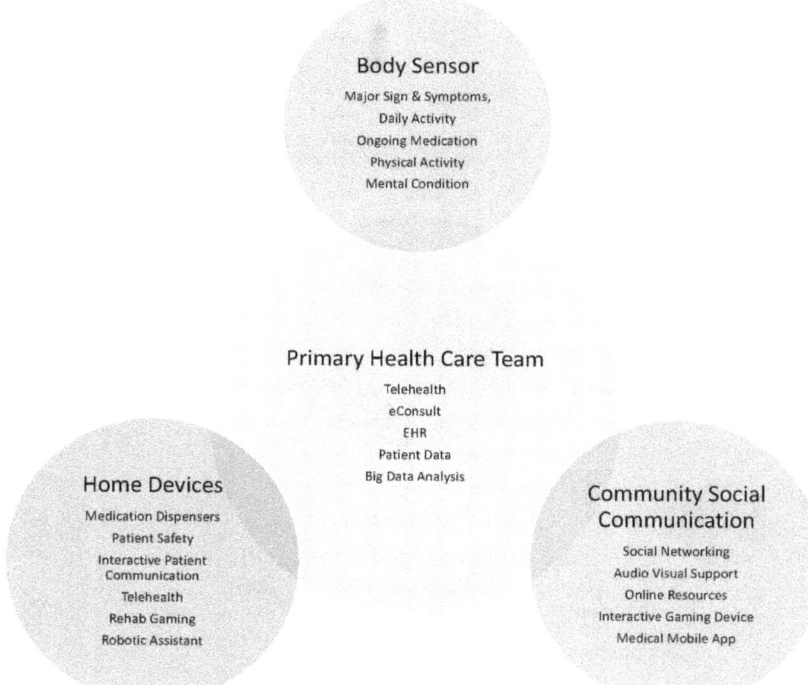

FIGURE 2.4 Technologies of primary care.

clinicians' capability to offer integrated, convenient care that channels know-how to the affected person and brings area-of-expertise consultations into the best care clinics. Furthermore, new technology offers possibilities to interact with patients in advancing their health via progressive conversations and more desirable self-control for persistent conditions [8].

2.3 HEALTHCARE MANAGEMENT

As its name suggests, healthcare management is a total management system for a healthcare facility. Healthcare management manages and organizes the total healthcare system step by step. This system is planned in such a way that it will be very helpful for healthcare providers. They can collect, store, retrieve, and exchange patient healthcare information in a more effective manner. By following this method, they can provide more care to the patient. This management system aims to help medical practitioners as well as the community. In this system, a person appointed as a manager handles the whole system and manages every system's operation. Some issues, like medical equipment and departmental budgets, are planned by the manager to meet their goals [9].

2.3.1 Technological Advancements in Healthcare Management

Technology plays a vital role in the healthcare management sector. Because healthcare management is a very complicated sector that includes different types of jobs, information and communication technology helps to solve many of these problems. This kind of technical knowledge is applicable in various healthcare sectors, like medical devices, medicines, vaccines, diagnostic and treatment procedures, systems, and so on. These are developed to gain health benefits and improve the quality of people's lives. Technology helps a patient monitor and self-help. A patient can monitor and capture real-time data about his or her own behavioral and physiological states using different technology. For this purpose, various mobile applications, wearable sensors, and smartphone sensors are used [10].

Technology also provides patients with a chance to avail themselves of integrated care. Technology-based care systems grounded in science-based approaches work for an array of chronic illnesses and behavioral health issues that respond positively to each patient's needs. This way, patients with specific diseases receive specific care and treatment. Also, we can say technology is part of a fundamental health structure. It also helps to capture data in detail and secure the correct examination outcome [11].

2.3.2 Information Technology in Healthcare

When technology is used to record, analyze, and share patient health-related data, it is called health information technology (Health IT). Different technical systems like health record systems and personal health tools like smart devices and app communities share information. Some of these techniques suggest a suitable diet for the patient or what preliminary steps to take for his or her disease. Health information technology aims to provide better service to the patient. This can be done by maintaining a record of patients and performing a detailed analysis. This information is used by practitioners and the Ministry of Health to provide better health options to the community and prevent disease. Quality of healthcare delivery and patient safety can be improved by information technology. It can also minimize medical errors and strengthen communication between patients and healthcare providers. An open-source electronic health record (EHR) and the Open Medical Record System (Open MRS) are very reliable and affordable solutions for maintaining patient records for low- and middle-income countries [12]. IT provides every patient's detailed record in other medical clinic health systems, helping doctors better understand a patient's medical history [13].

2.3.3 Requirements of Technological Advancement in Healthcare

For a long time, a paper chart was the standard procedure for tracking a patient's details. However, over time, problems arose with this system: Documents could only be accessed by one person at a time, it was not possible to access records from both the home and hospital, lots of manual work and human labor were needed to keep the records of clinical data, and it was challenging to keep a record of every past and present patient and track progress remotely after patients left [12].

By using IT, we can solve these problems very quickly and effortlessly. The following are some of those advancements:

1. *Electronic health records*: When a patient's health record is kept electronically, it becomes effortless to monitor that patient and access those data from different locations. Every piece of information is on a single platform. Different organizations have systems to maintain and control access to those data [14].
2. *mHealth*: mHealth, or mobile health, is a system that frees the whole system from wires and cords. By tablet or mobile, health staff can access data and transfer them freely. This system is used mainly for orders and documentation and to store more information for the patients. Patients can actively participate in this system; they directly send their health data to the physician [15, 16].
3. *Telemedicine or telehealth*: Telehealth is very useful in rural areas. Today, people in rural areas receive health benefits similar to the metropolitan population through this system. Telehealth is also very cost effective. It helps to reduce costs because no traditional office expenses are needed in this process [17].
4. *Portal technology*: In the current scenario, patients are becoming active participants in their healthcare. With doctors, they also take part in the treatment process. With portal technology, both patients and doctors access medical records and interact online.

5. *Self-service kiosks*: This is quite similar to portal technology. Using self-service kiosks, patients can register in a hospital or health center for treatment. Patients can use automated kiosks to pay co-pays, check identification, sign paperwork, and other registration requirements [18].
6. *Remote monitoring tools*: Monitoring a patient's health condition remotely can reduce costs and unnecessary visits to a doctor's office. If something goes wrong with a patient or the patient is in a severe condition, then that patient can contact the doctor immediately, and the doctor can also take immediate action [19].
7. *Sensors and wearable technology*: Sensors and wearable technology are worn by patients; from these, information goes directly to the doctor, and accordingly, they can take action. These systems can be of different types and as simple as an alert sent to a caretaker when a patient falls or a bandage that can detect skin pH levels to determine if a cut is becoming infected [20].
8. *Wireless communication*: Though wireless communication like walkie-talkies and instant messaging is widespread, it has recently been introduced in the medical sector [21]. Systems like Vocera Messaging allow users to send messages, like lab tests and alerts safely and securely to one another using smartphones, web-based consoles, or third-party clinical systems. These messaging systems can expedite the communication process while still tracking and logging sent and received information in a secure manner [22].
9. *Real-time location services*: This is also a growing technology in the healthcare field, such as monitoring equipment. Real-time location services help hospitals monitor effectiveness and immediately spot problem sectors. By tracking the movement of medical equipment or other things, anyone can detect that device's position in the hospital, so the chance of displacement is significantly less [23].
10. *Pharmacogenomics/genome sequencing*: Personalized medicine is becoming more popular day by day. To receive efficient healthcare and an accurate diagnosis, this has become very popular for treating certain diseases. Pharmacogenomics has also become popular because adverse drug events, misdiagnoses, readmissions, and other unnecessary costs can be avoided [24].

2.3.4 Internet of Things in Healthcare

The use of the Internet of Things (IoT) in the medical field is becoming more popular. IoT devices and applications are designed in such a manner that they are perfect for healthcare needs. They use sensors and apps that work, such as in remote healthcare monitoring, consultation, and delivery, very quickly. The IoT can be used in traditional medical equipment like inhalers and to monitor critical medical devices and receive alerts when they require maintenance or replacement. The

IoT can be beneficial not only for patients but also for their families, physicians, hospitals, and insurance companies [25].

1. *IoT for patients*: Wearable devices like a fitness band, blood pressure monitor, heart rate monitoring cuff, glucometer, and so on, give patients the opportunity for personal care. Through these devices, they can constantly monitor their health condition.
2. *IoT for doctors*: By using wireless and other IoT-based devices, doctors can monitor their patients remotely, and if required, they can take action accordingly. The IoT enables healthcare providers to be more watchful and connect with patients regularly. Data collected from the IoT help physicians provide the best treatment to patients, who expect the best results.
3. *IoT for hospitals*: As for patients and doctors, the IoT is also beneficial for hospitals or medical organizations. IoT devices are tagged with sensors to track the real-time location of medical equipment like wheelchairs, defibrillators, nebulizers, oxygen pumps, and so on. Not only the devices but medical staff can be monitored by the IoT system.
4. *IoT for insurance companies*: The IoT provides numerous opportunities for insurance companies with IoT-connected intelligent devices. Insurance companies can capture data from different devices for underwriting and claims policies. Underwriting, pricing, claims to handle, and risk assessment processes between insurers and customers become clear using IoT devices. Insurance companies can offer an interactive interface to the insurer through these IoT devices [26].

2.3.5 Virtual Reality and Augmented Reality in Healthcare

When a simulated environment is created through computer technology that makes us feel like a real-world virtual reality, users can also interact with this virtual 3D world. Virtual reality (VR) in healthcare can increase the effectiveness of medical services.

Augmented reality is an interactive experience of a real-world environment. In this system, objects in the real world are enhanced by information designed by computer. Sometimes these are generated across multiple sensory modalities, including visual, auditory, haptic, somatosensory, and olfactory [27]. Nowadays, virtual reality is a solution to many problems in the field of healthcare. It is used in different ways:

1. *Improved patient experience*: Virtual reality assists in patient engagement and also enables successful treatment. Augmented reality improves the overall patient experience and provides easier access by adding pop-up information and navigation features, among other things.
2. *Psychological relief and treatment*: The virtual reality environment is used for pain relief and betterment of sleep habits. It is also used to teach patients to overcome PTSD, which is very useful in the long run [28].

3. *Data visualization/body mapping/interactive patient information*: Through augmented reality, visualization of live patient data is possible. Using these live data, doctors can decide the patient's present condition or problem. Augmented reality (AR) can show the patient's body by diagnosing problematic points and the exact problem. This can be fitted into smart glasses and monitored by a smartphone. AR can do another important thing: Body mapping. When a doctor is physically unavailable, they can examine a patient's body using augmented reality.
4. *Accuracy of data*: Nevertheless, the main challenge of this system is the accuracy of incoming data and hardware configuration. Microsoft's HoloLens is an example. Using this lens, doctors can perform different types of checking and simulations with live stats, and they can also obtain valuable data for their research work [29].
5. *AR & VR in surgery*: An AR-VR model helps to plan any necessary surgery with maximum efficiency. It also helps to optimize the sequence and decide what action should be taken in that particular scenario. An AR surgery assistant also helps as a visual shorthand in a problematic situation and also looks after patient care, the patient's vital stats, critical information on a disease and its treatment, and so on. With the help of VR, surgeons can experience any critical operation beforehand. They can work with the scenario without dealing with a real-world situation [30].

2.4 HEALTHCARE MANAGEMENT IN INDIA

India's healthcare system is comprehensive, but there are many differences in management quality in rural, urban, and metropolitan areas, the same type of differences we can see in public and private healthcare [31].

2.4.1 History and Today

The Indian Health Ministry was established with India's Independence in 1947. After Independence, the Indian government put a high priority on the health sector in many of its 5-year plans. The state mainly governs healthcare. The Indian constitution takes care of the health of every person in India. If there is any lack in healthcare for people, the Health Ministry looks into it. This kind of lack inspired the Health Ministry to launch the National Rural Health Mission in 2005. This mission aims to provide adequate health service to every rural area [32].

2.4.2 Private and Public Sectors

The healthcare system in India is highly reputed. Healthcare between rural and urban areas is different. Rural areas suffer from lack of physicians; especially in low-income states, these types of problems are prominent. The state government

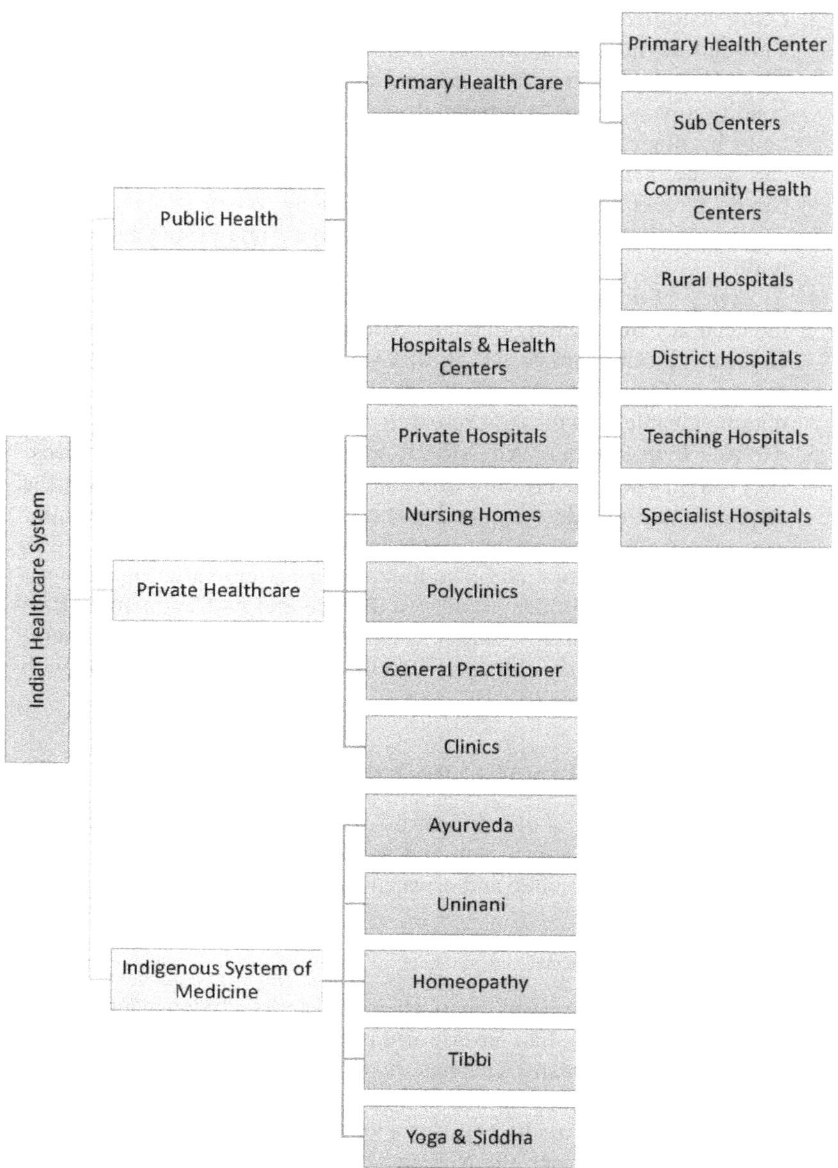

FIGURE 2.5 Structure of the healthcare system in India.

provides healthcare services, health education, and administrative and technical support from the central government.

Given inadequate support from the government, many people turn to the private health sector. Nevertheless, poor people do not have great access to this option. In some cases, employers provide healthcare costs, insurance, and so on. In many cases, they cannot bear the expense of medical treatment.

On the contrary, India's private health sector provides world-class health facilities to patients, but the price is relatively low compared to other developed countries, making India a favorite place for medical tourists. People searching for alternative medicine like Ayurveda and homoeopathy are also likely to travel to India. Ayurveda is a popular medication system in India and is an ancient medication procedure [31, 32].

2.5 CONCLUSION

A technologically sound healthcare system will put Indian society on a par with other developed countries. The government must increase the private and public healthcare sectors to be more beneficial with free-of-cost healthcare services. It is also necessary to increase public healthcare facilities in government hospitals. New schemes should be undertaken to provide quality care with good healthcare insurance schemes. Remote healthcare should act as an integrative hub for fitness care, helping patients' efforts, promoting collaboration with specialists, facilitating connections with nursing homes and domestic health, and advancing the population's fitness within a framework that improves the affected person's health with first-rate value. Achieving this could result in better guidance for patients and their circles of relatives and caregivers, extra schooling and professional improvement for clinicians, extra systematic deployment of the equipment itself, and coverage and compensation adjustments for the value of new equipment.

REFERENCES

[1] R. J. Holden and B.-T. Karsh, "The technology acceptance model: its past and its future in health care," *Journal of Biomedical Informatics*, vol. 43, pp. 159–172, 2010.

[2] J. Sivakumaran, *Technological Advancements in the Indian Healthcare Industry (India edition published from Bangalore).* Available: https://industry.siliconindia.com/viewpoint/cxoinsights/technological-advancements-in-the-indian-healthcare-industry-nwid-7678.html.

[3] T. Lang, "Advancing global health research through digital technology and sharing data," *Science*, vol. 331, pp. 714–717, Feb 11, 2011.

[4] D. Balabanova, A. Mills, L. Conteh, B. Akkazieva, H. Banteyerga, U. Dash, *et al.*, "Good health at low cost 25 years on: lessons for the future of health systems strengthening," *Lancet*, vol. 381, pp. 2118–2133, Jun 15, 2013.

[5] M. Chokshi, B. Patil, R. Khanna, S. B. Neogi, J. Sharma, V. K. Paul, *et al.*, "Health systems in India," *Journal of Perinatology*, vol. 36, pp. S9–S12, Dec 2016.

[6] *10 Essential Public Health Services*. Available: www.cdc.gov/publichealthgateway/publichealthservices/essentialhealthservices.html.

[7] P. A. Berman, "Rethinking health care systems: private health care provision in India," *World Development*, vol. 26, pp. 1463–1479, Jan 8, 1998.

[8] H. M. Young and T. S. Nesbitt, "Increasing the capacity of primary care through enabling technology," *Journal of General Internal Medicine*, vol. 32, pp. 398–403, Apr 2017.

[9] P. Keskinocak and N. Savva, "A review of the healthcare-management (modeling) literature published in manufacturing & service operations management," *Manufacturing & Service Operations Management*, vol. 22, pp. 59–72, 2020.
[10] J. Amlung, H. Huth, T. Cullen, and T. Sequist, "Modernizing health information technology: lessons from healthcare delivery systems," *JAMIA Open*, 2020.
[11] R. Baillieu, H. Hoang, A. Sripipatana, S. Nair, and S. C. Lin, "Impact of health information technology optimization on clinical quality performance in health centers: a national cross-sectional study," *PLoS ONE*, vol. 15, p. e0236019, 2020.
[12] N. Mor, "Information technology for primary healthcare in India," 2020. Available: https://www.medrxiv.org/content/10.1101/2021.02.15.21251723v1.full.
[13] H. Heathfield, D. Pitty, and R. Hanka, "Evaluating information technology in health care: barriers and challenges," *BMJ*, vol. 316, p. 1959, 1998.
[14] E. J. Layman, "Ethical issues and the electronic health record," *The Health Care Manager*, vol. 39, pp. 150–161, 2020.
[15] S. E. Bramwell, G. Meyerowitz-Katz, C. Ferguson, R. Jayaballa, M. McLean, and G. Maberly, "The effect of an mHealth intervention for titration of insulin for type 2 diabetes: A pilot study," *European Journal of Cardiovascular Nursing*, vol. 19, pp. 386–392, 2020.
[16] M. Nacinovich, *Defining mHealth*, Taylor & Francis, 2011.
[17] J. Kvedar, M. J. Coye, and W. Everett, "Connected health: a review of technologies and strategies to improve patient care with telemedicine and telehealth," *Health Affairs*, vol. 33, pp. 194–199, 2014.
[18] W. Liu, Y. Lu, C. Chen, Y. Du, F. Yan, and S. Xu, "UE-based optimization for self-service community healthcare kiosk," in *2012 IEEE 14th International Conference on e-Health Networking, Applications and Services (Healthcom)*, 2012, pp. 309–312.
[19] B. Celler, W. Earnshaw, E. Ilsar, L. Betbeder-Matibet, M. Harris, R. Clark, *et al.*, "Remote monitoring of health status of the elderly at home. A multidisciplinary project on aging at the University of New South Wales," *International Journal of Bio-medical Computing*, vol. 40, pp. 147–155, 1995.
[20] M. Y. Lee, H. R. Lee, C. H. Park, S. G. Han, and J. H. Oh, "Organic transistor-based chemical sensors for wearable bioelectronics," *Accounts of Chemical Research*, vol. 51, pp. 2829–2838, 2018.
[21] J. I. Rebstock and T. P. Rast, "Wireless healthcare communication system," Google Patents, 1999.
[22] J. Kuruzovich, C. M. Angst, S. Faraj, and R. Agarwal, "Wireless communication role in patient response time: a study of Vocera integration with a nurse call system," *CIN: Computers, Informatics, Nursing*, vol. 26, pp. 159–166, 2008.
[23] M. N. K. Boulos and G. Berry, "Real-time locating systems (RTLS) in healthcare: a condensed primer," *International Journal of Health Geographics*, vol. 11, pp. 1–8, 2012.
[24] V. Majhi, S. Paul, and R. Jain, "Bioinformatics for healthcare applications," in *2019 Amity International Conference on Artificial Intelligence (AICAI)*, 2019, pp. 204–207.
[25] S. R. Islam, D. Kwak, M. H. Kabir, M. Hossain, and K.-S. Kwak, "The Internet of Things for health care: a comprehensive survey," *IEEE Access*, vol. 3, pp. 678–708, 2015.
[26] A. S. Yeole and D. R. Kalbande, "Use of Internet of Things (IoT) in healthcare: a survey," in *Proceedings of the ACM Symposium on Women in Research 2016*, 2016, pp. 71–76.

[27] E. Zhu, A. Hadadgar, I. Masiello, and N. Zary, "Augmented reality in healthcare education: an integrative review," *PeerJ*, vol. 2, p. e469, 2014.

[28] V. Majhi, A. Saikia, A. Datta, A. Sinha, and S. Paul, "Comprehensive review on deep learning for neuronal disorders: applications of deep learning," *International Journal of Natural Computing Research (IJNCR)*, vol. 9, pp. 27–44, 2020.

[29] V. Majhi and S. Paul, "Application of content-based image retrieval in medical image acquisition," in *Challenges and Applications for Implementing Machine Learning in Computer Vision*, IGI Global, 2020, pp. 220–240.

[30] W. S. Khor, B. Baker, K. Amin, A. Chan, K. Patel, and J. Wong, "Augmented and virtual reality in surgery—the digital surgical environment: applications, limitations and legal pitfalls," *Annals of Translational Medicine*, vol. 4, 2016.

[31] J. Das and J. Hammer, "Location, location, location: residence, wealth, and the quality of medical care in Delhi, India: quality of care varied by neighborhood but not necessarily by patients' income level," *Health Affairs*, vol. 26, pp. w338–w351, 2007.

[32] L. V. Gangolli, R. Duggal, and A. Shukla, "Review of healthcare in India," Centre for Enquiry into Health and Allied Themes, Mumbai, 2005.

3 IoT Technologies for Smart Healthcare

Rehab A. Rayan and Christos Tsagkaris

CONTENTS

3.1 INTRODUCTION

Data analytics have grown into a critical tool because of ambiguous and disparate data worldwide. In healthcare, adapting approaches for data analytics is required for the routinely collected complex big data in many institutions. Examining such data could promote effective healthcare delivery at a lower cost. The entire world is challenged by critical public health issues regarding controlling fast-growing epidemics, chronically diseased populations and elderly people, maternal and infant death, poor livelihood factors with increased pollution, and poor drinking water quality and hygiene. Recently, however, despite the growing demand for more healthcare,

DOI: 10.1201/9781003207856-3

the conventional healthcare unit-oriented approach to mandating patients visiting a healthcare provider continues to predominate. For instance, to control chronic diseases, patients must visit a healthcare facility frequently, where the healthcare provider monitors the progress of the disease and changes therapy according to medical examinations. Healthcare facilities depend upon a dynamic, disease provider–oriented approach where the patient is missing as a key player in delivering healthcare (Firouzi et al. 2018). The chief limitations of this approach are as follows.

Time Constraints: While the quantities of ill and disabled individuals in the population are constantly growing, healthcare providers cannot devote adequate quality time to every case. Rapid examinations yield insufficient history about the patient's lifestyle involving diet, sleeping patterns, physical activity, and societal encounters, among other factors. Grasping such elements is vital to accurately diagnosing and managing patients.

Monitoring Compliance: Usually healthcare providers cannot monitor patients' adherence to prescribed therapies like special diets, medicines, or rehabilitation practices, resulting in more future hospital admissions, healthcare expenses, and economic load on patients (Sokol et al. 2005).

The Elderly Population: The global number of geriatric people, aged over 60 years, is expected to expand from 841 million individuals in 2013 to over 2 billion individuals by 2050 (over 200%); hence, more healthcare resources will be needed to care for this growing elderly population (Firouzi et al. 2018).

Urbanization: The World Health Organization (WHO) expects that 70% of the world's inhabitants will live in urban zones by 2015, showing that densely populated urban cities, potential epidemic centers promoting the rapid spread of infectious diseases, will demand more infrastructure for the healthcare of this growing population.

Lack of Health Personnel: The demand for healthcare services and hence providers keeps rising in both urban and rural settings, which requires adopting telemedicine interventions.

Healthcare Costs: The dramatically growing healthcare expenses are challenging. For instance, in 2017, the United States spent almost $327 billion on diabetes healthcare, up 26% since 2012 (American Diabetes Association 2018).

In recent years, healthcare has been increasingly using IT to deliver smart systems aimed at speeding up health diagnostics and treatment. These systems provide smart health monitoring and medical automation services in various contexts and environments (hospitals, workplaces, houses, on the go), allowing a major reduction in the cost of doctor visits and a general increase in the quality of patient care (Akmandor and Jha 2018). In this sense, the great proliferation of powerful embedded hardware, combined with the production of smart medical sensors and ubiquitous healthcare devices, has significantly altered the way the world approaches healthcare through the Internet of Medical Things (IoMT) (Alwan and Prahald Rao 2017).

Smart health (s-Health) is an area that has developed as a branch of two markets, smart cities, and e-Health (Solanas et al. 2014). Smart cities can be described as

> cities that are heavily focused on information and communication technologies that invest in human and social resources by fostering economic development,

> participatory governance, resource management, sustainability, and efficient mobility to enhance the quality of life of their people, while ensuring the dignity and safety of citizens.
>
> (Pérez-Martínez, Martínez-Ballesté, and Solanas 2013)

E-health can be defined as "an emerging area at the intersection of medical informatics, public health and business, with reference to the provision or improvement of health services and information via the Internet and related technologies." In a wider context, the word characterizes not just a technical advancement but also a state of mind, a way of thinking, an attitude, a contribution to the network, and global thinking, using information and communication technology to enhance treatment globally, regionally, and worldwide. There is overlap between s-Health and mobile health (m-Health).

3.2 IoT-BASED SMART HEALTH

Patient-centered care (PCC) is a growing health framework tailored to the patient's personal healthcare needs that was initially designed by the Picker Institute in 1988 and introduced by the Picker/Commonwealth Program. In 2001, the Institute of Medicine described PCC in a landmark report as healthcare based on recognized collaboration between providers, patients, and families valuing patient's preferences, informing and engaging patients in decision-making regarding their care (Institute of Medicine [US] Committee on the National Quality Report on Health Care Delivery 2001).

PCC was evidently successful on small scales; however, it is promising for a larger one despite competing with hospital-centered care. PCC will not cancel clinics or hospitals, but it would integrate such organizations in a mutual framework for patients' healthcare via the IoT. The IoT offers services through a network of sensors, actuators, telecommunication, cloud computing, and big data via the Internet. The IoT could be tailored to address the current limitations in health by providing timely and effective services at lower expense, leading to a sustainable healthcare setting. The healthcare setting could be classified into big healthcare organizations such as hospitals, small ones such as clinics or pharmacies, and non-clinical settings such as homes or communities (Farahani et al. 2018).

Many patients seek hospitals for healthcare, especially operations, where hospitals can apply innovative technologies. An IoT-connected intelligent ambulance enables diagnosing cases, so the hospital and healthcare providers can efficiently prepare prior to the arrival of the patient at the hospital. Intelligent ambulances need clinical diagnostic sensors, a protected connection to the hospital, and techniques to smartly manage processes and devices, for instance, applying the IoT in operation rooms and intensive or primary care units for efficiently transferring data and harmonizing tasks among the medical personnel and devices (Farahani, Firouzi, and Chakrabarty 2020).

Primary healthcare (PHC) providers are major healthcare givers to several patients. The IoT can secure PHC physicians' two-way communication for reserving appointments without phone calls and remotely logging into laboratory findings before patient encounters. The IoT would serve as an affordable and time-saving option for screening patients remotely prior to face-to-face interaction with a physician. The IoT could facilitate timely confirmation of insurance coverage and prescription of cost-effective home IoT self-monitoring devices.

Globally mobile clinics are attracting more attention. In rural African areas, mobile clinics deliver affordable and high-quality care with no need to approach official healthcare-providing organizations. For the minimal infrastructure of a mobile clinic, the IoT could highly enhance its care-delivering capacity by communicating distantly with hospitals for more specialized diagnoses or therapeutic services (Hill et al. 2014).

Nowadays, telemedicine is a major IoT representative, with an expected global market worth $45.5 billion in 2019, along with estimated expansion by 2026 to reach approximately $175.5 billion (Mikulic 2020). Smartphones are in almost all hands worldwide, enabling networking via IoT with other sensors for future tele-screening. Using smartphones, patients could monitor their own health and produce data, which could predict upcoming health-related events. Meanwhile, patients could visit healthcare providers virtually via teleconferencing; hence, growing remote healthcare services would decrease health systems' medical personnel.

Now more individuals are aware of the significance of early prevention and maintaining good health over requiring clinical care later. People are benefiting from IoT networking in self-monitoring medical devices, sports technologies, and fitness-tracking wearables, which allow ongoing monitoring of health. The IoT could build an economic structure to minimize expenses of health insurance by using health monitoring to incentivize wellness, creating a more effective, patient-oriented framework and motivating active patient engagement in healthcare.

Telemedicine services could limit the elderly, disabled, and chronically diseased people's number of visits to healthcare facilities. Yet a technology infrastructure at home could support them effectively and invisibly, facilitating patients in living more freely with better quality and well-being. Ambient-assisted life, a European model for an intelligent home, could enhance personal abilities via sensitive and responsive automated settings. Now, the IoT exists in digital home marketplaces such as home-controlling systems and devices through a smartphone; hence, the IoT could serve elderly patients needing healthcare. For instance, intelligent toilets could routinely analyze urine without visiting the physician. Intelligent homes could adjust noise and lights, satisfying the sensory needs of autistic patients (Rashidi and Mihailidis 2013).

Globally, people are moving toward cities, adding to the load on the infrastructure there. Smart cities and connected societies are rising via linking and merging infrastructures to render cities more proficient, affordable, and sustainable. IoT models could supply timely data, enabling individuals' rapid and informed decisions. Health is a key system in cities; therefore, it will be integrated in the smart cities' infrastructure. For instance, broad ecological sensors could send data to central sites to be accessed via the health system. Ecological data on contaminants, temperature, humidity, polluted water, or allergens could be disseminated in a timely way to people to avoid health threats. For instance, asthma patients could be alerted to avoid sites high in dust or pollen counts. The IoT could merge smart traffic lights to help in routing ambulances, saving lives via collaboration with transportation infrastructure, yet the IoT needs smart settings allowing connectivity between stakeholders, including healthcare providers, patients, healthcare facilities, cities, and societies.

3.3 ADVANTAGES OF APPLYING THE IoT IN HEALTH

The healthcare industry is in a desperate state. Healthcare services are more expensive than ever, the global population has increased, and the incidence of chronic problems is increasing as healthcare technology promotes consumer engagement and encourages health issues. In such a situation, the possibility of remote care is welcomed more than ever. However, existing health frameworks are not incorporated into technologies that can improve the quality of care by updating them in proper time with patient data and enabling them to take steps in treatment. Novel patient tracking solutions enable physicians to improve the quality of care while focusing on overall cost reduction (Zineldin 2006). What we are approaching is a world where basic healthcare will be out of reach for most people, a large part of society will be unproductive because of old age, and people will be more prone to chronic illness. Can we assume that this is not the end of the matter, no matter what development of electronic gateways people have undertaken? Although automation will never prevent the population from aging or remove serious diseases, it can, in terms of versatility, try to do health benefits conveniently.

Medical diagnostics consume a large part of hospital costs. Technology can move medical control routines to the patient's home (home-centered) from a hospital (hospital-centered). The right diagnosis also reduces the need to stay in hospital. The IoT has wide application in many areas, including telecommunications (Suri et al. 2016). A common expectation is the complete implementation of this model in the healthcare sector, as it enables healthcare facilities to function more efficiently and clinics to provide excellent treatment (Hassanalieragh et al. 2015). There are unmatched benefits of using this technology-based treatment system that can improve the speed and affordability of treatments and improve patients' health (Alansari et al. 2018). The actual world is connected by the IoT to the virtual world of the Internet. Household appliances (such as air purifiers, thermostats, etc.), vehicles, heavy machinery, building, medical devices, and the human body are part of the physical environment (Greengard 2015). Applying IoT technology to healthcare aims to improve the quality of life of patients, the level of treatment of chronic illnesses, hazard warnings, and life-saving treatments.

There are several uses of the IoT for healthcare: (1) *Health tracking.* Current portable devices can detect basic human body movements, evaluate human actions, and assess health status. Smart portable devices can reduce patient anxiety and reduce resource waste (such as smartwatches) (Abawajy and Hassan 2017). In traditional hospitals, this adds to other responsive health monitoring systems. (2) *Patient help for health records.* Clinics can remind patients to take medication on time through certain IoT devices. Network devices such as electrocardiograms, blood oxygen, and blood pressure will strengthen the continuous structure of assessment, monitoring, and support for patients and caregivers, thus enhancing clinical results (Fernandes and Lucena 2017). (3) *Service enhancement.* The IoT can help link cars with network systems. When a vehicle is involved in an accident, by submitting the location and address of the accident, the device can determine the seriousness of the accident and assist the traffic control department and the health center. This will encourage the injured to receive treatment quickly (Thomas and Rad 2017). (4) *Resource collection for large-scale data analysis.* Large amounts of health data can be produced by the health IoT. Health data collection, mining, and usage will further encourage and enhance the production of IoT health (Mahdavinejad et al. 2018).

Recently, there has been increasing interest in architectures that recognize the partnership between cloud, fog, and edge computing. The key objective is to take full advantage of the capacity for managing not only usable data but also data processing, analysis, correlation, and inference of low-level edge nodes and fog levels. As intelligent mapping of computational and resource management data across nodes is able to meet the stringent requirements of IoMT systems. Such approaches represent a promising response to integrating efficient distributed healthcare applications and services.

3.4 SIGNIFICANT FEATURES AND APPLICATIONS OF THE IoT IN HEALTH

The main applications of the IoT in healthcare pertain to mobile health, ambient assisted living (AAL), medications, and implants. IoT applications in mHealth can be vaguely divided in two categories: Apps developed for healthcare professionals and institutions and apps developed for patients, carers, and healthcare workers. Their key features for patients are continuous real-time remote monitoring, prevention of chronic diseases, early diagnosis of complications (aided by wearables), and proper documentation of health records. Carers, defined here as relatives of patients or third individuals involved in patients' care at home, can enjoy the benefits of IoT smart healthcare through AI-assisted help lines and tracking systems. Employing these modalities can prioritize carers facing an urgent situation. This can also provide carers with educational resources and ad hoc information (Genet et al. 2011; Vizer et al. 2019). Regarding healthcare workers, the advantages of IoT-based mHealth include flexible staff mobility and performance; sped up collection and processing of patient data; mitigation of the risk of mistakes; decrease of human error risk; and cost-effective treatment, considering the direct and indirect cost of healthcare in the long run (Raju et al. 2020; Zhang et al. 2018).

IoT technologies for ambient assisted living include but are not limited to smart homes and smart environments, agent-based pervasive computing and decision-making methods, and IoT sensing technologies (wireless sensor networks, smart sensors, gateways, etc.). The purpose of these modalities is the creation of smart services and automation features in private and public space. The IoT and smart systems' infrastructures comprise intelligent personal assistants, cloud computing, and smart environment paradigms. Easing the lives of older or disabled people can be one of the first goals of the use of this technology in the community (Memon et al. 2014; Sadoughi, Behmanesh, and Sayfouri 2020). The constant measurement of vitals with patient-friendly devices can help both in detecting emergencies and in properly monitoring patients. For example, wearable glucose calculators can not only warn a patient with diabetes about low levels of glucose, they can also detect asymptomatic incidents of hypoglycemia or spikes in blood glucose following certain food intake. Once the patient or the physician connects the wearable to a smartphone, a full record of this information will be available, optimizing the course of treatment (Rghioui et al. 2019, 201; Sharma, Singh, and Singh 2013). Gradually, wearables may effectively process their input, leading to essential decision-making output. In machine learning, widespread collection of patients' data can act as a multiplier of capacity (Cox, Lane, and Volchenboum 2018; Dimitrov 2016).

For medicine, the IoT has great potential both in research and in everyday clinical practice. Drug repurposing has been improved with IoT systems that are capable of compiling and comparing data regarding the chemical structure and the clinical features of existing medicines. Regarding research, IoT applications can speed up the collection and processing of data from laboratory experiments to clinical trials. Mokou et al. (2020) have described a model of IoT-based drug repurposing for bladder cancer, which can be applied to other neoplastic diseases as well (Mokou et al. 2020). In terms of clinical practice, the IoT can transform the logistics of pharmacies of drug administration within clinics. Jara, Zamora, and Skarmeta (2014) proposed a model of interconnecting patients, physicians, pharmaceutical companies, and regulatory bodies for the timely detection of adverse events. Although confidentiality and anonymization concerns need to be taken into consideration, this is an example of the potential of IoT-based smart healthcare in contemporary medical practice. Tracking or enhancing patients' compliance with pharmaceutical treatments with wearables has also been attempted (Madanian and Parry 2019; Reinhardt, Oliveira, and Ring 2020).

The concept of implants is not new in medicine. From pacemakers to neuromodulation–pain management devices, biomedical technology has devised solutions enhancing or replacing physiological functions of the human body. Essentially, what medical implants and the IoT have in common is wearables. Implants are the penultimate version of wearable devices. In most cases, they require interventional placement methods, and they are expected to remain on the patient for a considerable amount of time. What the IoT brings to conventional implants is interconnectivity. So far, patients would visit a healthcare professional to collect and assess the measurements of an implanted device. IoT-based implants provide real-time monitoring thorough data collection and storage in (mostly) online/cloud-based databases (Andreu-Perez et al. 2015; Dimitrov 2016). Implants pose greater risks than wearables, which can be removed in case of dysfunction. Researchers and manufacturers have issued concerns regarding the interaction between implantable devices, particularly pacemakers, with IoT signals (Stachel et al. 2013). A growing body of evidence is focusing on tackling this challenge through electromagnetic filters and standard electromagnetic compatibility tests (Trigano et al. 2005).

3.4.1 Simultaneous Monitoring and Reporting

Real-time monitoring via mobile networks can save lives in the event of a medical emergency, such as heart failure, diabetes, asthma attacks, and so on (Shaw et al. 2020). With real-time diagnostic monitoring with a smart healthcare device connected to a mobile app, connected sensors are used to collect necessary medical data and use the mobile network to provide doctors with the information. A study released by the Center for Linked Health Policy showed that there was a 50% reduction in 30-day readmission because of remote monitoring of patients with heart failure. The IoT system retrieves and transmits health data: Blood pressure, oxygen and blood sugar levels, weight, and ECG (Ali et al. 2020). This information is stored in the cloud and can be shared with an accredited doctor, an insurance agent, a participating healthcare provider, or an external consultant to access the information collected, regardless of time, place, or unit.

3.4.2 End-to-End Connectivity and Affordability

With the help of mobile healthcare technology and other new developments and next-generation treatment facilities, the IoT will simplify the emergency management experience. Compatibility, network-to-network connectivity, data availability, and information sharing to determine quality healthcare services are supported by the IoT for socialized care. Link technology such as Bluetooth technology, Wi-Fi, Z-wave, ZigBee, and other creative methods can facilitate the diagnosis of diseases and illnesses in patients and can also bring creativity to healthcare professionals' treatments (Ghamari et al. 2016). By minimizing unnecessary visits, using high-quality facilities, and optimizing distribution and planning, technology-driven installation thus reduces costs.

3.4.3 Data Analysis

According to its real-time use, the enormous amount of knowledge of a biomedical front gains in a brief time is difficult to store and manage if access to the cloud is not convenient. It is also a tough investment for caregivers to collect and manually review data collected from various devices and sources. IoT devices can capture, report, and analyze information in real time and reduce the need to store raw data (Provost and Murray 2011). We can do all this over the cloud with only access to final graph reports from vendors. In addition, healthcare practices enable organizations to gain vital health research and data-driven insights that speed up decision-making and are less susceptible to error.

3.4.4 Tracking, Alerts, and Remote Medical Care

In life-threatening situations, time is critical. Medical embedded systems collect useful information and send data for real-time monitoring to physicians while sending texts via smartphone devices and other community facilities to individuals on important aspects. Reports and warnings provide a strong insight into the patient's status, regardless of location and time. It also helps to build alternatives that are well known and provide fast treatment. In this way, the IoT facilitates real-time warning, reporting, and monitoring; facilitates practical treatments; enhances physicians' accuracy and effective interventions; and improves the overall performance of patient care.

Providers of healthcare will call a doctor who is in an immediate situation several kilometers away with smart smartphone devices. Doctors will review patients easily with healthcare transportation solutions and identify diseases when they are on the move. Via linked systems that expect the construction of machines that can transmit drugs based on patient medications and disease-related data, many healthcare supply chains are also available. The IoT will improve hospital patient treatment. This would decrease the comprehensive health treatment of people.

3.4.5 Research

The IoT for health can also be used for research as it allows researchers to gain an enormous amount of data about the patient's condition, which may have taken several years if they had collected it individually. Such recorded information can be used for prior results that can assist scientific research. Thus, the IoT can not only save time but also research money. In medical research, therefore, the IoT has an important influence. It facilitates the introduction of major and expanded medical treatments. The IoT is used in several techniques that improve the quality of treatment that patients receive. The IoT is now also updating existing devices by using intelligent software embedding chips. This chip improves the care and treatment for a patient.

3.4.6 Patient-Generated Health Data

All health-related information created or reported by patients or caregivers is patient-generated health information. Patient-generated health data (PGHD) contains information that relates to the patient's health or care history, lifestyle choices, and symptoms that are reported by patients or accessed from smartphones and medical devices that are compatible with the Internet. The major difference between PGHD and the data that doctors receive is that patients are primarily educated and can share the previous information.

Remote control of patients is a blessing for people living in day care or hospitals. Small IoT-based devices can monitor PGHD and can be modified directly by educators and physicians. If an experimental treatment appears to be ineffective, this is an effective way of maintaining the patient's health and proposing changes to the method. Some other benefits of remote monitoring of patients include diagnosis of acute illnesses before they become too severe and detection of drug and alcohol problems with digital drugs in patients seeking care for heart problems.

3.4.7 Management of Chronic Diseases and Preventative Care

Diseases such as diabetes, heart attack, cancer, obesity, arthritis, and stroke, among others, are becoming more common. It is often necessary for individuals affected by these conditions to take better care of themselves between their medical appointments, and they will benefit from IoT-based devices. Besides other devices, such as glucometers, test equipment, and asthma instruments, flexible instruments can help patients keep track of their health. In addition, Internet-enabled devices store their health-related data in the cloud, and it can then be accessed by professionals.

In the medical industry, introducing the IoT will also be beneficial for overweight people who are not recovering from illness and want to avoid problems in the future. Health information can be obtained regularly from anyone and can be shared with caregivers. This will help recognize even a mild issue and stop long-term illness.

3.4.8 Home-Based and Short-Term Care

Caregivers can also recognize those who are able to stay in their own homes and monitor their well-being with IoT-based technology. By tracking their condition in real time using data obtained by these devices, they can instantly take care of those who need it. Short-term treatment can be provided to patients who have already been discharged from the hospital after an operation or after recovery from an emergency. This treatment method eliminates the need to visit the hospital during the recovery process, enabling patients outside the facility to receive high-quality healthcare.

3.5 CASE STUDY: CYBERMED AS AN IoT-BASED SMART HEALTH MODEL

CyberMed was founded in 2016 and is described as an innovative addition to the telehealth market. CyberMed's products and services merge the IoT and telemedicine, enabling people to use medical devices such as digital stethoscopes or pulse oximeters. Patients can use these items during their telemedicine appointments. The collected data are transmitted to the cloud and become instantly available to the doctor, who cannot perform the physical examination otherwise. The major challenge that CyberMed addresses is the inability of physicians to thoroughly assess a patient with conventional telecommunication means such as telephone or video calls. The lack of means and experience prolongs the struggle of the patient, increases the risk of mismanagement, and may cause higher expenses if the patient is unnecessarily transported to a hospital (Makin 2018).

CyberMed offers a comprehensive telehealth approach with real-time modalities and data storing capacity. Healthcare professionals have more means to assess the patient and a detailed record of each consultation. CyberMed's app is known as CDoc. It is compatible with Windows, iOS, and Android, allowing patients to have a doctor visit without leaving their home. Its principal success is the active involvement of patients in the management of their own health. In a patient-centric communication context, the patient becomes responsible for the accuracy of their vitals and assists the doctor in examining them and making a diagnosis. CyberMed is currently nationwide in the United States. It is the first company to bring medical records, telemedicine, and IoT devices together, given that it owns and develops all its own components (Tian et al. 2019).

3.6 LIMITATIONS OF ADOPTING THE IoT IN HEALTH

Many countries around the world have increasingly tried to integrate new technology into different areas of life. Mobile computer applications have become popular in many areas, such as smart homes, e-health, green infrastructure, intelligent network devices, and many more. Some industry watchdogs noted in 2018 that IoT adoption was still in its infancy in Southeast Asia, with just 8% adopting the technology. Why is IoT adoption not more rapid and widespread, with this much hype? However rapid the proliferation of actual applications on the Internet, they cannot address many of the security constraints and issues that have recently become a priority for most researchers in this field. IoT, with online patient health monitoring and the use of recently conducted clinical trials, continues to rise in cases of care use (Kang et al. 2018). In healthcare, the risks and disadvantages of using smart devices are shown in the following.

3.6.1 Data Security and Privacy

IoT devices can pose a threat to users' security and privacy. Unauthorized access to IoT computers will put people's treatment and private data at extreme risk (Zeadally and Bello 2019), such as replication, capture, organization, and transmittal of health data to the cloud via wireless networks, especially clinical networks and smartphones. Prefix replication, impersonation attack, wavelength interference, and cloud monitoring are available for the device layer. Traffic is redirected through a man-in-the-middle attack during cloud browsing to allow command to be given directly to a device. A direct link attack is proposed using a service discovery protocol such as universal plug and play or Bluetooth low energy (BLE) features for locating and targeting IoT devices.

The main problem and danger with IoT technology in general and in the health sector seem to be the security of patient information and confidentiality. Using purpose and configuration, IoT devices collect and transmit cloud information in real time for data processing. The infrastructure for receiving and processing data will be designed and optimized to be scalable to collect, process, and store data in real time from millions of research model units to gain insights. However, most

IoT devices that receive data suffer from a lack of data standards and protocols. In addition, there is still a significant amount of confusion concerning legislation on data ownership and privacy issues. Cybercriminals who may use stolen data or information for medical identity fraud or extortion are sensitive to patient information collected by various connected devices or portable devices. A hacker or criminal can use patient data to establish a false identity or to purchase drugs or diagnostic supplies that can be resold. Harmful hackers can also make false compensation claims on behalf of the individual (Varadharajan and Bansal 2016).

Telco's infrastructure, equipment suppliers, hospitals, and other participants must take constructive measures to ensure that their communities are safe. When buying, for instance, devices or stuff for healthcare, especially devices that hospitals need to use, hospitals and other healthcare providers must be extremely picky. Hospitals and IT providers need to discuss how best to host large and complex infrastructure given these limitations in IoT technology.

3.6.2 Connectivity

To authenticate, authorize, and connect various nodes on a network, today's IoT ecosystems depend on a centralized client/server paradigm. Networks will become bottlenecks as they expand to join billions of users, though they are adequate now. A potential solution can involve pushing certain tasks to the limit, for example, fog computing: An architecture that uses edge devices to conduct a large amount of local computing, storage, communication, and routing across the backbone of the Internet. Edge devices are usually routers that provide quicker and more powerful backbones and exchanges with authenticated access. The trend is to make the peripheral device smart and the core device as described dumb and fast. Here, smart devices such as IoT centers take over mission-critical tasks and data processing, and analytical roles are taken over by cloud servers. Peer-to-peer communications are other options, where devices directly recognize and authenticate each other and share information without a central server. This model will have its own set of challenges, like security, but with emerging technologies such as blockchain, that can be met.

3.6.3 Compatibility and Data Integration

There is currently no international standard for device identification and tracking efficiency. There is no consensus on IoT standards and requirements, so products made by different vendors do not fit well with each other. The lack of precision prevents large-scale integration of the IoT, reducing its possible effectiveness. Security and integrity remain important and prohibit users from using artificial intelligence for therapeutic purposes, as there is a risk of violating or hacking remote healthcare strategies. The leakage of confidential information about the health and location of the patient and the manipulation of sensor data can have important implications, which outweigh the benefits of IoT (Stergiou et al. 2018). This limitation is the easiest to address. Manufacturers of this technology, such as

Bluetooth, USB, and so on, only need to recognize one standard. There is nothing innovative or revolutionary needed.

3.6.4 Implementation Costs

While IoT aims to reduce healthcare costs in the long term, the cost of clinical integration and employee training is very high. Has the IoT been the solution to the increase in the cost of medicines? Let us summarize why a currency's value or financial costs are a major crisis for the IoT. The growing prevalence of care is more influential today than ever. Technical advancements in the IoT have never been seen to cover rising medical costs; on the contrary, they are becoming more expensive (Lee and Lee 2015).

3.6.5 Complexity and Risk of Errors

The performance of compatible detection devices can be affected by disk failures, anomalies, or even power outages, putting healthcare facilities at risk. Also, skipping a scheduled software update can be much more dangerous than skipping a medical check-up. As in all complex systems, there are many more possibilities for failure. With the IoT, things are going to go wrong. For example, let us say both you and your spouse get a message that you have run out of milk, you both buy milk on the way home. As a result, you and your partner have bought twice the amount of milk you need. Or maybe a software bug automatically prevents your printer's new ink cartridge from being imported every hour for a few days, or, at worst, there might be a power failure when all you need is a replacement (Kai Zhang, Dahai Han, and Hongping Feng 2010).

3.7 FUTURE INSIGHTS

The IoT will be further established in healthcare in the future. The IoT market in medicine is constantly growing and is expected to reach $158 billion by 2022. This technology can be applied in a wide variety of healthcare settings to remotely monitor patients and guide the right diagnosis. Apart from a standard in the healthcare industry, the IoT tends to become a trend among patients. According to recent analyses, wearables alone would attain $222 million in 2021 starting from a volume of $113.2 million in 2017. Within ten years, the existing 10 billion devices are expected to reach 50 billion (Baker, Xiang, and Atkinson 2017; Tian et al. 2019).

Currently, physicians may assume that IoT devices cannot be suggested or prescribed to older adult patients because of their low level of digital literacy. Accumulating evidence from emergency care suggests that older people are willing and, in most cases, capable of trying telemedicine. As time passes, the digital gap will be filled with patients more and more knowledgeable about smart devices. Accumulating experience with these modalities will make physicians more confident (Gopal et al. 2019). Moreover, novel IoT research offers the chance of monitoring patients' residential environments, providing a more comprehensive approach to disease and the factors creating or sustaining it. In this context, Islam et al. (2020) have used a set of sensors collecting information about the heartbeat and body temperature and at the same time about the room temperature and the CO and CO_2 levels (Islam, Rahaman, and Islam 2020).

The notion of IoT smart healthcare seems to be compatible with new trends in the perception of health. During the last years, the classical definition of health by the WHO, as being a state of complete physical, mental, and social wellbeing, has been criticized (Bohn Stafleu van Loghum 2013). Modern researchers recognize that this status of welfare is not applicable to most of the population. Consequently, they focus on functionality, highlighting the coping mechanisms developed by systems and individuals. This perception suggests a tendency of de-escalating illness to disease. In this context, IoT smart healthcare is expected to transform disease management in a way that increases the functionality and the independence of the patient nearly up to the level of a healthy individual (Salvador-Carulla and Garcia-Gutierrez 2011).

3.8 CONCLUSIONS

A significant representative of the modern age of information technology is the Internet of Things. The IoT is growing, with more innovative potential. It results from the recent evolution in wireless communications and is a network that is expanding across the Internet. To understand the "Internet of Everything," we should link different information-sensing devices to the Internet. The IoT has commonly been used in different fields at present, such as smart cities, smart houses, smart logistics, smart transport, and so on. Among them, one of its significant fields of operation is smart health. Every year, countless individuals lose their lives because of different illnesses or health issues. People are gradually paying more attention to health problems. Therefore, a promising research domain in smart health has been applying IoT techniques to address health problems.

Techniques like wearable biosensors and innovations in big data, particularly regarding proficient analyzing of huge, multidisciplinary, disseminated, and diverse datasets, have enabled personalized e-Health and m-Health services. Yet the IoT has the potential for better availability and accessibility, individualized and customized services, and enhanced return on investments. As IoT-based e-Health expands, supporting current healthcare demands, there still exist some key challenges prior to coherent, secure, adaptable, and proficient interventions that could be adopted to solve several healthcare issues. Overall, IoT applications can contribute significantly to the management and monitoring of chronic conditions, in the early detection of complications, and in various levels of disease prevention. The lack of globally standardized IoT processes and concerns about safety and confidentiality as well as various implementation costs have been obstacles to the deployment of such solutions. This chapter discussed IoT-based e-Health settings along with their applications. It also presented the key opportunities and challenges like managing data, scalability, interoperability, legislation, device-network-human interfaces, privacy, and security.

REFERENCES

Abawajy, J. H., and M. M. Hassan. 2017. "Federated Internet of Things and Cloud Computing Pervasive Patient Health Monitoring System." *IEEE Communications Magazine* 55 (1): 48–53. doi:10.1109/MCOM.2017.1600374CM.

Akmandor, A. O., and N. K. Jha. 2018. "Smart Health Care: An Edge-Side Computing Perspective." *IEEE Consumer Electronics Magazine* 7 (1): 29–37. doi:10.1109/MCE.2017.2746096.

Alansari, Zainab, Safeeullah Soomro, Mohammad Riyaz Belgaum, and Shahaboddin Shamshirband. 2018. "The Rise of Internet of Things (IoT) in Big Healthcare Data: Review and Open Research Issues." In *Progress in Advanced Computing and Intelligent Engineering*, edited by Khalid Saeed, Nabendu Chaki, Bibudhendu Pati, Sambit Bakshi, and Durga Prasad Mohapatra, 675–685. Advances in Intelligent Systems and Computing. Singapore: Springer. doi:10.1007/978-981-10-6875-1_66.

Ali, Farman, Shaker El-Sappagh, S. M. Riazul Islam, Daehan Kwak, Amjad Ali, Muhammad Imran, and Kyung-Sup Kwak. 2020. "A Smart Healthcare Monitoring System for Heart Disease Prediction Based on Ensemble Deep Learning and Feature Fusion." *Information Fusion* 63 (November): 208–222. doi:10.1016/j.inffus.2020.06.008.

Alwan, Omar S., and K. Prahald Rao. 2017. "Dedicated Real-Time Monitoring System for Health Care Using ZigBee." *Healthcare Technology Letters* 4 (4): 142–144. doi:10.1049/htl.2017.0030.

American Diabetes Association. 2018. "Economic Costs of Diabetes in the U.S. in 2017." *Diabetes Care* 41 (5): 917–928. doi:10.2337/dci18-0007.

Andreu-Perez, J., D. R. Leff, H. M. D. Ip, and G. Yang. 2015. "From Wearable Sensors to Smart Implants—Toward Pervasive and Personalized Healthcare." *IEEE Transactions on Biomedical Engineering* 62 (12): 2750–2762. doi:10.1109/TBME.2015.2422751.

Baker, Stephanie Edwards, Wei Xiang, and Ian M. Atkinson. 2017. "Internet of Things for Smart Healthcare: Technologies, Challenges, and Opportunities." *IEEE Access*. doi:10.1109/ACCESS.2017.2775180.

Bohn Stafleu van Loghum. 2013. "Towards a New Definition of Health?" *Tijdschrift voor gezondheidswetenschappen* 91 (3): 138. doi:10.1007/s12508-013-0050-3.

Cox, Suzanne M., Ashley Lane, and Samuel L. Volchenboum. 2018. "Use of Wearable, Mobile, and Sensor Technology in Cancer Clinical Trials." *JCO Clinical Cancer Informatics* 2: 1–11. doi:10.1200/CCI.17.00147.

Dimitrov, Dimiter V. 2016. "Medical Internet of Things and Big Data in Healthcare." *Healthcare Informatics Research* 22 (3): 156–163. doi:10.4258/hir.2016.22.3.156.

Farahani, Bahar, Farshad Firouzi, and Krishnendu Chakrabarty. 2020. "Healthcare IoT." In *Intelligent Internet of Things: From Device to Fog and Cloud*, edited by Farshad Firouzi, Krishnendu Chakrabarty, and Sani Nassif, 515–545. Cham: Springer International Publishing. doi:10.1007/978-3-030-30367-9_11.

Farahani, Bahar, Farshad Firouzi, Victor Chang, Mustafa Badaroglu, Nicholas Constant, and Kunal Mankodiya. 2018. "Towards Fog-Driven IoT EHealth: Promises and Challenges of IoT in Medicine and Healthcare." *Future Generation Computer Systems* 78 (January): 659–676. doi:10.1016/j.future.2017.04.036.

Fernandes, Chrystinne Oliveira, and Carlos José Pereira De Lucena. 2017. "A Software Framework for Remote Patient Monitoring by Using Multi-Agent Systems Support." *JMIR Medical Informatics* 5 (1): e9. doi:10.2196/medinform.6693.

Firouzi, Farshad, Amir M. Rahmani, K. Mankodiya, M. Badaroglu, G. V. Merrett, P. Wong, and Bahar Farahani. 2018. "Internet-of-Things and Big Data for Smarter Healthcare: From Device to Architecture, Applications and Analytics." *Future Generation Computer Systems* 78 (January): 583–586. doi:10.1016/j.future.2017.09.016.

Genet, Nadine, Wienke GW Boerma, Dionne S. Kringos, Ans Bouman, Anneke L. Francke, Cecilia Fagerström, Maria Gabriella Melchiorre, Cosetta Greco, and Walter Devillé. 2011. "Home Care in Europe: A Systematic Literature Review." *BMC Health Services Research* 11 (1): 207. doi:10.1186/1472-6963-11-207.

Ghamari, Mohammad, Balazs Janko, R. Simon Sherratt, William Harwin, Robert Piechockic, and Cinna Soltanpur. 2016. "A Survey on Wireless Body Area Networks for EHealthcare Systems in Residential Environments." *Sensors (Basel, Switzerland)* 16 (6). doi:10.3390/s16060831.

Gopal, Gayatri, Clemens Suter-Crazzolara, Luca Toldo, and Werner Eberhardt. 2019. "Digital Transformation in Healthcare—Architectures of Present and Future Information Technologies." *Clinical Chemistry and Laboratory Medicine (CCLM)* 57 (3). De Gruyter: 328–335. doi:10.1515/cclm-2018-0658.

Greengard, Samuel. 2015. *The Internet of Things*. Cambridge, MA: The MIT Press.

Hassanalieragh, Moeen, Alex Page, Tolga Soyata, Gaurav Sharma, Mehmet Aktas, Gonzalo Mateos, Burak Kantarci, and Silvana Andreescu. 2015. "Health Monitoring and Management Using Internet-of-Things (IoT) Sensing with Cloud-Based Processing: Opportunities and Challenges." In *2015 IEEE International Conference on Services Computing*, 285–292. doi:10.1109/SCC.2015.47.

Hill, Caterina F., Brian W. Powers, Sachin H. Jain, Jennifer Bennet, Anthony Vavasis, and Nancy E. Oriol. 2014. "Mobile Health Clinics in the Era of Reform." *The American Journal of Managed Care* 20 (3): 261–264.

Institute of Medicine (US) Committee on the National Quality Report on Health Care Delivery. 2001. *Envisioning the National Health Care Quality Report*. Edited by Margarita P. Hurtado, Elaine K. Swift, and Janet M. Corrigan. Washington, DC: National Academies Press (US). www.ncbi.nlm.nih.gov/books/NBK223318/.

Islam, Md. Milon, Ashikur Rahaman, and Md. Rashedul Islam. 2020. "Development of Smart Healthcare Monitoring System in IoT Environment." *SN Computer Science* 1 (3): 185. doi:10.1007/s42979-020-00195-y.

Jara, Antonio J., Miguel A. Zamora, and Antonio F. Skarmeta. 2014. "Drug Identification and Interaction Checker Based on IoT to Minimize Adverse Drug Reactions and Improve Drug Compliance." *Personal and Ubiquitous Computing* 18 (1): 5–17. doi:10.1007/s00779-012-0622-2.

Kang, Minhee, Eunkyoung Park, Baek Hwan Cho, and Kyu-Sung Lee. 2018. "Recent Patient Health Monitoring Platforms Incorporating Internet of Things-Enabled Smart Devices." *International Neurourology Journal* 22 (Suppl 2): S76–82. doi:10.5213/inj.1836144.072.

Lee, In, and Kyoochun Lee. 2015. "The Internet of Things (IoT): Applications, Investments, and Challenges for Enterprises." *Business Horizons* 58 (4): 431–440. doi:10.1016/j.bushor.2015.03.008.

Madanian, Samaneh, and Dave Parry. 2019. "IoT, Cloud Computing and Big Data: Integrated Framework for Healthcare in Disasters." *Studies in Health Technology and Informatics* 264 (August): 998–1002. doi:10.3233/SHTI190374.

Mahdavinejad, Mohammad Saeid, Mohammadreza Rezvan, Mohammadamin Barekatain, Peyman Adibi, Payam Barnaghi, and Amit P. Sheth. 2018. "Machine Learning for Internet of Things Data Analysis: A Survey." *Digital Communications and Networks* 4 (3): 161–175. doi:10.1016/j.dcan.2017.10.002.

Makin, Cheryl. 2018. "Telehealth: CyberMed in East Brunswick Aims to Carry Healthcare Evolution to the Next Step." *MyCentralJersey.Com*. July 13. www.mycentraljersey.com/story/news/health/2018/07/13/telehealth-next-steps-cybermed-east-brunswick/749334002/.

Memon, Mukhtiar, Stefan Rahr Wagner, Christian Fischer Pedersen, Femina Hassan Aysha Beevi, and Finn Overgaard Hansen. 2014. "Ambient Assisted Living Healthcare Frameworks, Platforms, Standards, and Quality Attributes." *Sensors (Basel, Switzerland)* 14 (3): 4312–4341. doi:10.3390/s140304312.

Mikulic, Matej. 2020. "Telemedicine Market Size Worldwide 2019 vs 2026." *Statista*. May 12. www.statista.com/statistics/671374/global-telemedicine-market-size/.

Mokou, Marika, Vasiliki Lygirou, Ioanna Angelioudaki, Nikolaos Paschalidis, Rafael Stroggilos, Maria Frantzi, Agnieszka Latosinska, et al. 2020. "A Novel Pipeline for Drug Repurposing for Bladder Cancer Based on Patients' Omics Signatures." *Cancers* 12 (12). doi:10.3390/cancers12123519.

Pérez-Martínez, P., A. Martínez-Ballesté, and A. Solanas. 2013. "Privacy in Smart Cities—A Case Study of Smart Public Parking." In *PECCS*. doi:10.5220/0004314700550059.

Provost, Lloyd P., and Sandra Murray. 2011. *The Health Care Data Guide: Learning from Data for Improvement*. 1st edition. San Francisco, CA: Jossey-Bass.

Raju, Bharath, Fareed Jumah, Omar Ashraf, Vinayak Narayan, Gaurav Gupta, Hai Sun, Patrick Hilden, and Anil Nanda. 2020. "Big Data, Machine Learning, and Artificial Intelligence: A Field Guide for Neurosurgeons." *Journal of Neurosurgery* 1 (aop). American Association of Neurological Surgeons: 1–11. doi:10.3171/2020.5.JNS201288.

Rashidi, Parisa, and Alex Mihailidis. 2013. "A Survey on Ambient-Assisted Living Tools for Older Adults." *IEEE Journal of Biomedical and Health Informatics* 17 (3): 579–590. doi:10.1109/JBHI.2012.2234129.

Reinhardt, Ingrid Carla, Dr Jorge C. Oliveira, and Dr Denis T. Ring. 2020. "Current Perspectives on the Development of Industry 4.0 in the Pharmaceutical Sector." *Journal of Industrial Information Integration* 18 (June): 100131. doi:10.1016/j.jii.2020.100131.

Rghioui, Amine, Jaime Lloret, Lorena Parra, Sandra Sendra, and Abdelmajid Oumnad. 2019. "Glucose Data Classification for Diabetic Patient Monitoring." *Applied Sciences* 9 (20). Multidisciplinary Digital Publishing Institute: 4459. doi:10.3390/app9204459.

Sadoughi, Farahnaz, Ali Behmanesh, and Nasrin Sayfouri. 2020. "Internet of Things in Medicine: A Systematic Mapping Study." *Journal of Biomedical Informatics* 103 (March): 103383. doi:10.1016/j.jbi.2020.103383.

Salvador-Carulla, L., and Carlos Garcia-Gutierrez. 2011. "The WHO Construct of Health-Related Functioning (HrF) and Its Implications for Health Policy." *BMC Public Health*. doi:10.1186/1471-2458-11-S4-S9.

Sharma, M., G. Singh, and R. Singh. 2018. "An Advanced Conceptual Diagnostic Healthcare Framework for Diabetes and Cardiovascular Disorders." *ICST Transactions on Scalable Information Systems* 5 (18): 154828. doi:10.4108/eai.19-6-2018.154828.

Shaw, Ryan J., Q. Yang, A. Barnes, D. Hatch, M. J. Crowley, A. Vorderstrasse, J. Vaughn, et al. 2020. "Self-Monitoring Diabetes with Multiple Mobile Health Devices." *Journal of the American Medical Informatics Association: JAMIA* 27 (5): 667–676. doi:10.1093/jamia/ocaa007.

Sokol, Michael C., Kimberly A. McGuigan, Robert R. Verbrugge, and Robert S. Epstein. 2005. "Impact of Medication Adherence on Hospitalization Risk and Healthcare Cost." *Medical Care* 43 (6): 521–530. doi:10.1097/01.mlr.0000163641.86870.af.

Solanas, A., C. Patsakis, M. Conti, I. S. Vlachos, V. Ramos, F. Falcone, O. Postolache, et al. 2014. "Smart Health: A Context-Aware Health Paradigm within Smart Cities." *IEEE Communications Magazine* 52 (8): 74–81. doi:10.1109/MCOM.2014.6871673.

Stachel, J. R., E. Sejdić, A. Ogirala, and M. H. Mickle. 2013. "The Impact of the Internet of Things on Implanted Medical Devices Including Pacemakers, and ICDs." In *2013 IEEE International Instrumentation and Measurement Technology Conference (I2MTC)*, 839–844. doi:10.1109/I2MTC.2013.6555533.

Stergiou, Christos, Kostas E. Psannis, Byung-Gyu Kim, and Brij Gupta. 2018. "Secure Integration of IoT and Cloud Computing." *Future Generation Computer Systems* 78 (January): 964–975. doi:10.1016/j.future.2016.11.031.

Suri, N., M. Tortonesi, J. Michaelis, P. Budulas, G. Benincasa, S. Russell, C. Stefanelli, and R. Winkler. 2016. "Analyzing the Applicability of Internet of Things to the Battlefield Environment." In *2016 International Conference on Military Communications and Information Systems (ICMCIS)*, 1–8. doi:10.1109/ICMCIS.2016.7496574.

Thomas, M. J., and B. Rad. 2017. "Reliability Evaluation Metrics for Internet of Things, Car Tracking System: A Review." doi:10.5815/IJITCS.2017.02.01.

Tian, Shuo, Wenbo Yang, Jehane Michael Le Grange, Peng Wang, Wei Huang, and Zhewei Ye. 2019. "Smart Healthcare: Making Medical Care More Intelligent." *Global Health Journal* 3 (3): 62–65. doi:10.1016/j.glohj.2019.07.001.

Trigano, Alexandre, Olivier Blandeau, Christian Dale, Man-Fai Wong, and Joe Wiart. 2005. "Reliability of Electromagnetic Filters of Cardiac Pacemakers Tested by Cellular Telephone Ringing." *Heart Rhythm* 2 (8): 837–841. doi:10.1016/j.hrthm.2005.03.011.

Varadharajan, Vijayaraghavan, and Shruti Bansal. 2016. "Data Security and Privacy in the Internet of Things (IoT) Environment." In *Connectivity Frameworks for Smart Devices: The Internet of Things from a Distributed Computing Perspective*, edited by Zaigham Mahmood, 261–281. Computer Communications and Networks. Cham: Springer International Publishing. doi:10.1007/978-3-319-33124-9_11.

Vizer, Lisa M., Jordan Eschler, Bon Mi Koo, James Ralston, Wanda Pratt, and Sean Munson. 2019. "'It's Not Just Technology, It's People': Constructing a Conceptual Model of Shared Health Informatics for Tracking in Chronic Illness Management." *Journal of Medical Internet Research* 21 (4): e10830. doi:10.2196/10830.

Zeadally, Sherali, and Oladayo Bello. 2019. "Harnessing the Power of Internet of Things Based Connectivity to Improve Healthcare." *Internet of Things*, July, 100074. doi:10.1016/j.iot.2019.100074.

Zhang, Kai, Dahai Han, and Hongping Feng. 2010. "Research on the Complexity in Internet of Things." In *2010 International Conference on Advanced Intelligence and Awareness Internet (AIAI 2010)*, 395–398. doi:10.1049/cp.2010.0796.

Zhang, Peng, Douglas C. Schmidt, Jules White, and Shelagh Mulvaney. 2018. "Towards Precision Behavioral Medicine with IoT: Iterative Design and Optimization of a Self-Management Tool for Type 1 Diabetes." *2018 IEEE International Conference on Healthcare Informatics (ICHI)*. doi:10.1109/ICHI.2018.00015.

Zineldin, Mosad. 2006. "The Quality of Health Care and Patient Satisfaction: An Exploratory Investigation of the 5Qs Model at Some Egyptian and Jordanian Medical Clinics." *International Journal of Health Care Quality Assurance Incorporating Leadership in Health Services* 19 (1): 60–92. doi:10.1108/09526860610642609.

4 A Novel Design of Digital Circuits Using Reversible Logic Synthesis

Shruti Jain

CONTENTS

4.1 INTRODUCTION

Digital techniques are beneficial because they have readable output instead of reproducing a continuous series of values. Digital circuits are designed from large assemblies of electronic illustrations of Boolean logic functions [1]. These circuits use transistors to create logic gates in succession to execute Boolean logic, which led to the basis of digital electronics. Digital electronic circuits are based upon switching ON (1) or OFF (0). Energy loss is an important aspect in digital design. Power, or energy, is the essence of every circuit or any activity that can be imagined [2]. The main problem arises from Landauer's principle (LP), for which there is no solution. LP relates to the minimum energy for computation that requires clarifying what explanatory values we are looking for. It does not provide any explanation as to why the big bang banged as big as it did. With dark energy and dark matter making up the majority of the energy in the universe and no detailed understanding of what these are, there seems to be plenty more to learn and discover [3]. Landauer's principle doesn't associate energy with a bit. Rather, it sets the minimum amount of energy required to change a bit (about 0.0172 eV, 2.76×10^{-21} joules). The bit itself has no energy; it just sits there. It is essential to conserve power in the best possible way so that human beings can survive in an efficient and sustainable manner [4, 5]. In digital circuits, energy and power

DOI: 10.1201/9781003207856-4

dissipation is the main concern. Loss of information is rendered in the form of heat that results in power dissipation. In digital system design, many gates are not reversible, like AND, OR, XOR, and so on, or it can be said that a number of gates used in digital electronics are irreversible gates [6]. Design that does not result in a loss of information is known as reversible logic. The different types of logic are irreversible and reversible [7].

Energy dissipates whenever switching occurs in irreversible logic. To overcome this issue, reversible logic has been introduced [8, 9]. For reversible logic, loss of information in every bit produces $kT \ln 2$ joules of heat energy, where T is the temperature and k is Boltzmann's constant. The energy dissipated in a system results in a direct relationship to the number of bits wiped out during computation [10, 11]. Reversible logic is used mainly in quantum computers. In recent years, reversible logic has been used in low-power very large scale integration design because it helps reduce power dissipation. A reversible logic gate will convert an input to the opposite at the output; for example, if the input is 1, the output is 0. If the input is 1, then the output is 0. Of the different digital gates, only the NOT gate is reversible. Compared to irreversible logic, reversible logic (RL) [12, 13, 14] has the ability to minimize power dissipation, the major concern in digital circuit designing, and hence contribute to the conservation of energy [15, 16, 17]. RL is finding promising and profound applications in recent fields like DNA computing, computer graphics, low-power complementary metal oxide semiconductor (CMOS), nanotechnology, communication, and so on [18, 19]. This logic supports two-way processing forward and backward. There is one-to-one mapping between the input and output values. This signifies not only that output can be differentiated from input, but input can also be recuperated from output [20, 21, 22]. The computational complexity of each kind of RL is different, so its optimization is not great, and this will have varying quantum cost (QC) and delay. The QC for 1×1 reversible gates is zero, and the QC for 2×2 reversible gates (RGs) is one. In RL, feedback and fan-out are not considered, which makes the synthesis essentially different [23, 24, 25].

The lessening of parameters makes up the bulk of the work engaged in the design of reversible circuits. The authors implemented different universal gates using reversible gate logic with respect to its preceding counterparts. There are a lot of arithmetic operations that are executed on a computer arithmetic and logic unit through the use of adders and subtractors [26, 27]. The proposed implementation of digital circuits using reversible logic considers access to future computing technology. There are six diverse types of reversible gates, out of which three gates based on simulation using Verilog coding are shortlisted based on their performance parameters. The three gates simulated in SPICE and Toffoli gates show remarkable results based on different electrical parameters. Using the final selected gate (Toffoli), different combinational circuits are designed and simulated. The circuits are simulated using both types of logic (reversible and irreversible), but the results using reversible logic are outstanding.

In this chapter, Section 4.2 explains the proposed methodology, including the design of different digital circuits using Toffoli reversible logic, and Section 4.3 presents the results and provides a discussion of the different designed digital circuits, followed by concluding remarks.

4.2 PROPOSED METHODOLOGY

The authors simulated and analyzed different digital circuits consisting of combinational and sequential circuits using reversible logic, as shown in Figure 4.1. Out of six different reversible gates, three showed remarkable performance on the basis of different evaluation parameters. Based on electrical parameters, the Toffoli gate was chosen, with the help of which other digital circuits were implemented. Last, the results of reversible and irreversible gates were compared, and it was found that circuits designed using the Toffoli gate showed remarkable performance.

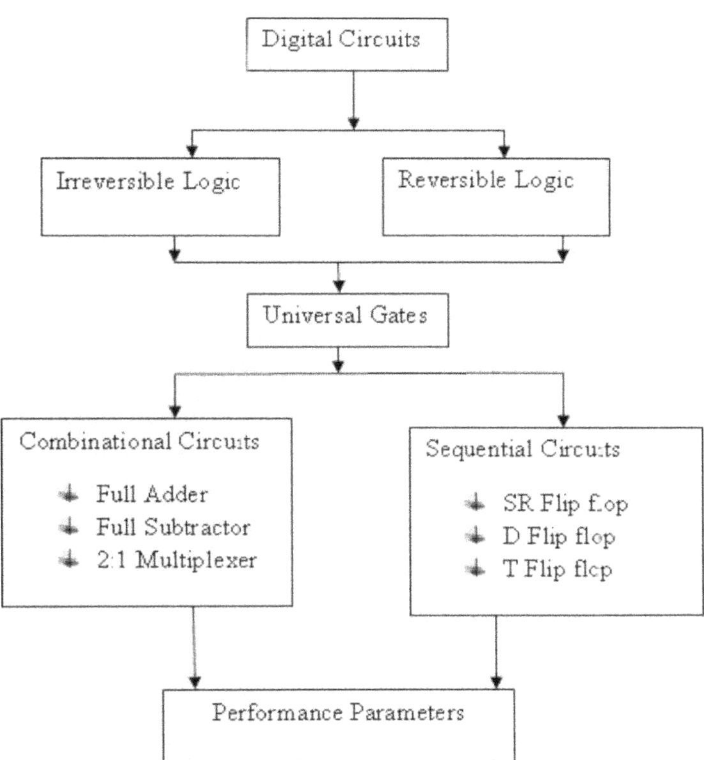

FIGURE 4.1 Methodology for designing different digital circuits.

1. *Reversible Gates Using Different Gates*: There are various types of RGs, which are classified as the Feynman gate (shown in Figure 4.2a) [28, 29], Toffoli gate (shown in Figure 4.2b) [30], Fredkin gate (shown in Figure 4.2c) [31, 32], Peres gate (shown in Figure 4.2d) [33], TR gate (shown in Figure 4.2e), and a new gate (shown in Figure 4.2f).

The input/output, corresponding equations, and QC values are shown in Table 4.1.

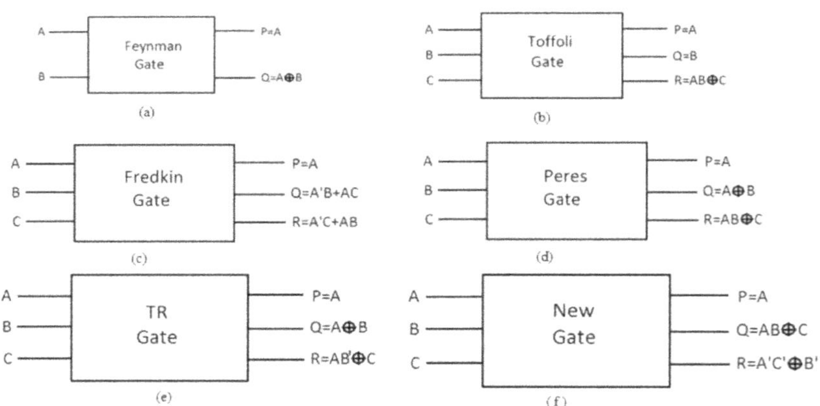

FIGURE 4.2 Types of different reversible gates.

TABLE 4.1
Different Reversible Gates and Their Equations

Gates	Input/Output	Equations	QC
Feynman Gate (FeG)	Two-input (*A* and *B*) and two-output (*P* and *Q*)	$P = A,\ Q = A \oplus B$	1
Toffoli Gate	Three-input (*A*, *B*, and C) and three-output (*P*, *Q*, and R)	$P = A,\ Q = B,$ $R = AB \oplus C$	5
Fredkin Gate (FrG)	*A*, *B*, and C (three-input) and *P*, *Q*, and R (three-output)	$P = A$ $Q = \bar{A}B + AC$ $R = AB + \bar{A}C$	5
Peres Gate (PG)	*A*, *B*, and C (three-input) and *P*, *Q*, and R (three-output)	$P = A$ $Q = A \oplus B$ $R = AB \oplus C$	4
TR Gate	*A*, *B*, and C (three-input) and *P*, *Q*, and R (three-output)	$P = A$ $Q = A \oplus B$ $R = A\bar{B} \oplus C$	4
New Gate	*A*, *B*, and C (three-input) and *P*, *Q*, and R (three-output)	$P = \mathrm{A}$ $Q = AB \oplus C$ $R = \bar{A}\bar{C} \oplus \bar{B}$	

2. *Universal Gates (NAND and NOR Gates)*: If universal gates are designed, then any Boolean expression of digital circuits can be designed. There are two universal gates: NAND and NOR [34, 35].
3. *Digital Logic*: Using reversible and irreversible logic, various combinational and sequential circuits can be designed. In a combinational logic circuit (CLC), the output is dependent on the combination of inputs. A CLC has 'timing', 'no memory', or 'feedback loops' within its design. In this chapter, only three CLCs are considered: Full adder, full subtractor, and 2:1 multiplexer. In a sequential logic circuit (SLC), output not only depends on the present value, it also depends on past values. Sequential circuits have a memory element which stores value [34]. SLCs consist of latches and flip flops (FFs), which is a one-bit memory element. There are different types of FFs, but the authors only designed set rest (SR), D, and T FFs using IrL and RL [36, 37].
4. *Performance Parameters*: The different gates were simulated in a simulation program with integrated circuit emphasis (SPICE), and the various electrical parameters, namely slew rate, power dissipation (*PD*), output resistance (R_o), input resistance (R_i) and common mode rejection ratio (*CMRR*) [34], were calculated. The authors also used the VIVADO 2018 tool using Verilog coding to calculate different parameters like transistor count, delay, and power dissipation.

4.3 RESULTS AND DISCUSSION

The authors used reversible logic concepts in designing the different digital circuits. Initially, different reversible gates were implemented on VIVADO, XILINX ISE using Verilog coding. The transistor count, delay, and power dissipation were calculated and are shown in Table 4.2.

Based on the different parameters like delay and power, it was observed that the Feynman, Toffoli and Peres gates resulted in the minimum values among the six gates. The Feynman gate exhibited a 75.5-ns delay and 28.71-mW power dissipation, the Toffoli gate showed a 50-ns delay and 26.91-mW power dissipation, and the Peres gate demonstrate a 60-ns delay and 29.32-mW power dissipation.

TABLE 4.2
Comparison of Different RGs

Gate	Transistor Count	Delay (ns)	Power Dissipation (mW)
Feynman	6	**75.5**	**28.71**
Toffoli	12	**50**	**26.91**
Peres	18	**60**	**29.32**
Fredkin	16	80	30
TR	18	88.67	38.44
New	20	98.237	33.5

To further validate the enhanced reversible gates, the implementation of three gates (Feynman, Toffoli, and Peres) was done using CMOS technology [16] in the SPICE tool. The FeG can be implemented using CMOS technology using IrL and RL and is demonstrated in Figures 4.3a and 4.3b, respectively. The Toffoli gate (shown in Figure 4.4) and Peres gate (shown in Figure 4.5) can be implemented using CMOS technology using reversible logic.

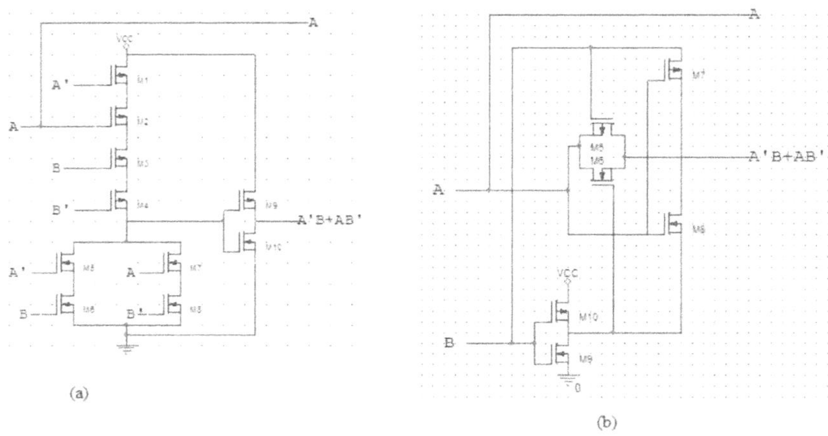

FIGURE 4.3 Execution of Feynman gate using (a) irreversible; (b) reversible logic.

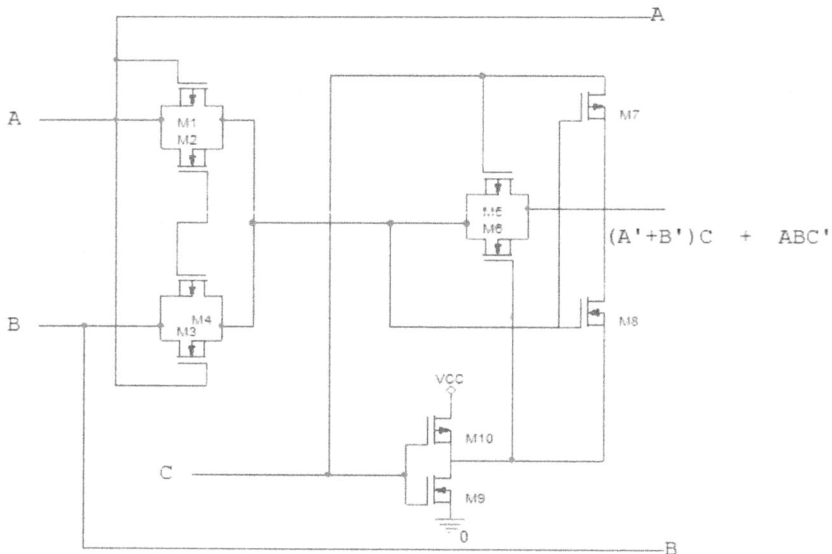

FIGURE 4.4 Execution of Toffoli gate using reversible logic.

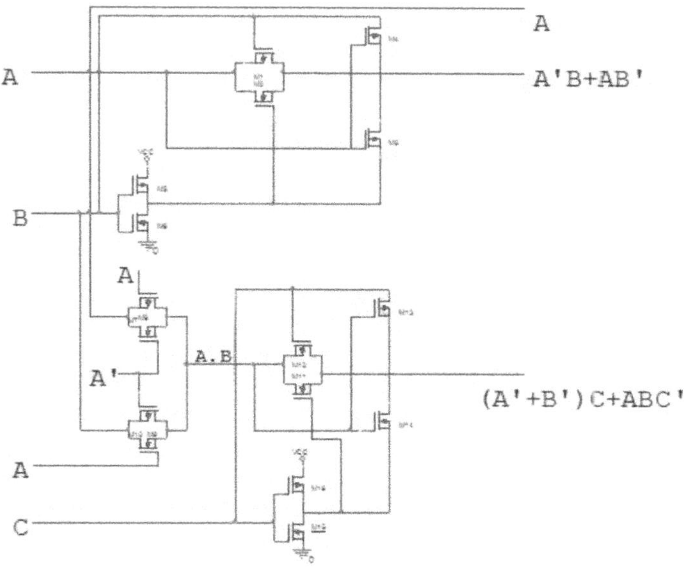

FIGURE 4.5 Execution of Peres gate using reversible logic.

TABLE 4.3
Performance Parameters of Three Gates

	Parameters	Voltage Gain (dB)	Slew Rate (V/μsec)	CMRR (dB)	Input Resistance (Ω)	Output Resistance (kΩ)
FeG	Irreversible	50.55	13×10^6	140.747	1020	0.805
	Reversible	26.5	1.2×10^3	1.6065	7.529×10^3	0.9189
TG	Irreversible	67.79	9.8×10^4	103.365	1020	0.9285
	Reversible	44.222	6×10^4	347.82	1.626×10^5	0.9643
PG	Irreversible	51.78	3×10^{-7}	0.478	1020	0.3725
	Reversible	0	2×10^3	—	7.53×10^3	5×10^8

Based on the simulation of the three gates using irreversible and reversible logic, different electrical parameters were evaluated and are shown in Table 4.3.

Table 4.3 shows the different electrical parameters like voltage gain, input impedance, output impedance, slew rate, and CMRR. Among the different gates, the Toffoli gate showed the best results. With the help of the Toffoli gate, different universal gates were implemented. Figures 4.6a and 4.6b show the NAND and NOR gates using reversible gates, respectively.

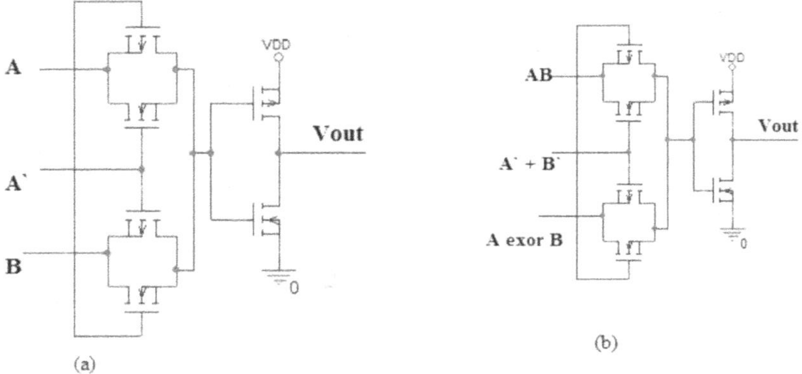

FIGURE 4.6 Implementation of reversible gates: (a) NAND gate; (b) NOR gate.

TABLE 4.4
Performance Parameters of Irreversible and Reversible Universal Gates

	Parameters	Voltage Gain (dB)	Slew Rate (V/μsec)	CMRR (dB)	Power Dissipation (mW)	Input Resistance (Ω)	Output Resistance (kΩ)
NAND Gate	**Irreversible**	81.168	9×10^3	113.23	8.06	1020	0.807
	Reversible	76.31	410	85.45	7.8	64.03×10^3	0.697
NOR Gate	**Irreversible**	71.79	17×10^3	109.3	20.3	1020	0.4534
	Reversible	51.876	8.5×10^4	71.345	10.8	64.07	0.322

The different universal gates were simulated using irreversible and reversible logic. The various electronic parameters were evaluated and are shown in Table 4.4.

Table 4.4 shows the different electrical parameters of NAND and NOR gates for both irreversible and reversible logic. It has been seen that the NAND gate dissipates only 7.80 mW, and the NOR gate dissipates only 10.8 mW power. Based on Table 4.3, the authors concluded that reversible logic shows the better results. Using universal gate logic, the authors designed different digital circuits using both reversible and irreversible logic.

4.3.1 Combinational Circuits

When two or more logic gates are combined together in order to produce precise outputs for different combinations of gate variables, with no storage involved, then such circuits are termed combinational logic circuits. In these circuits, the output is always dependent on the input. For combinational circuits, the authors implemented a full adder, full subtractor, and 2:1 multiplexer.

1. Full Adder: A full adder adds two binary numbers (A and B), considering previous output C_{in}, which results in a sum (S) and carry out (C_{out}) [10]. Figures 4.7 and 4.8 show the execution of a full adder circuit using irreversible and reversible logic, respectively.

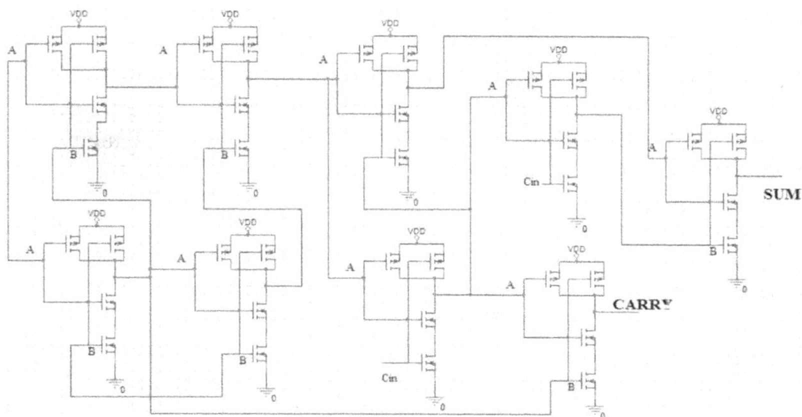

FIGURE 4.7 Realization of full adder using irreversible logic.

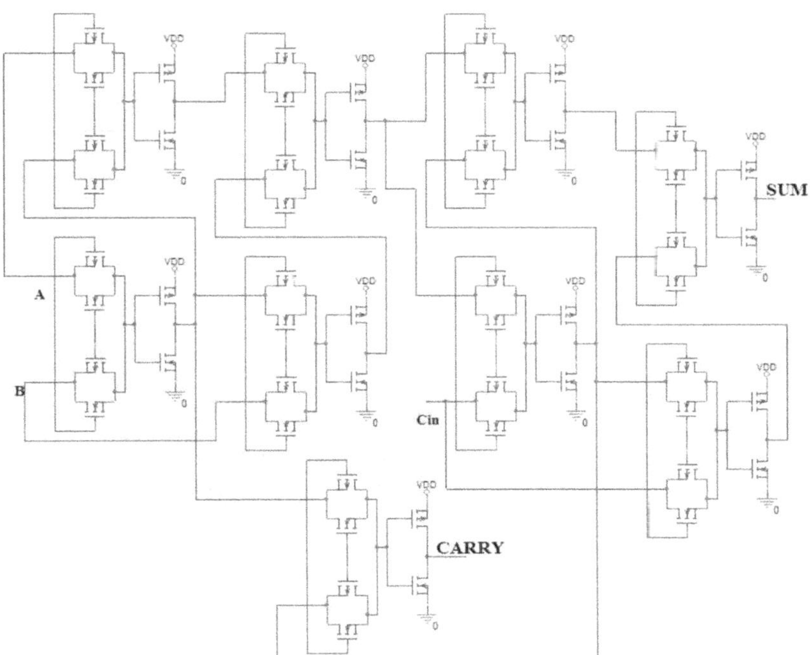

FIGURE 4.8 Realization of full adder using reversible logic.

The full adder circuit was simulated using irreversible and reversible logic, and the various electronic parameters were evaluated and are shown in Table 4.5.

The advantage of the adder circuit is in simulation and usage in various applications like up-counters, multipliers, and arithmetic programmable-state machines.

2. Full Subtractor: Its circuit is used for subtraction of three bits, A, B, and B_{in} (previous borrow), resulting in two outputs, D_i (difference) and B_o (borrow). Figures 4.9 and 4.10 show the implementation of a full subtractor circuit using irreversible and reversible logic, respectively.

TABLE 4.5
Evaluation of Performance Parameters for Full Adder Circuit

Parameters		Voltage Gain (dB)	Slew Rate (V/μsec)	CMRR (dB)	Power Dissipation (mW)	Input Resistance (kΩ)	Output Resistance (kΩ)
Reversible	SUM	222.097	14×10^6	320.51	0.118	82.885	0.7143
	CARRY	71.12	30×10^6	20.772	0.118	76.43	0.5587
Irreversible	SUM	115.5	115×10^3	98.96	6.98	79.65	0.755
	CARRY	73.22	3.75×10^3	9.068	6.98	68.98	0.7147

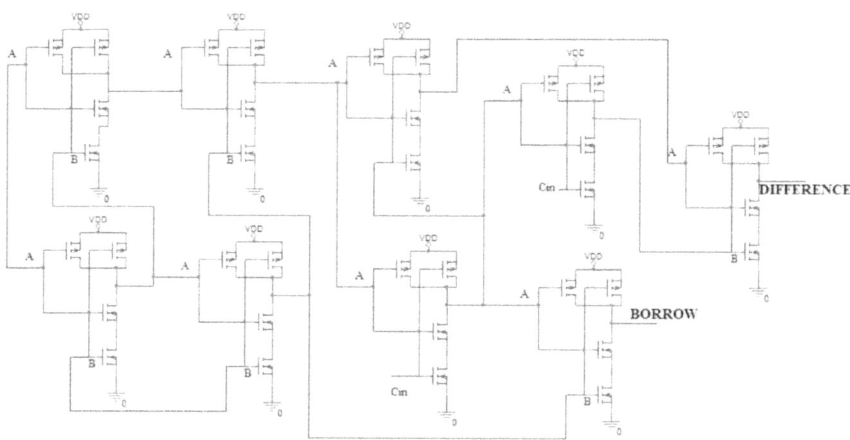

FIGURE 4.9 Execution of full subtractor using irreversible logic.

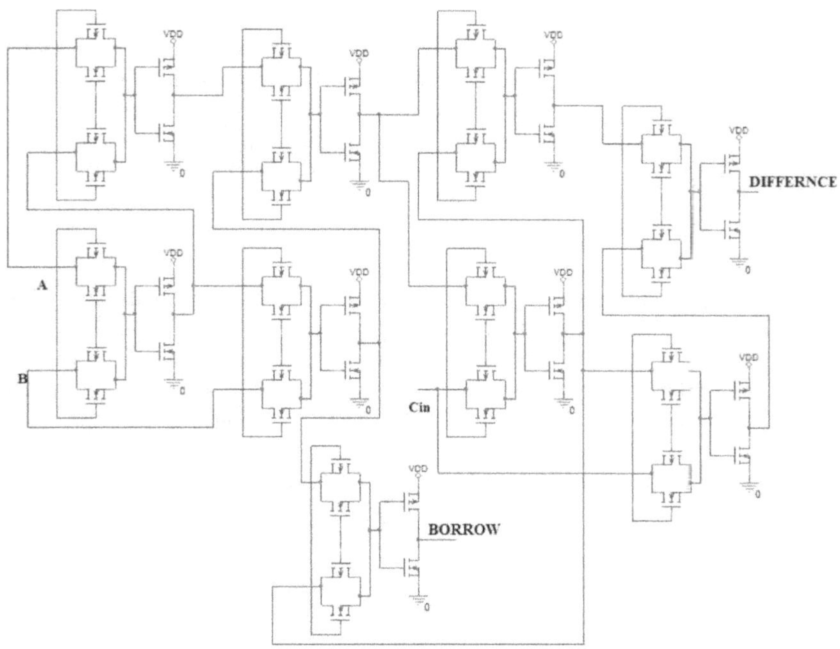

FIGURE 4.10 Execution of full subtractor using reversible logic.

TABLE 4.6
Evaluation of Performance Parameters for Full Subtractor Circuit

Parameters		Voltage Gain (dB)	Slew Rate (V/μsec)	CMRR (dB)	Power Dissipation (mW)	Input Resistance (kΩ)	Output Resistance (kΩ)
Reversible	**Difference**	216.65	13.5×10^6	325.95	0.119	88.64	0.7143
	Borrow	62.117	4.9×10^6	351.226	0.119	74.32	0.5726
Irreversible	**Difference**	119.32	115×10^3	100.352	7	81.44	0.755
	Borrow	51.794	52×10^3	27.44	7	75.65	0.7215

The full subtractor circuit was simulated using irreversible and reversible logic, and the various electronic parameters were evaluated and are shown in Table 4.6.

From Table 4.6, it can be observed that reversible logic shows the maximum voltage gain: 216.65 dB difference and 62.117 dB borrow. Likewise, considering the other parameters, reversible logic shows the better results.

3. 2:1 Multiplexer: A multiplexer is a CLC with many inputs and one output. Multiplexing, or MUX, is the act of compressing a wide data bus, like 16 bits of data, onto a single line for transmission. The value of multiplexing is that we can send 16 bits of data on a single pair of wires by cleverly encoding the data on the sending end. There are $2n$ inputs, which have n select lines. Figures 4.11 and 4.12 show the realization of a 2:1 multiplexer circuit using irreversible and reversible logic, respectively.

A 2:1 multiplexer was simulated using irreversible and reversible logic, and the various electronic parameters were evaluated and are shown in Table 4.7.

From Table 4.7, it can be observed that reversible logic shows the maximum voltage gain: 59.91 dB, slew rate, 104×10^3 V/µsec, 63.81 kΩ input resistance, and 10.44 dB CMRR. This signifies that reversible logic shows the better results.

After combinational circuits, different sequential circuits were simulated.

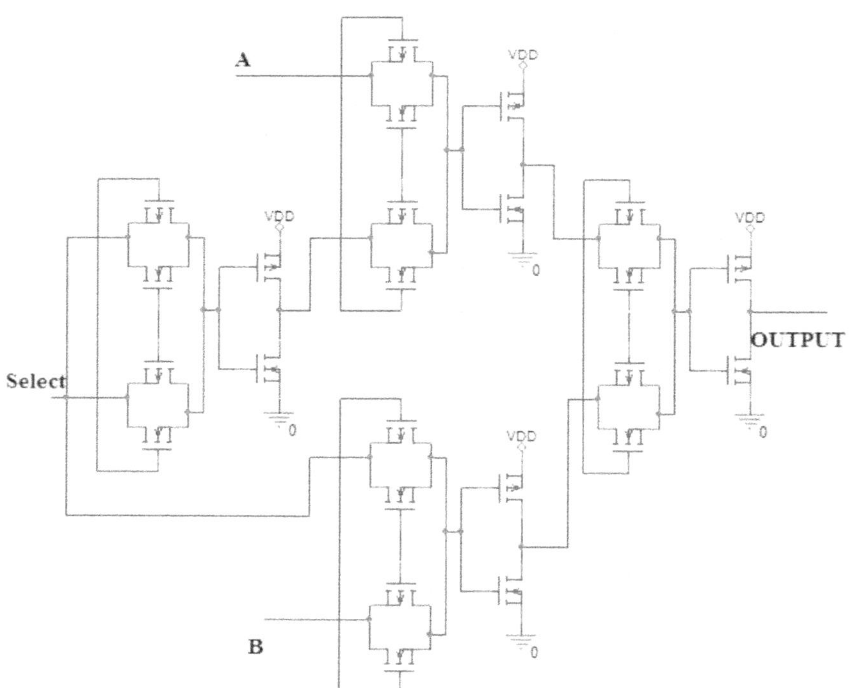

FIGURE 4.11 Realization of 2:1 multiplexer using irreversible logic.

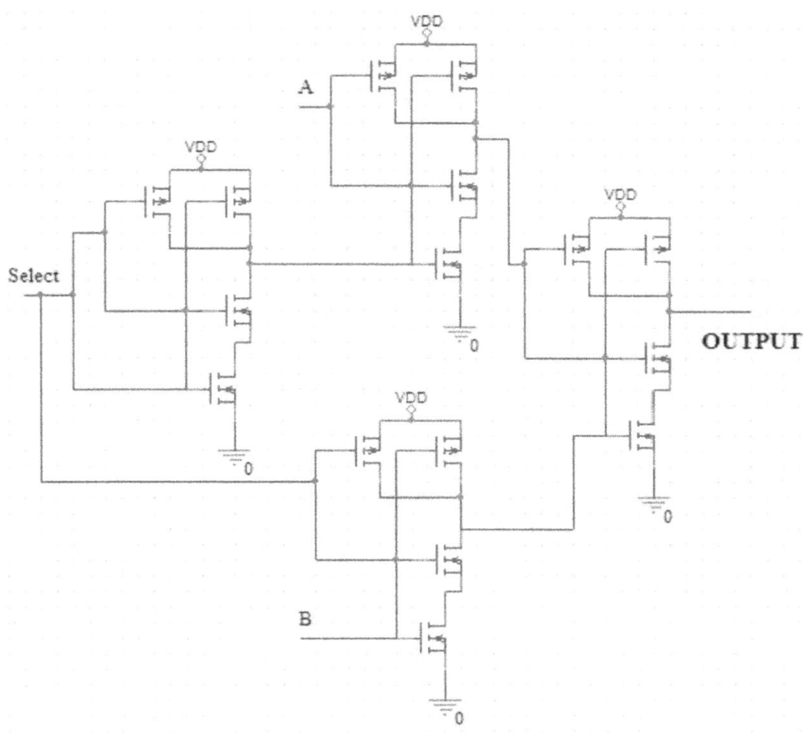

FIGURE 4.12 Realization of 2:1 multiplexer using reversible logic.

TABLE 4.7
Electronic Parameter Comparison of 2:1 Multiplexer Circuit Using IrL and RL

Parameters	Voltage Gain (dB)	Slew Rate (V/μsec)	CMRR (dB)	Power Dissipation (mW)	Input Resistance (kΩ)	Output Resistance (kΩ)
Reversible	59.91	104×10^3	10.44	0.101	63.81	0.7175
Irreversible	52.28	12.8×10^3	1.292	2.92	58.77	0.983

4.3.2 Sequential Circuits

Sequential circuits are digital logic circuits that work in accordance with timing signal inputs. They have inherent memory and retain their state as SET (1) and RESET (0) indefinitely until a subsequent timing pulse or any other input trigger signal is applied to change the state of storage. They are usually expressed as bistable devices signifying two states, SET (1) and RESET (0). The authors considered *SR*, *D*, and *T* flip flops.

1. The *SR flip-flop*, or SR latch, has two inputs, one SET or S (1) and another RESET or R (0), and two outputs, *Q* and complement (not) *Q*. The basic single-bit *SR* FF is designed by cross-coupling of two input NAND gates. Figure 4.13 shows the implementation of a gated *SR* latch using reversible gates.

An SR latch was simulated using irreversible and reversible logic, and the various electronic parameters were evaluated and are shown in Table 4.8.

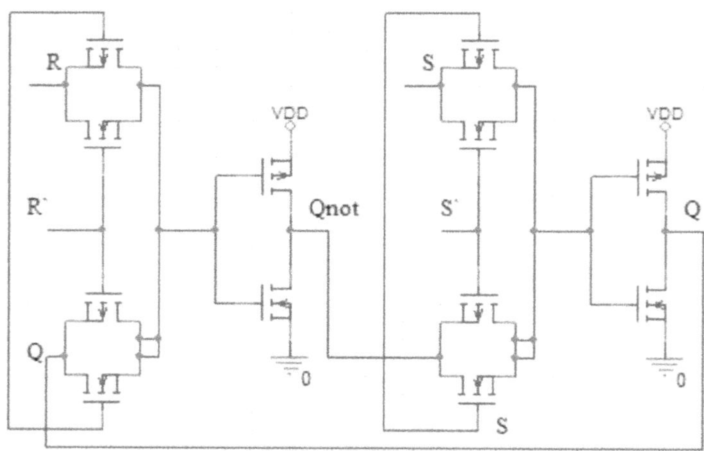

FIGURE 4.13 Reversible gated SR latch.

TABLE 4.8
Electronic Parameter Comparison of SR Latch Circuit Using IrL and RL

Parameters		Voltage Gain (dB)	Slew Rate (V/μsec)	CMRR (dB)	Power Dissipation (mW)	Input Resistance (kΩ)	Output Resistance (kΩ)
Reversible	Q	**12.825**	**360 × 10³**	**12.88**	**0.148**	**8.364**	**0.7631**
	$\bar{Q}$	11.2	11 × 10³	5.74	0.148	1.265	0.1256
Irreversible	Q	8.127	182 × 10³	8.666	0.177	6.654	0.8663
	$\bar{Q}$	3.925	1.42 × 10³	5.23	0.177	1.108	0.425

From Table 4.8, it can be observed that 12.825 dB voltage gain, 360 × 10^3 V/μsec slew rate, and 12.88 dB CMRR are the highest among the values. In an SR FF, if 1 is applied to both S and R inputs, it results in unpredictable output. The limits of the SR-flip flop are overcome by cascading a second stage in the circuit, which is arranged with a clock/clock line to cause an edge triggering option. The most basic version is called a D-flip flop, where D stands for data.

2. The *data* or *delay (D) flip flop* is a sequential circuit that has two stable states, and it can store one bit of state information. It can be considered a basic memory cell, and it also ensures that the inputs of S and R in an SR latch would never be equal to 1 at the same time. It is mostly used in digital electronics. *D*-FFs are usually considered zero-order hold elements or delay line elements. Figure 4.14 shows the implementation of a *D*-FF using reversible logic.

A D-flip flop was simulated using irreversible and reversible logic, and the various electronic parameters were evaluated and are shown in Table 4.9. The

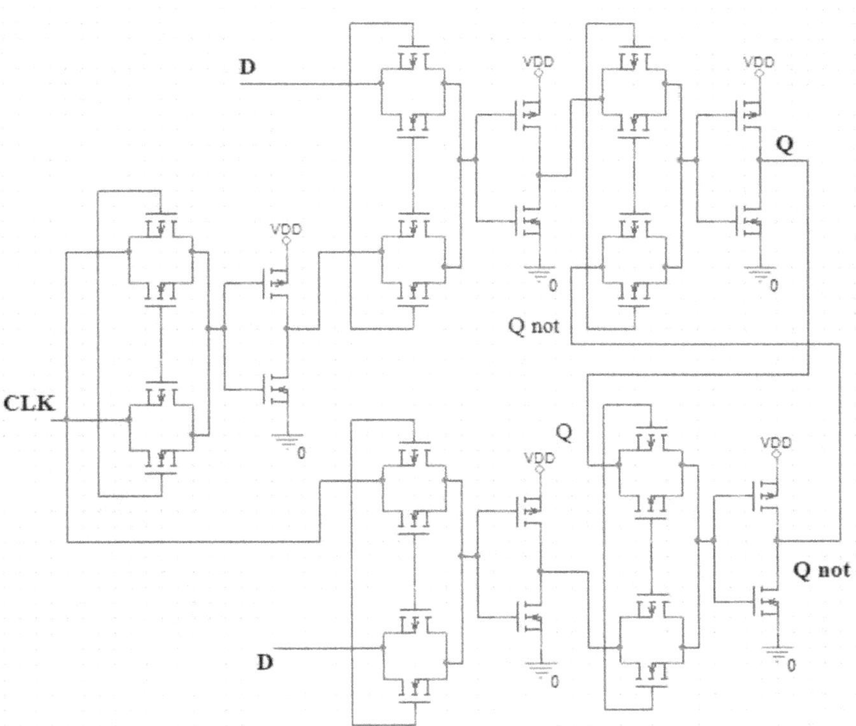

FIGURE 4.14 Reversible *D*-FF.

TABLE 4.9
Electronic Parameter Comparison of D-Flip Flop Circuit Using IrL and RL

Parameters		Voltage Gain (dB)	Slew Rate (V/μsec)	CMRR (dB)	Input Resistance (kΩ)	Output Resistance (kΩ)
Reversible	Q	112.15	2.58×10^3	68.77	50×10^7	1.525
	$\bar{Q}$	92.062	2×10^3	69.28	4.98×10^7	1.621
Irreversible	Q	16.4	1.25×10^3	65.91	1.2×10^4	3.232
	$\bar{Q}$	15.9	0.5×10^3	67.901	0.34×10^4	3.915

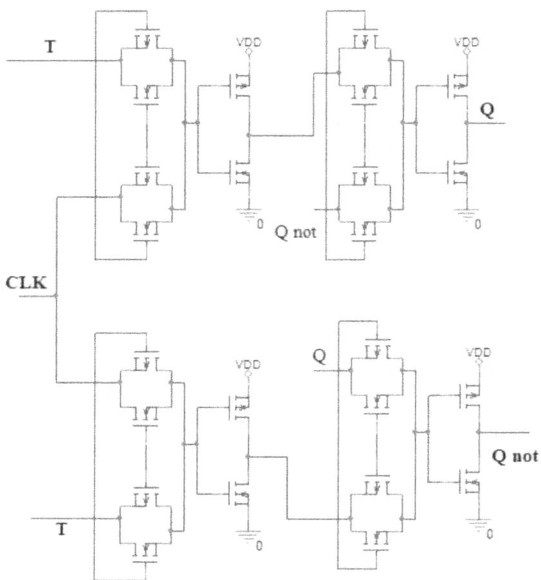

FIGURE 4.15 Reversible *T*-FF.

advantage of D-flip flops is their simplicity, and the input and output are fundamentally indistinguishable but relocated in time by one clock period.

After simulation, it was observed that 23.9 mW and 37.6 mW power were dissipated using reversible and irreversible logic, respectively. Also, it was observed that 112.15 dB voltage gain, 2.58×10^3 V/μsec slew rate, and 68.77 dB CMRR were achieved using reversible logic. A *D* FF simply passes the input to the output when clocked. They are usually used for simple latched registers.

3. There are many ways of designing a *toggle (T) flip flop* (*T*-FF). It can be designed using an *SR* or *D* flip flop. Figure 4.15 shows the implementation of a *T*-FF using reversible logic.

TABLE 4.10
Electronic Parameter Comparison of T-Flip Flop Circuit Using IrL and RL

Parameters	Voltage Gain (dB)	Slew Rate (V/μsec)	Power Dissipation (mW)	CMRR (dB)	Input Resistance (kΩ)	Output Resistance (kΩ)
Reversible	72.42	3.82×10^{15}	25.5	240.036	10.99	0.668
Irreversible	55.43	2.25×10^{15}	34.58	176.23	5.21	0.863

A T-flip flop was simulated using irreversible and reversible logic, and the various electronic parameters were evaluated and are shown in Table 4.10.

After simulation, it was observed that 25.5 mW and 34.58 mW power were dissipated using reversible and irreversible logic, respectively. Also, it was observed that 72.42 dB voltage gain, 3.82×10^{15} V/μsec slew rate, and 240.036 dB CMRR were achieved using reversible logic.

4.4 CONCLUSION

In a fast processing environment, the main goal is to achieve high accuracy and less energy consumption. A reversible logic circuit dissipates less power as it recovers energy loss and prevents bit error. Reversible computing has many applications in different areas which require speed, high energy efficiency, and performance. Computers are based on reversible logic that can reuse a portion of the signal energy. In this chapter, the authors have discussed irreversible and reversible logic and how reversible logic is better than traditional irreversible gates. Different types of digital circuits using reversible logic were designed. Initially, six different types of reversible gates were simulated. Out of six gates, the Toffoli gate showed the best results, and busing this gate, NAND and NOR gates were simulated in SPICE with the help of universal gates. The different digital circuits were designed and simulated, and it was observed that reversible logic outperformed the other results. In the future, the authors will try other circuits like multipliers, arithmetic programmable-state machines, and so on.

REFERENCES

[1] C.C. Tripathi, Nikihil Maraiwalla, Dinesh Kumar, Shruti Jain, "Mobile Radio Communications and 5G Networks", Springer, Singapore (2020).

[2] Shruti Jain, Sudip Paul, "Recent Trends in Image and Signal Processing in Computer Vision", Springer, Singapore (2020).

[3] Michael P. Frank, "Reversibility for Efficient Computing", Ph.D. Thesis (May 1999).

[4] Shruti Jain, Meenakshi Sood, Sudip Paul, "Advances in Computational Intelligence Techniques", Springer, Singapore (2020).

[5] M. Frank, "Introduction to Reversible Computing: Motivation, Progress, and Challenges", ACM Inc., New York (2005), pp. 385–390.

[6] M.S. Islam et al., "Low cost quantum realization of reversible multiplier circuit", Information Technology Journal, 8 (2008), p. 208.
[7] D. Krishnaveni, M. Geeta Priya, "Design of an efficient reversible 8*8 Wallace tree multiplier", Submitted for IEEE Transactions on Circuits and Systems I.
[8] H.R. Bhagyalakshmi, M.K. Venkatesha, "Optimized reversible BCD adder using new reversible logic gates", Journal of Computing, 2 (Feb 2010).
[9] D. Samtani, N.K. Patel, A. Gupta, S. Jain, "Design of universal gates based on reversible logic", International Journal of Emerging Technologies in Computational and Applied Sciences (IJETCAS), 11(2) (Dec 2014– Feb 2015), pp. 174–178.
[10] H.R. Bhagyalakshmi, M.K. Venkatesha, "An improved design of a multiplier using reversible logic gates", International Journal of Engineering Science and Technology, 2(8) (2010), pp. 3838–3845.
[11] A.P. Chandrakasan, R.W. Broderson, "Low Power Digital CMOS Design", Kluwer Academic Publishers, Boston, MA (1995).
[12] Yibin Ye, K. Roy, "Energy recovery circuits using reversible and partially reversible logic", in IEEE Transactions on Circuits and Systems I: Fundamental Theory and Applications, 43(9) (1996), pp. 769–778.
[13] Dai Hongyu, Zhou Runde, "Improved energy recovery logic for low power computation", in IEEE 2002 International Conference on Communications, Circuits and Systems and West Sino Expositions, 2 (2002), pp. 1740–1743.
[14] Kirti Singh, Madhu Singh, "Reversible full adder design with reduced quantum cost", International Journal of Electrical, Electronics and Computer Engineering, 4(2) (2015), pp. 146–153.
[15] V. Anantharam, M. He, K. Natarajan, H. Xie, and M.P. Frank, "Driving fully-adiabatic logic circuits using custom high-Q MEMS resonators", in Proceedings of International Conference on Embedded Systems & Applications, CSREA (2004), pp. 5–11.
[16] W.C. Athas, L.J. Svensson, J.G. Koller, N. Tzartzanis, E.Y.-C. Chou, "Low-power digital systems based on adiabatic switching principles", in IEEE Transactions on Very Large Scale Integration (VLSI) Systems, 2(4) (Dec. 1994), pp. 398–407.
[17] D.J. Frank, "Power constrained CMOS scaling limits", IBM Journal of Research and Development, 46(2/3) (2002), pp. 235–244.
[18] C.H. Bennett, "The thermodynamics of computation—A review", International Journal of Theoretical Physics, 21(12) (1982), pp. 905–940.
[19] M. Shams, M. Haghparast, K. Navi, "Novel reversible multiplier circuit in nanotechnology", World Applied Science Journal, 3(5) (2008), pp. 806–810.
[20] Fateme Naderpour, Abbas Vafaei, "Reversible multipliers: Decreasing the depth of the circuit", in ICECE 2008 (20–22 Dec 2008).
[21] M. Haghparast, S. Jafarali Jassbi, K. Navi, O. Hashemipour, "Design of a novel reversible multiplier circuit using HNG gate in nanotechnology", World Applied Science Journal, 3(6) (2008), pp. 974–978.
[22] M.S. Islam et al., "Low cost quantum realization of reversible multiplier circuit", Information Technology Journal, 8 (2009), p. 208.
[23] Anindita Banerjee, Anirban Pathak, "An analysis of reversible multiplier circuits", arXiv:0907.3357 (2009), pp. 1–10.
[24] H. Thapliyal, M.B. Srinivas, "Novel reversible multiplier architecture using reversible TSG gate", in Proceedings of IEEE International Conference on Computer Systems and Applications (Mar 2006), pp. 100–103.
[25] C.H. Bennett, "Time/space trade-offs for reversible computation", SIAM Journal on Computing, 18(4) (1989), pp. 766–776.

[26] H. Buhrman, J. Tromp, P. Vitanyi, "Time and space bounds for reversible simulation", Journal of Physics A: Mathematical and General, 34 (2001), pp. 6821–6830.
[27] C.H. Bennett, "Logical Reversibility of Computation", IBM Journal of Research and Development (Nov 1973), pp. 525–532.
[28] R. Feynman, "Quantum mechanical computers", Optic News, 11 (1985), pp. 11–20.
[29] R.P. Feynman, "Quantum mechanical computers", Foundations of Physics, 16(6) (1986), pp. 507–531.
[30] T. Toffoli, "Reversible computing", Tech Memo MIT/LCS/TM-151, MIT Lab for Computer Science (1980).
[31] E.F. Fredkin, T. Toffoli, "Design principles for achieving high-performance submicron digital technologies," In A. Adamatzky, eds., *Collision-Based Computing*, Springer, London (2002). https://doi.org/10.1007/978-1-4471-0129-1_2.
[32] E. Fredkin, T. Toffoli, "Conservative logic", International Journal of Theory of Physics, 21 (1982), pp. 219–253.
[33] A. Peres, "Reversible logic and quantum computers", Physical Review A, 32 (1985), pp. 3266–3276.
[34] S.M. Kang, Y. Leblebici, "CMOS Digital Integrated Circuit", 3rd edition, Tata McGraw Hill (2006).
[35] J.S. Hall, "An electroid switching model for reversible computer architectures", in PhysComp '92: Proceedings of the Workshop on Physics and Computation, Oct 2–4, 1992, Dallas, Texas, IEEE Computer Society Press (1992), pp. 237–247.
[36] R. Landauer, "Irreversibility and heat generation in the computational process", IBM Journal of Research and Development, 5 (1961), pp. 183–191.
[37] Md. M.H. Azad Khan, "Design of full adder with reversible gate", in International Conference on Computer and Information Technology, Dhaka, Bangladesh (2002), pp. 515–519.

5 Denoising of Biomedical Images Using Two-Dimensional Fourier-Bessel Series Expansion-Based Empirical Wavelet Transform

Pradeep Kumar Chaudhary and Ram Bilas Pachori

CONTENTS

5.1 INTRODUCTION

Biomedical images are used for automatic diagnosis of many diseases. Some of the common biomedical images used for research are fundus images (photographic image), magnetic resonance imaging (images of the brain), mammograms (X-ray images of the breast), skin lesion images (photographic images), and many more. Before processing these images for diagnostic purpose, they undergo many steps, like image acquisition and image transmission, which lead to the introduction of noise in the images.

Noise in images can be either in additive or multiplicative form. An additive noise in an image can be expressed as $V(x, y) = I(x, y) + N(x, y)$, while multiplicative noise satisfies $V(x, y) = I(x, y) \times N(x, y)$, where $I(x, y)$ is the original

DOI: 10.1201/9781003207856-5

image, $N(x, y)$ denotes the noise introduced to the image, and $V(x, y)$ denotes the corrupted image due to the introduction of noise in the original image [1]. The most common noise introduced in biomedical images is Gaussian noise (additive noise), in which each pixel in the noisy image is the sum of the true pixel value and a random Gaussian distributed noise value.

The introduction of noise will create distortion in the image and cause problems in further processing, such as object detection, classification, and segmentation [2]. Image denoising is the process of removing noise to try to recover the image in its original form. In the literature, various methods have been proposed for denoising images, such as averaging [3], median filtering [4], fractional filtering [2], convolution neural network-based denoising [5], patch-based denoising [6], sparse filtering-based denoising [7], and wavelet thresholding-based denoising [8–16]. This chapter focuses on a wavelet thresholding-based approach. Wavelet thresholding uses the concept that the small-value coefficients in a sub-image are most likely considered noise, and the large-value coefficients are considered significant values of the image. The thresholding operation is a non-linear approach, and it is carried out on one coefficient at a time. If the coefficient value is less than a set threshold value (T), then it is set to zero; this is known as hard thresholding. Figure 5.1 shows a plot of the hard thresholding function $F(x)$, which is used in this work. After thresholding, an inverse wavelet transform is applied on the resultant coefficients, leading to an image with less noise. In this chapter, an optimal thresholding estimation technique for image denoising is used. The threshold value depends on coefficients present in the sub-image; that is, for each sub-image, a different threshold value is estimated.

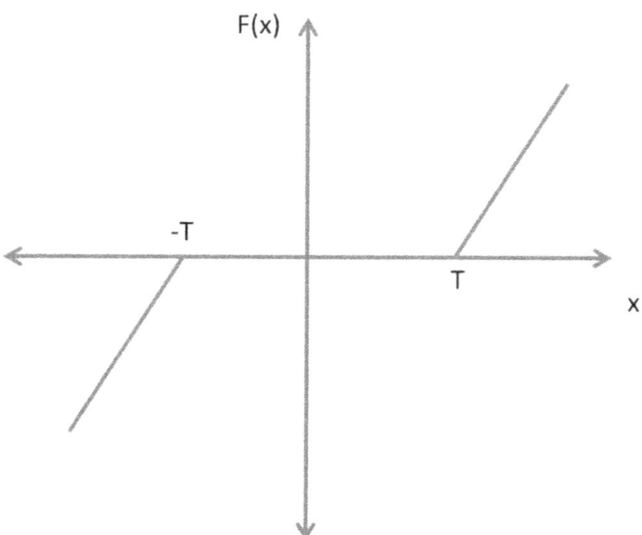

FIGURE 5.1 Plot of thresholding function.

Wavelet analysis has proven to be one of the best methods for image denoising [17]. The drawback of the wavelet transform is that it is a non-adaptive method; that is, the method is independent of signal characteristics. So in this chapter, adaptive algorithms called order-zero and order-one two-dimensional (2D)-Fourier-Bessel series expansion (FBSE)-based empirical wavelet transform (2D-FBSE-EWT) approaches are used for denoising. Next, a brief introduction to FBSE is provided, followed by the advantages of using FBSE and its applications in signal and image processing.

FBSE transforms the time-domain signal into the order-domain. It uses Bessel functions as a basis function set. Bessel functions are obtained by solving the second-order ordinary differential equation of the form [18, 19],

$$x^2\ddot{y}+x\dot{y}+\left(x^2-m^2\right)y=0 \tag{5.1}$$

It is also known as the Bessel equation, where m in Equation (5.1) is known as the order of the Bessel equation. The solution of Equation (5.1) is as follows:

$$y=AJ_m\left(x\right)+BY_m\left(x\right) \tag{5.2}$$

where A and B are arbitrary constants, and $J_m\left(x\right)$ $Y_m\left(x\right)$ are kind one and kind two Bessel functions. Bessel functions of kind one follow the property of orthogonality and can be stated as "For each fixed nonnegative integer m, the sequence of Bessel functions of the first kind $J_m\left(k_{m,1}x\right)$, $J_m\left(k_{m,2}x\right)$, $J_m\left(k_{m,3}x\right)$, . . ., $J_m\left(k_{m,n}x\right)$ forms an orthogonal set on the interval $0\le x\le R$ with respect to the weight function x"; that is, $\int_{x=0}^{R}xJ_m\left(k_{m,p}x\right)J_m\left(k_{m,q}x\right)dx=0$, where $q\neq p$, $k_{m,p}=\mathcal{E}_{m,p}/R$, and $\mathcal{E}_{m,p}$ is the pth positive root of the Bessel function of order m [19].

The advantages of using FBSE over Fourier transform (FT) are as follows:

1. FT uses sine and cosine as basis functions, which are stationary in nature, so it is suitable for representing stationary signals, whereas, FBSE uses Bessel functions as basis functions, which are non-stationary in nature, so it is suitable for representing non-stationary signals. It can also be said that the basis functions of FT are periodic and non-converging in nature and, on the other hand, the FBSE basis functions are aperiodic and converging in nature. Figure 5.2 shows the basis function of FT and FBSE. The sine and cosine functions are shown in Figure 5.2a, and the Bessel functions of order-zero and order-one are shown in Figure 5.2b.
2. FT represents the real signal in terms of complex exponential functions, and FBSE represents the real signal in terms of real Bessel basis functions.
3. FT represents the real signal in terms of positive and negative frequencies, whereas, FBSE represents the real signal only in terms of positive frequencies.

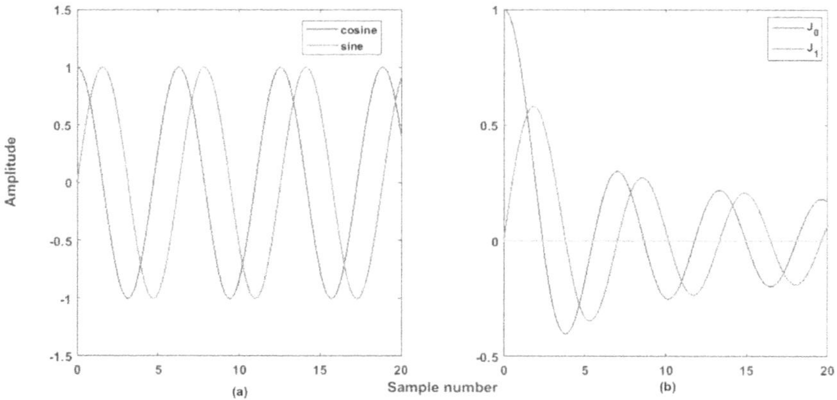

FIGURE 5.2 Plot of basis functions for (a) FT (sine and cosine); and (b) FBSE (Bessel functions of orders zero and one).

4. The spectrum based on FT provides *N*/2 unique coefficients, whereas FBSE provides *N* unique coefficients, where *N* is the length of the signal.
5. For a wide-band signal, FBSE provides compact representation as compared to FT. The Bessel functions decay with time and are amplitude modulated (AM) in nature. Due to this reason, the Bessel functions contribute to AM bandwidth and provide compact representation.

To understand points 2, 3, and 4, let us consider an example of a real signal with two frequency components: f1 = 50 Hz and f2 = 120 Hz, with sampling frequency = 1000 Hz. Figure 5.3a shows the plot of the considered signal with samples = 50. FT is implemented for the signal using the fast Fourier transform (FFT) algorithm, as FT provides complex representation of a real signal so it will give both the magnitude and phase information of the obtained spectrum. The magnitude of the FT is shown in Figure 5.3b. From Figure 5.3b, we can say that FT provides only 25 unique coefficients (the length of the signal is 50 samples). The coefficients after sample number 25 in Figure. 5.3b correspond to negative frequencies, and before sample number 25, they represent positive frequencies (which is the mirror image of the negative frequencies). Figures 5.3c and 5.3d show the amplitude and magnitude of the FBSE coefficients, respectively, and from Figure 5.3d, it can be said that FBSE provides 50 unique coefficients (the length of the signal is 50 samples) and has only positive frequencies and real coefficients. To understand point 5, we have considered a kind one Bessel function of order 150, that is, a $J_0\left(\frac{\varepsilon_{150} l}{L}\right)$ signal, where $L = 500$, $l = 0, 1, 2, \ldots, 499$, and ε_{150} is the 150th positive root of the equation $J_0(.) = 0$. The signal $J_0\left(\frac{\varepsilon_{150} l}{L}\right)$ is an AM signal whose plot is shown Figure 5.4a. Figures 5.4b and 5.4c show the Fourier spectrum and

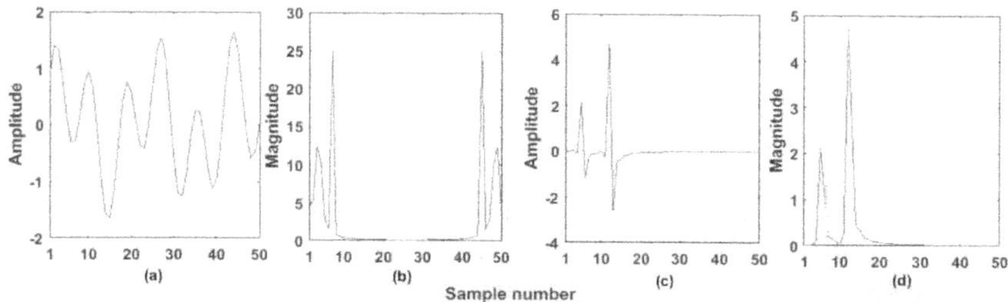

FIGURE 5.3 (a) Real signal; (b) magnitude of FT; (c) FBSE coefficients; and (d) magnitude of FBSE coefficients.

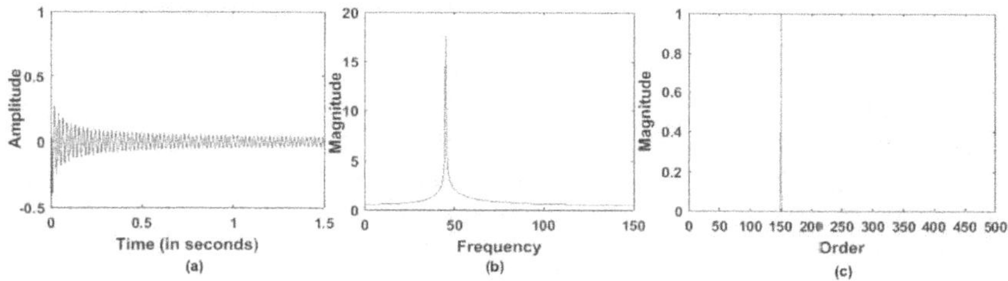

FIGURE 5.4 Plots of (a) signal $J_0\left(\frac{\mu_{150} l}{L}\right)$; (b) magnitude of FT (single sided); and (c) real FBSE coefficients of the signal.

magnitude of FBSE coefficients for the signal in Figure 5.4a. It can be concluded from Figures 5.4b and 5.4c that for modulated signals, FBSE can provide compact representation.

FBSE has been used in signal and image analysis in the literature due to its various advantages over FT. FT provides complex coefficients, whereas FBSE provides real coefficients. This advantage of FBSE is used in the Fourier-Bessel expansion-based discrete energy separation algorithm (FB-DESA) for component separation from amplitude-modulated and frequency-modulated (AM-FM) signal [20]. In the discrete energy separation algorithm, it was found that due to the filtering operation, there will be changes in the amplitude and frequency functions of the filtered signal. To compensate for this, FBSE is used for component separation using grouping operations, and as FBSE provides real coefficients, there is no change in the amplitude and frequency functions of the filtered signal. Inspired by the grouping operation of FB-DESA, the FBSE-based dyadic decomposition (FBD) method is used for X-ray image decomposition and was used for the diagnosis of COVID-19 [21]. FBD is a discrete wavelet transform (DWT) type of implementation in the FBSE domain using grouping operations. DWT decomposes the signal in terms of a scaled and translation version of a mother wavelet, and in the frequency-domain, its implementation is like dyadic decomposition [22]. The advantage of the FBD method over DWT is that any level of decomposition can be obtained in a single step, and it provides one extra level of decomposition. FBD and DWT can be considered constant-Q dyadic decomposition methods. Flexible time-frequency coverage wavelet transform (FAWT) provides a constant Q-factor transform but provides flexibility to select a desirable Q-factor, redundancy, and dilation factor for designing filter banks [23]. FAWT uses FT for implementation, and FT represents a real signal in both positive and negative frequencies. So, in order to ensure flexible control over filter design, two separate channels are used in high-pass filtering operations: One for positive frequencies and the other for negative frequencies. Since FBSE represents the signal only in positive frequencies, implementation of FAWT in the FBSE domain is easier based on this concept of FBSE-based flexible time-frequency coverage wavelet transform (FBSE-FAWT) has been developed [24]. FBD and FBSE-FAWT are constant-Q decomposition methods and are non-adaptive in nature. With the introduction of empirical mode decomposition (EMD), the problem of non-adaptive decomposition of the signal was solved. EMD decomposes the signal into meaningful intrinsic mode functions (IMFs) [25]. An IMF must satisfy two conditions: (1) in all the data of the IMF, the number of extrema (maxima and minima) and the number of zero crossings must either be equal or differ at most by one, and (2) at any point, the mean value of the envelope defined by the local maxima and the envelope defined by the local minima must be zero. However, there are a few drawbacks of EMD, such as a lack of theoretical background, no robust stopping criterion for sifting processes, and a problem of mode mixing, whereas empirical wavelet transforms (EWTs) provide both good time-frequency localization and adaptiveness with mathematical explanation [26]. But still, EWT has problems like interference and redundancy due to improper segmentation of the image spectrum. FBSE-EWT uses the FBSE spectrum instead of an FT-based spectrum for better segmentation of image spectra in the EWT algorithm. The FT-based spectrum provides poor segmentation performance when frequency components are closely spaced. FBSE provides better (twice) spectrum resolution than FT, so by using FBSE in place of FT in EWT, better boundary segmentation can be obtained [26, 27]. Inspired by the advantage of FBSE-EWT, the 2D version of FBSE-EWT, that is, 2D-FBSE-EWT, is used for glaucoma detection using fundus images [28]. Other applications in which FBSE is used are electroencephalogram signal analysis [29–36], electrocardiogram signal analysis [36–38], photoplethysmogram signal analysis [27], speech processing [39, 40], and cross-term reduction in Wigner-Ville distribution [41].

In this chapter, order-zero 2D-FBSE-EWT and order-one 2D-FBSE-EWT based wavelet thresholding methods are used for image denoising. The wavelet thresholding method calculates the optimal thresholding value for each sub-image obtained after decomposing the image using 2D-FBSE-EWT in order to remove noise. For analysis purposes, three types of biomedical images are used: Fundus, mammogram, and skin lesion. We have compared our proposed order-zero 2D-FBSE-EWT and order-one 2D-FBSE-EWT based image denoising methods with an existing 2D-EWT-based image denoising method [42]. The performance parameter used is peak signal-to-noise ratio (PSNR) [43]. The term

PSNR is expressed as the ratio between the maximum possible value (power) of a signal and the power of distorting noise that affects the quality of its representation. The mathematical expression for PSNR is as follows:

$$\mathrm{PSNR} = 20\log_{10}\left(\frac{I_{\max}}{\sqrt{\mathrm{MSE}}}\right) \tag{5.3}$$

where mean square error (MSE) can be expressed as

$$\mathrm{MSE} = \frac{1}{XY}\sum_{x=0}^{X-1}\sum_{y=0}^{Y-1}\left[I(x,y) - \hat{I}(x,y)\right]^2 \tag{5.4}$$

In Equations (5.3) and (5.4), $I(x,y)$ represents the original image of size $X \times Y$, $\hat{I}(x,y)$ is an image obtained after denoising, and $I_{\max}$ is the maximum pixel value of image $I(x,y)$.

The rest of the chapter is organized as follows. The "Databases" section briefly describes the databases used in this study. The "Methodology" section discusses the 2D-FBSE-EWT-based denoising operation. Experimental results and discussion related to the obtained results are provided in the "Results" and "Discussion" sections, respectively. Finally, a summary of the chapter is presented in the "Conclusion" section.

5.2 DATABASES

In this chapter, three databases are used, which are listed in Table 5.1. The table shows the references of the database used, the name of the database, the number of images in that database, and a link to the database.

5.3 METHODOLOGY

The flow chart for the 2D-FBSE-EWT (same for order-zero and order-one) method is shown in Figure 5.5. First, FBSE is applied to the image $I(x, y)$ of size $X \times Y$ row-wise to get the row FBSE coefficient matrix $\overline{I(x,y)}$; then, the average is taken along the column to get the average column FBSE spectrum $\overline{\tilde{I}(1,y)}$, which is shown in Figure 5.6a. Similarly, the column FBSE coefficient matrix $Ir(x,y)$

TABLE 5.1
Image Count per Database

Reference	Database	Count	Website
[44]	Retinal image	169	http://medumrg.webs.ull.es/research/retinal-imaging/rim-one/
[45]	Skin lesion	10,015	www.kaggle.com/kmader/skin-cancer-mnist-ham10000
[46]	Mammogram	2,620	www.eng.usf.edu/cvprg/Mammography/Database.html

and average row FBSE spectrum $\widetilde{Ir}(x,1)$ are obtained, shown in Figure 5.6b. In order to obtain the average order-zero and order-one FBSE spectra, order-zero and order-one FBSEs are used. The mathematical expressions of order-zero and order-one FBSE for a 1D signal $x(l)$ of length L are as follows:

$$x(l)=\sum_{m=1}^{L} C_m J_0\left(\frac{\varepsilon_m l}{L}\right), \quad l=0,1,2,\ldots,L-1 \text{ (order-zero)} \tag{5.4}$$

$$x(l)=\sum_{m=1}^{L} B_m J_1\left(\frac{\varepsilon_m l}{L}\right), \quad l=0,1,2,\ldots,L-1 \text{ (order-one)} \tag{5.5}$$

where C_m and B_m are order-zero and order-one FBSE coefficients, expressed as follows [47–48]:

$$C_m=\frac{2}{L^2\left(J_1\left(\varepsilon_m\right)\right)^2}\sum_{l=0}^{L-1} l\,x(l)\,J_0\left(\frac{\varepsilon_m l}{L}\right), \quad m=1,2,3,\ldots,L \tag{5.6}$$

$$B_m=\frac{2}{L^2\left(J_0\left(\varepsilon_m\right)\right)^2}\sum_{l=0}^{L-1} l\,x(l)\,J_1\left(\frac{\varepsilon_m l}{L}\right), \quad m=1,2,3,\ldots,L \tag{5.7}$$

In these equations, $J_0(.)$ and $J_1(.)$ are Bessel functions of orders zero and one, respectively. The parameter ε_m denotes the mth positive roots of the equation $J_0(.)=0$. The initial roots of Bessel functions can be obtained by using the relation $\varepsilon_m=\varepsilon_{m-1}+\pi$ [19]. After obtaining the initial roots, other roots are computed using the Newton-Raphson method. The root k can be obtained using the Newton-Raphson method by setting $J_0(k)=0$, and it is derived using the Taylor series approach [19]. The order m can be directly mapped in the frequency domain ω_m using the relation $\varepsilon_m=\omega_m L$, where $\varepsilon_m\approx m\pi$. The value of L will be equal to X if FBSE is applied row-wise, and it will be equal to Y if FBSE is applied column-wise. The matrix obtained after applying Equation (5.6) row-wise on the image $I(x,y)$ will give the order-zero row FBSE coefficient matrix $\overline{I(x,y)}$. Similarly, if Equation (5.6) is applied column-wise on the image $I(x,y)$, it will give the order-zero column FBSE coefficient matrix $\overline{Ir(x,y)}$. Averaging the order-zero row FBSE coefficient matrix $\overline{I(x,y)}$ along the column and the order-zero column FBSE coefficient matrix $\overline{Ir(x,y)}$ along the row will provide the order-zero average column FBSE spectrum $\tilde{I}(1,y)$ and order-zero average row FBSE spectrum $\widetilde{Ir}(x,1)$, respectively. In the same way, the order-one average column FBSE spectrum and order-one average row FBSE spectrum can be obtained just by replacing order-zero FBSE with order-one FBSE.

After obtaining the average row and column FBSE spectrum, meaningful boundaries are calculated using the scale-space approach [49]. From those boundaries, filter banks are designed. If *Nrow* and *Ncol* are the number of boundaries detected in the average row and column spectrum, respectively, then

$\gamma_{row} = \left[\varphi_1, \left[\alpha_n\right]_{n=1}^{Nrow-1}\right]$ represents the row filter bank, and $\gamma_{col} = \left[\varphi_1, \left[\alpha_n\right]_{n=1}^{Ncol-1}\right]$ represents the column filter bank. The scaling function φ and wavelet function α in terms of order *m* can be expressed as follows [50]:

$$\varphi_1(m) = \begin{cases} 1, if\ |m| \leq (1-\sigma)m_1 \\ \cos\left[\dfrac{\pi\rho(\sigma, m_i)}{2}\right], if\ (1-\sigma)m_1 \leq |m|(1+\sigma)m_1 \\ 0, \text{ otherwise.} \end{cases} \tag{5.8}$$

$$\alpha_i(m) = \begin{cases} 1, \text{if } (1+\sigma)m_i \leq |m| \leq (1-\sigma)m_{i+1} \\ \cos\left[\dfrac{\pi\rho(\sigma, m_{i+1})}{2}\right], \text{if } (1-\sigma)m_{i+1} \leq |m| \leq (1+\sigma)m_{i+1} \\ \sin\left[\dfrac{\pi\rho(\sigma, m_i)}{2}\right], \text{if } (1-\sigma)m_i \leq |m| \leq (1+\sigma)m_i \\ 0, \text{ otherwise} \end{cases} \tag{5.9}$$

where m_i represents the *i*th boundary in order (*m*) axis and function ρ, defined as

$$\rho(\sigma.m_i) = \phi\left[\frac{|m| - (1-\sigma)m_i}{2\sigma m_i}\right] \tag{5.10}$$

and

$$\phi(n) = \begin{cases} 0, & \text{if } n \leq 0 \\ \phi(n) + \phi(1-n), & \forall n \varepsilon [01] \\ 1, & \text{if } n \geq 1 \end{cases} \tag{5.11}$$

To design a tight frame for the scaling and wavelet function, σ must satisfy the following condition:

$$\sigma < \min_i \left(\frac{m_{i+1} - m_i}{m_{i+1} + m_i}\right) \tag{5.12}$$

After designing the filter banks, image *I(x,y)* is filtered with the filter bank γ_{row} row-wise. Its output is then filtered with the filter bank γ_{col} column-wise [49]. Filtering of the image can be performed in the frequency domain by multiplying filter banks with the FT coefficients of image, followed by the inverse FT, or in the time domain by convolving the image with filter banks. The result will give the total (*Nrow* + 1) × (*Ncol* + 1) sub-images. The variables *Nrow* and *Ncol* can

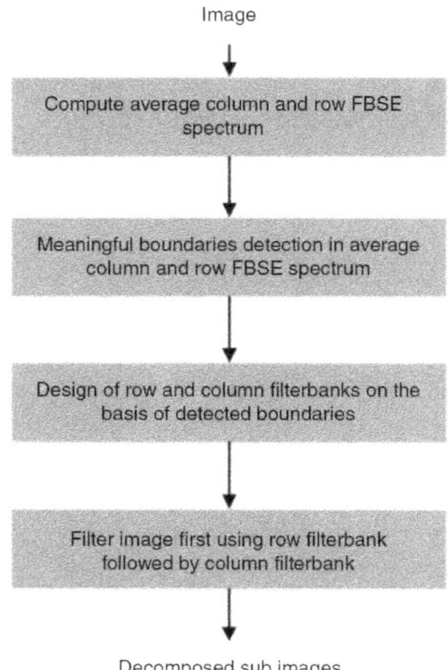

FIGURE 5.5 Steps for the 2D-FBSE-EWT method.

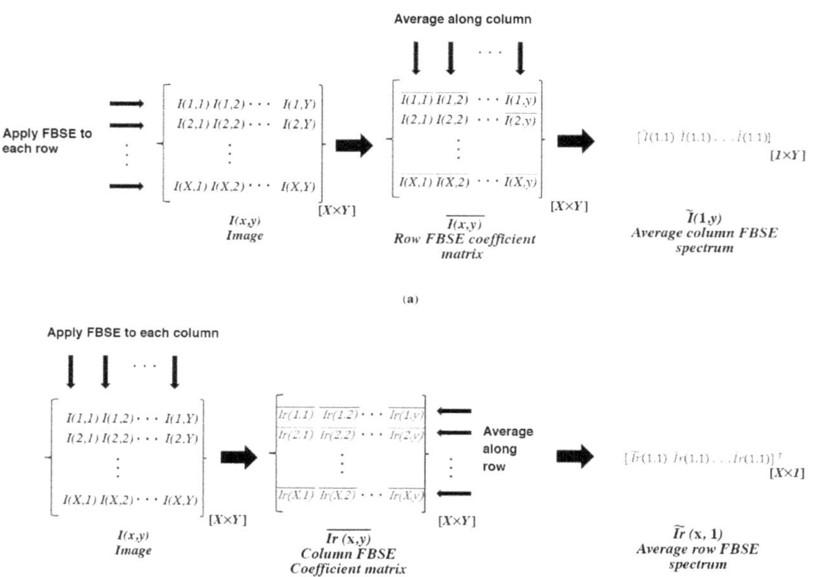

FIGURE 5.6 Steps for calculating (a) average column; and (b) average row FBSE spectrum.

be selected automatically or manually. The original image (or inverse 2D-FBSE-EWT) can be obtained by adding all sub-images.

After obtaining sub-images using 2D-FBSE-EWT method, the wavelet thresholding algorithm is applied. The threshold value depends on the coefficient values of the sub-images. The steps involved in the wavelet thresholding algorithm are as follows [42]:

1. Apply 2D-FBSE-EWT to decompose the noisy image into sub-images.
2. The threshold value of each sub-image coefficient (*A*) is computed using Equation (5.13):

$$T_A = \sigma\sqrt{2\log(M)} \tag{5.13}$$

where *M* is the number of pixels in the image, and the estimated noise level (σ) is calculated using the following relation:

$$\sigma = \text{median}\left(\text{abs}\left(A - \text{median}(A)\right)\right) \times 0.6745 \tag{5.14}$$

3. Perform hard thresholding for each sub-image coefficient, that is, the estimated coefficient: $\tilde{A} = A$ if *A* is more than T_A, else $\tilde{A} = 0$.
4. Apply inverse 2D-FBSE-EWT in order to get back the denoised image.

If the number of channels of the image is more than one, for example, an RGB image (three-channel), then 2D-FBSE-EWT is applied to each channel, which will result in sub-images in each channel. For each sub-image of each channel, wavelet thresholding is applied. After thresholding, inverse 2D-FBSE-EWT is applied to the sub-images of each channel in order to get the denoised channels. Then all three denoised channels are combined together to get the denoised RGB image.

5.4 RESULTS

In this chapter, three databases, fundus, mammogram, and skin images, are used for studying the denoising ability of order-zero and order-one 2D-FBSE-EWT methods. A total of 30 images from each database are considered in the experiment. The performance of order-zero and order-one 2D-FBSE-EWT is compared with 2D-EWT methods. The number of channels in the fundus, mammogram, and skin images were three, one, and three, respectively.

Biomedical images are first added with additive Gaussian noise of standard deviations 10, 20, 30, and 40, respectively. Then order-zero and order-one 2D-FBSE-EWT and 2D-EWT are applied on noisy images to get sub-images. By using the wavelet threshold algorithm, thresholds are calculated for each sub-image coefficient separately. Hard thresholding is done on coefficients of each sub-image, and finally reconstruction is performed to obtain the denoised image. In Figure 5.7a, the first image is an original fundus image, the second is a noisy image (additive Gaussian noise of standard deviation 20), the third is a denoised image obtained using 2D-EWT, the fourth is a denoised image obtained using order-zero 2D-FBSE-EWT, and the last is a denoised image obtained using order-one 2D-FBSE-EWT. Similarly, Figures 5.7b and 5.7c are original, noisy, and denoised images obtained using 2D-EWT, order-zero 2D-FBSE-EWT, and order-one 2D-FBSE-EWT of mammogram and skin images, respectively.

To compare the denoising performance of order-zero 2D-FBSE-EWT, order-one 2D-FBSE-EWT, and 2D-EWT, *Nrow* and *Ncol* are set automatically. Figure 5.8a,b,c provides the average PSNR vs. standard deviation plots for fundus, mammogram, and skin images, respectively. From each database, a total of 30 images are used in the study, so the average PSNR is calculated for each database for a different standard deviation.

5.5 DISCUSSION

The denoising ability of order-zero and order-one 2D-FBSE-EWT is analyzed in this work, and the results are compared with the 2D-EWT method. Three databases (30 images from each) namely fundus, mammogram, and skin images, are used for analysis. The standard deviation of additive Gaussian noise is set as 10, 20, 30, and 40. In the experiment, the number of boundaries is automatically selected, and comparison is done between order-zero 2D-FBSE-EWT, order-one 2D-FBSE-EWT, and EWT. From Figure 5.8a,b,c, it can be seen that order-zero 2D-FBSE-EWT had better performance than order-one 2D-FBSE-EWT and 2D-EWT.

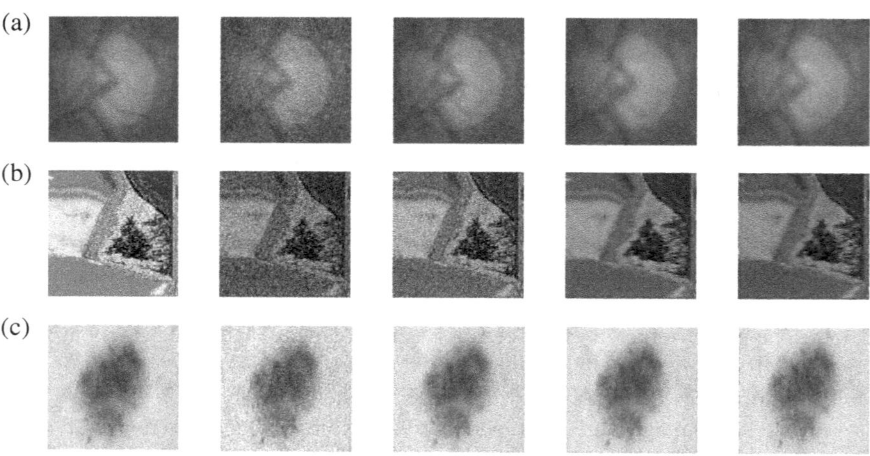

FIGURE 5.7 (Left–right) Original image, noisy image (standard deviation = 20), denoised image using 2D-EWT, denoised image using order zero 2D-FBSE-EWT, and order-one 2D-FBSE-EWT of (a) fundus; (b) mammogram; and (c) skin image.

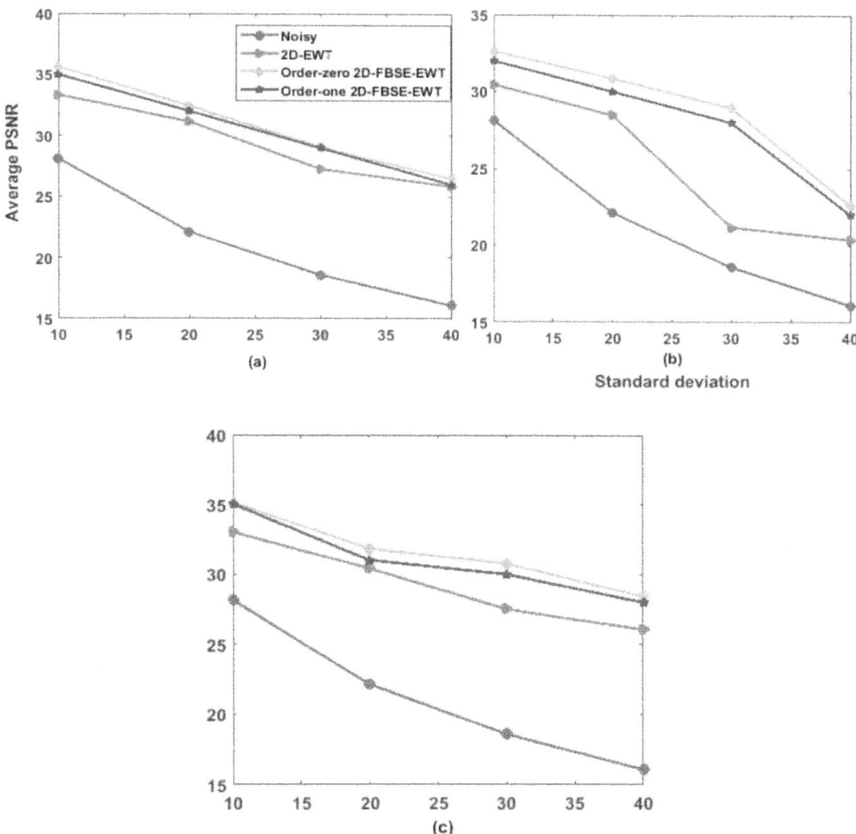

FIGURE 5.8 Average PSNR versus standard deviation plot for (a) fundus; (b) mammogram; and (c) skin image.

5.6 CONCLUSION

This chapter discusses the advantage of using FBSE over FT. Various FBSE-based approaches are discussed in the introduction. Adaptive order-zero and order-one 2D-FBSE-EWT have been used in the work for denoising using a wavelet thresholding approach.

This work studied the denoising ability of order-zero and order-one 2D-FBSE-EWT and compared it with 2D-EWT. For study, three databases are used, fundus, mammogram, and skin lesion. Results show that order-zero 2D-FBSE-EWT outperformed order-one 2D-FBSE-EWT and 2D-EWT. Thus, the 2D-FBSE-EWT technique is a promising method that can be used for the analysis of biomedical images.

REFERENCES

[1] C. Boncelet, "Image noise models", in *The Essential Guide to Image Processing*, Cambridge, MA: Academic Press, Elsevier (2009): 143–167.

[2] A.K. Shukla, R.K. Pandey, and P.K. Reddy, "Generalized fractional derivative based adaptive algorithm for image denoising", *Multimedia Tools and Applications* (2020): 1–24.

[3] R.C. Gonzalez, and R.E. Woods, *Digital Image Processing*, Upper-Saddle River, NJ: Prentice-Hall (2002).

[4] B.I. Justusson, "Median filtering: Statistical properties", in *Two-Dimensional Digital Signal Processing II*, Berlin, Heidelberg: Springer (1981): 161–196.

[5] V. Jain, and H.S. Seung, "Natural image denoising with convolutional networks", *Advances in Neural Information Processing Systems,* 21 (2008): 769–776.

[6] C. Kervrann, and J. Boulanger, "Optimal spatial adaptation for patch-based image denoising", *IEEE Transactions on Image Processing,* 15, no. 10 (2006): 2866–2878.

[7] K. Dabov, A. Foi, V. Katkovnik, and K. Egiazarian, "Image denoising by sparse 3-D transform-domain collaborative filtering", *IEEE Transactions on Image Processing,* 16, no. 8 (2007): 2080–2095.

[8] D.L. Donoho, "De-noising by soft thresholding", *IEEE Transactions on Information Theory,* 43 (1993): 933–936.

[9] S.G. Chang, B. Yu, and M. Vattereli, "Adaptive wavelet thresholding for image denoising and compression", *IEEE Transactions on Image Processing,* 9 (Sept. 2000): 1532–1546.

[10] D.L. Donoho, and I.M. Johnstone, "Adapting to unknown smoothness via wavelet shrinkage", *Journal of American Statistical Association,* 90, no. 432 (Dec. 1995): 1200–1224.

[11] S.G. Chang, B. Yu, and M. Vattereli, "Wavelet thresholding for multiple noisy image copies", *IEEE Transactions Image Processing*, 9 (Sept. 2000): 1631–1635.

[12] S.G. Chang, B. Yu, and M. Vattereli, "Spatially adaptive wavelet thresholding with context modeling for image denoising", *IEEE Transactions Image Processing,* 9 (Sept. 2000): 1522–1530.

[13] M. Vattereli, and J. Kovacevic, *Wavelets and Subband Coding*, Englewood Cliffs, NJ: Prentice Hall (1995).

[14] M. Jansen, *Noise Reduction by Wavelet Thresholding*, New York: Springer-Verlag Inc. (2001).

[15] D.L. Donoho, and I.M. Johnstone, "Ideal spatial adaptation via wavelet shrinkage", *Biometrica,* 81 (1994): 425–455.

[16] D.L. Donoho, and I.M. Johnstone, "Wavelet shrinkage: Asymptopia?", *Journal of the Royal Statistical Society, Series B,* 57, no. 2 (1995): 301–369.

[17] L. Kaur, S. Gupta, and R.C. Chauhan, "Image denoising using wavelet thresholding", *The Indian Conference on Computer Vision, Graphics and Image Processing (ICVGIP),* 2 (2002): 16–18.

[18] K. Martin, "Bessel functions", *Lecture Notes, Penn State-Göttingen Summer School on Number Theory,* 82 (2012): 161–162.

[19] W. Johnson, "Advanced engineering mathematics: E. Kreyszig John Wiley. 856 pp., 79s." *International Journal of Mechanical Sciences,* 5 (1963): 423–424.

[20] R.B. Pachori, and P. Sircar, 2010, "Analysis of multicomponent AM-FM signals using FB-DESA method", *Digital Signal Processing,* 20(1): 42–62.

[21] P.K. Chaudhary, and R.B. Pachori, "Automatic diagnosis of COVID-19 and pneumonia using FBD method", *2020 IEEE International Conference on Bioinformatics and Biomedicine (BIBM)* (2020): 2257–2263.

[22] I. Daubechies, and B.J. Bates, *Ten Lectures on Wavelets*, Philadelphia, PA: Society for Industrial and Applied Mathematics (1992).

[23] I. Bayram, "An analytic wavelet transform with a flexible time-frequency covering", *IEEE Transactions on Signal Processing,* 61(5): 1131–1142.

[24] V. Gupta and R. B Pachori, "Classification of focal EEG signals using FBSE based flexible time-frequency coverage wavelet transform", *Biomedical Signal Processing and Control,* 62 (2020): 102124.

[25] N. E. Huang, Z. Shen, S.R. Long, M.C. Wu, H.H. Shih, Q. Zheng, N.C. Yen, C.C. Tung, and H.H. Liu, "The empirical mode decomposition and the Hilbert spectrum for nonlinear and non-stationary time series analysis", *Proceedings of the Royal Society of London. Series A: Mathematical, Physical and Engineering Sciences,* 454, no. 1971 (1998): 903–995.

[26] A. Bhattacharyya, L. Singh, and R.B. Pachori, "Fourier–Bessel series expansion based empirical wavelet transform for analysis of non-stationary signals", *Digital Signal Processing,* 78 (2018): 185–196.

[27] R. Katiyar, V. Gupta, and R.B. Pachori, "FBSE-EWT-based approach for the determination of respiratory rate from PPG signals", *IEEE Sensors Letters,* 3, no. 7 (2019): 1–4.

[28] P.K. Chaudhary, and R.B. Pachori, "Automatic diagnosis of glaucoma using two-dimensional Fourier-Bessel series expansion based empirical wavelet transform", *Biomedical Signal Processing and Control,* 64 (2021): 102237.

[29] R.B. Pachori and P. Sircar, "EEG signal analysis using FB expansion and second-order linear TVAR process", *Signal Processing,* 88, no. 2 (Feb. 2008): 415–420.

[30] V. Gupta and R.B. Pachori, "Epileptic seizure identification using entropy of FBSE based EEG rhythms", *Biomedical Signal Processing and Control,* 53, no. 101569 (Aug. 2019): 1–11.

[31] T. Siddharth, P. Gajbhiye, R.K. Tripathy, and R.B. Pachori, "EEG based detection of focal seizure area using FBSE-EWT rhythm and SAE-SVM network", *IEEE Sensors Journal*, 20, no. 19 (Oct. 2020): 11421–11428.

[32] A. Bhattacharyya, R.K. Tripathy, L. Garg, and R.B. Pachori, "A novel multivariate-multiscale approach for computing EEG spectral and temporal complexity for human emotion recognition", *IEEE Sensors Journal*, 21, no. 3 (Feb. 2021): 3579–3591.

[33] V. Gupta and R.B. Pachori, "FBDM based time-frequency representation for sleep stages classification using EEG signals", *Biomedical Signal Processing and Control,* 64, no. 102265 (Feb. 2021): 1–16.

[34] A. Anuragi, D. Sisodia, and R.B. Pachori, "Automated alcoholism detection using Fourier-Bessel series expansion based empirical wavelet transform", *IEEE Sensors Journal,* 20, no. 9 (May 2020): 4914–4924.

[35] P. Gajbhiye, R.K. Tripathy, and R.B. Pachori, "Elimination of ocular artifacts from single channel EEG signals using FBSE-EWT based rhythms", *IEEE Sensors Journal,* 20, no. 07 (Apr. 2020): 3687–3696.

[36] V. Gupta, A. Bhattacharyya, and R.B. Pachori, "Automated identification of epileptic seizures from EEG signals using FBSE-EWT method", in G.R. Naik (Ed.), *Biomedical Signal Processing-Advances in Theory, Algorithms and Applications,* Singapore: Springer, (2019).

[37] R.K. Tripathy, A. Bhattacharyya, and R.B. Pachori, "Localization of myocardial infarction from multi lead electrocardiogram signals using multiscale convolution neural network", *IEEE Sensors Journal,* 19, no. 23 (Dec. 2019): 11437–11448.

[38] R.K. Tripathy, A. Bhattacharyya, and R.B. Pachori, "A novel approach for detection of myocardial infarction from ECG signals of multiple electrodes", *IEEE Sensors Journal*, 19, no. 12 (June 2019): 4509–4517.

[39] P. Jain and R.B. Pachori, "Event-based method for instantaneous fundamental frequency estimation from voiced speech based on eigenvalue decomposition of Hankel matrix", *IEEE/ACM Transactions on Audio, Speech and Language Processing,* 22, no.10 (Oct. 2014): 1467–1482.

[40] A.S. Hood, R.B. Pachori, V.K. Reddy, and P. Sircar, "Parametric representation of speech employing multi-component AFM signal model", *International Journal of Speech Technology,* 18, no. 3 (Sept. 2015): 287–303.

[41] R.B. Pachori, and P. Sircar, "A new technique to reduce cross terms in the Wigner distribution", *Digital Signal Processing,* 17, no. 2 (Mar. 2007): 466–474.

[42] C.A. Nair, and R. Lavanya, "Enhanced empirical wavelet transform for denoising of fundus images", in *International Conference on Soft Computing Systems*, Singapore: Springer (Apr. 2018): 116–124.

[43] J. Korhonen, and J. You, "Peak signal-to-noise ratio revisited: Is simple beautiful?", in *2012 Fourth International Workshop on Quality of Multimedia Experience*, IEEE (2012): 37–38.

[44] Rim-One-Medical Image Analysis Group, available from April, 2017, http://medumrg.webs.ull.es/research/retinal-imaging/rim-one/.

[45] P. Tschandl, C. Rosendahl, and H. Kittler, "The HAM10000 dataset, a large collection of multi-source dermatoscopic images of common pigmented skin lesions", *Scientific Data,* 5, no. 1 (2018): 1–9.

[46] K. Bowyer, D. Kopans, W.P. Kegelmeyer, R. Moore, M. Sallam, K. Chang, and K. Woods, "The digital database for screening mammography", *Third International Workshop on Digital Mammography,* 58 (1996): 27.

[47] J. Schroeder, "Signal processing via Fourier-Bessel series expansion", *Digital Signal Processing,* 3, no. 2 (1993): 112–124.

[48] K. Gopalan, T.R. Anderson, and E.J. Cupples, "A comparison of speaker identification results using features based on cepstrum and Fourier-Bessel expansion", *IEEE Transactions on Speech and Audio Processing,* 7, no. 3 (1999): 289–294.

[49] J. Gilles, and K. Heal, "A parameterless scale-space approach to find meaningful modes in histograms—Application to image and spectrum segmentation", *International Journal of Wavelets, Multiresolution and Information Processing,* 12, no. 6 (2014): 1450044.

[50] J. Gilles, G. Tran, and S. Osher, "2D empirical transforms. Wavelets, ridgelets, and curvelets revisited", *SIAM Journal on Imaging Sciences,* 7, no. 1 (2014): 157–186.

6 Alert System for Epileptic Seizures

R. Reena Roy and G.S. Anandha Mala

CONTENTS

6.1 INTRODUCTION

The human brain consists of neurons, which send a constant level of electronic signals. But in the case of abnormality in the body, the brain continues to send electrical signals, a state that is medically termed an electrical storm. Using that, seizures can be detected. Many researchers have cooperated to use this method to detect seizures that occur within a few moments in epilepsy. A slight variation in a patient's electrical activity (disruption) is more than enough to detect. Using multiple detection helps obtain more accurate results. A micro-electromechanical system (MEMS) is a suitable sensor for detecting muscular convolutions and is compact and easily attachable. This accelerometer notes seizures with accurate values. It doesn't cause discomfort to the patient.

DOI: 10.1201/9781003207856-6

6.2 LITERATURE SURVEY

Earlier systems had many drawbacks, as they reported many false seizures, were not economically suitable for middle-class people to use, failed to detect seizures in some cases and also produced high false alarm rates. The new system has new techniques and strategies as follows:

1. The brain signal is decomposed into five frequency sub-bands, and 80 features can be extracted. Among those 80, 7 high-quality features are extracted that can be fed into an enlightened data transport (EDT). The EDT is capable of detecting various types of epileptic seizures [1].
2. EEG signals are used to separate two to five classes. Various methods of epileptic seizure detection just by visual examination are time consuming and inaccurate. Automatic detection of non-convulsive status epilepticus (NCSE), which is a more significant event for doctors to detect [2], can be done.
3. Early detection of focal seizure is done using microelectrodes. The microelectrodes record intra-cortical neural signals. This signal may help to diagnose seizures [3].
4. A single accelerometer sensor is capable of detecting seizures with 10-sec duration. This algorithm detected 40 (86–95%) of 46 convulsive seizures, psychogenic non-epileptic seizures (PNESs) and complex partial seizures (CPSs). Among 20 patients, there was a total rate of 270 false alarms. It detects seizures in clinical and non-clinical environments. A higher false alarm rate is the major disadvantage, which creates panic in patients as well as caretakers [4].

6.3 PROPOSED SYSTEM

The proposed technology will help epilepsy patients lead better and more secure lives. The idea of the system is to clearly address and solve their problems. If even a single seizure goes unnoticed, it may lead to drastic problems for the patient's health. A heart rate sensor and MEMS sensor detect seizures. Once a seizure is detected, the system continues monitoring the patient and alerts the caretaker. The MQ telemetry transport (MQTT) protocol is used to send a message to the caretaker to track the location when the patient is outside. A call for an ambulance is made if the seizure lasts too long or the person has repeated seizures. A special application is created to call for an ambulance and to track the live location of the patient. The mobile application helps to record the type and duration of the seizure event. It also includes reminders for medicine. Reports for the particular patient can be generated and viewed. Emergency contacts can be added through the mobile application. This device is connected to a mobile application via Bluetooth. When a seizure is confirmed, a message is transmitted to the surroundings to initiate the necessary protective measures for the patient. The device is designed as wireless, wearable personal equipment. Using a heart rate sensor, the heartbeat can be accurately monitored. Muscular convulsions are collected using micro-electro-mechanical sensors. The sensors used are small in size and can be firmly attached to the body. The objective of this project is to develop a low-cost, portable generalized seizure alert device which can notify nearby family or caregivers when a seizure occurs through alarms, phone calls or text alerts and can be used by all people.

6.4 SYSTEM ARCHITECTURE

Figure 6.1 is an architecture diagram which represents how the project works. The epileptic patient wears a handband which contains a heart rate sensor and MEMS sensor. The MEMS sensor is connected to an MCP3206 converter. Both sensors are connected to NodeMCU, which is connected to the mobile application through the MQTT protocol.

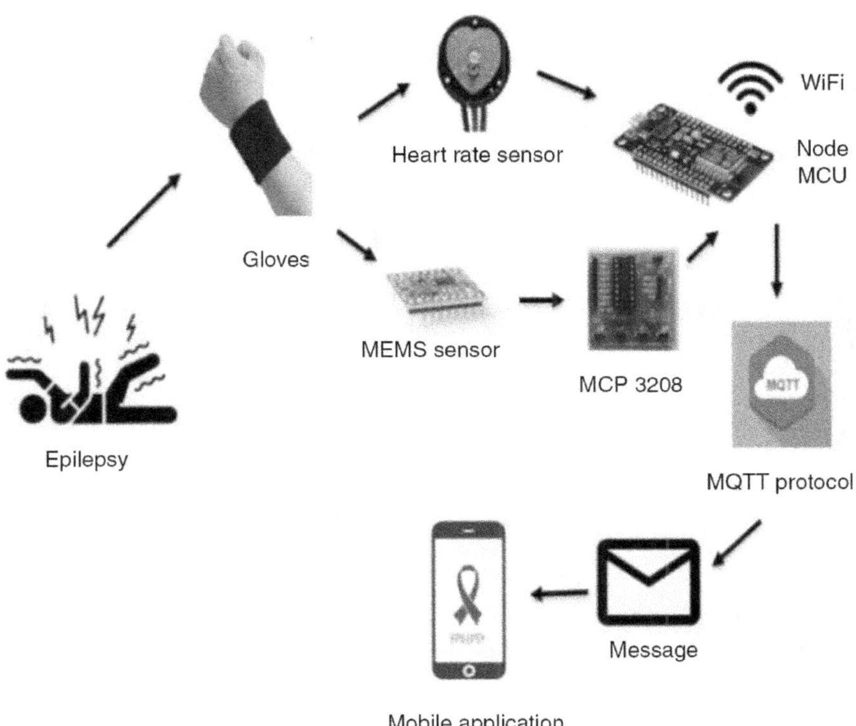

FIGURE 6.1 Architectural design.

6.5 SCOPE OF THE PROJECT

When a seizure is detected for an epileptic patient, the system generates an SMS alert to the caretaker with the live location. The system also alerts an ambulance if a prolonged seizure occurs. An application with many features for the epileptic patient has been developed.

- In the future, advanced Internet of Things (IoT) concepts will be implemented.
- Detection of seizures using multiple sensors is a smart way to reduce false reports.
- Using the MQTT protocol, alerting can be done faster.
- This system acts as a lifesaver and additional caretaker for epileptic patients.
- In the future, the system can be further modified and used as a caretaker for epileptic patients.

6.6 HARDWARE REQUIREMENTS

6.6.1 Heart Rate Sensor

Heart rate is measured using an electronic device called a heart rate sensor. When a finger is placed on it, it provides digital output of the heartbeat. The beat LED flashes in unison with each heartbeat when the heartbeat detector is working. The digital output is connected to a microcontroller to measure the beats per minute (BPM) rate.

6.6.2 MEMS Sensor

MEMS sensors are used to detect and measure external stimuli like acceleration. They consist of a micro-machined proof mass suspended between two parallel plates. The proof mass moves when acceleration is applied: one air gap decreases, and the other gap increases, which creates a change in capacitance proportional to acceleration.

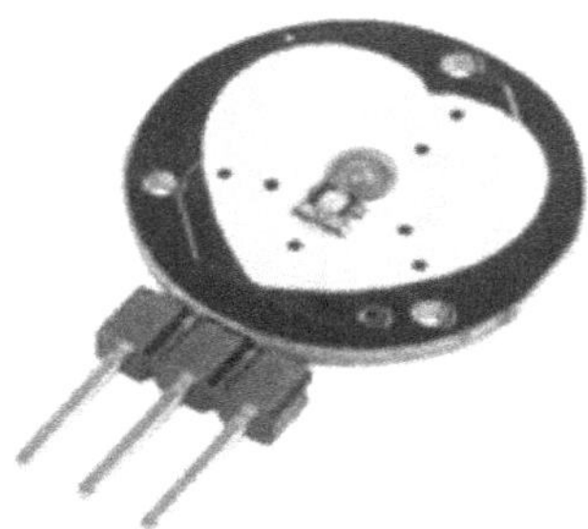
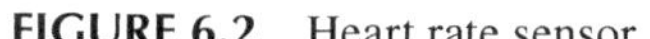

FIGURE 6.2 Heart rate sensor.

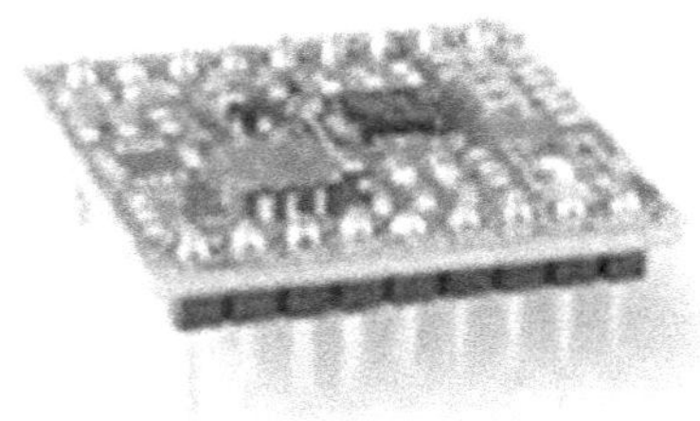

FIGURE 6.3 MEMS sensor.

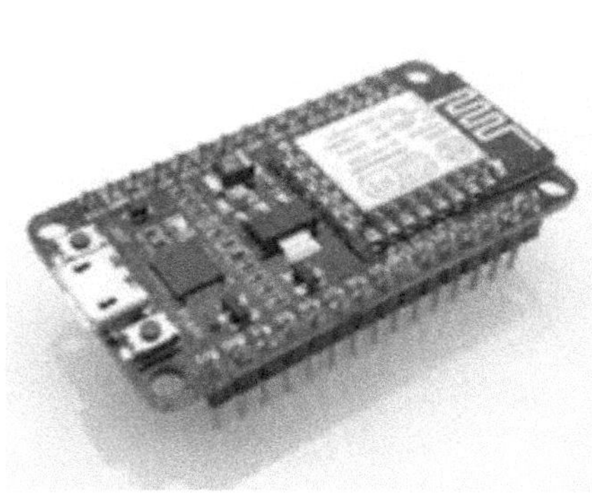

FIGURE 6.4 NodeMCU.

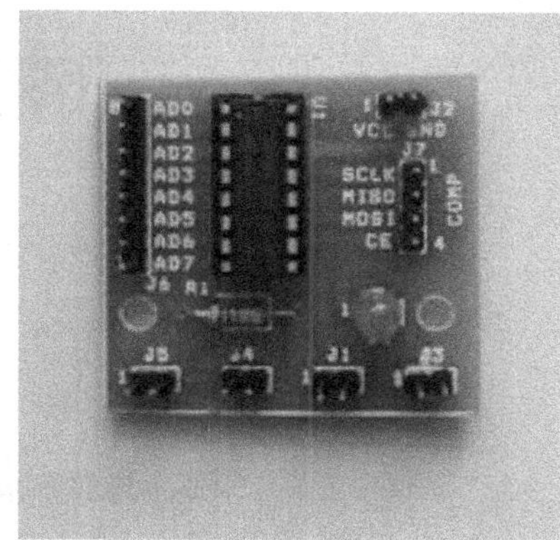

FIGURE 6.5 MCP3208.

6.6.3 NodeMCU

NodeMCU is an open-source IoT platform which includes firmware that works on the ESP8266 Wi-Fi SoC from Espressif Systems and hardware based on the ESP-12 module. It is breadboard friendly and can be powered via a micro-USB port.

6.6.4 MCP3208

The MCP3008 is a low-cost, eight-channel, 10-bit analog-to-digital converter which combines high performance and low power consumption in a small package [4]. It is ideal for embedded control applications. The MCP3008 includes successive approximation register (SAR) architecture and a serial peripheral interface. It allows 10-bit ADC capability to be added to any peripheral interface microcontroller. The MCP3008 provides 200k samples/second and is available in 16-pin payload data interface panel and small outline integrated circuit packages.

6.7 SOFTWARE REQUIREMENTS

6.7.1 Arduino Compiler

The open-source Arduino software (IDE) creates a simple code to write and upload to the panel. It runs on Linux, Mac OS X and Windows. Nature is written in Java and founded on managing and other open-source software.

6.7.2 MQTTBox

MQTTBox is a helper program to develop and test MQTT-based clients, brokers, devices, clouds and apps. It helps to maximize development and testing

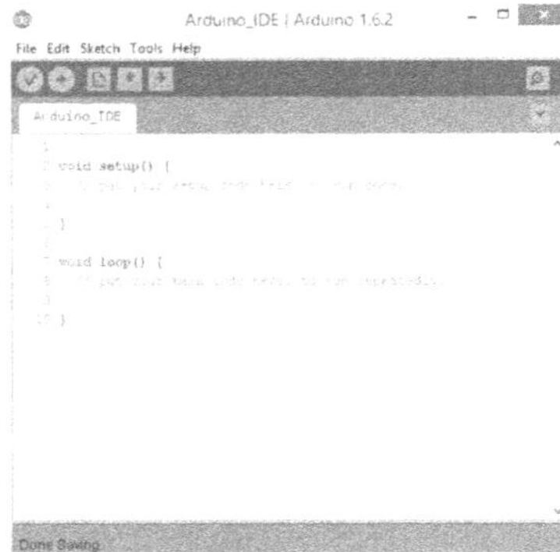

FIGURE 6.6 Arduino IDE.

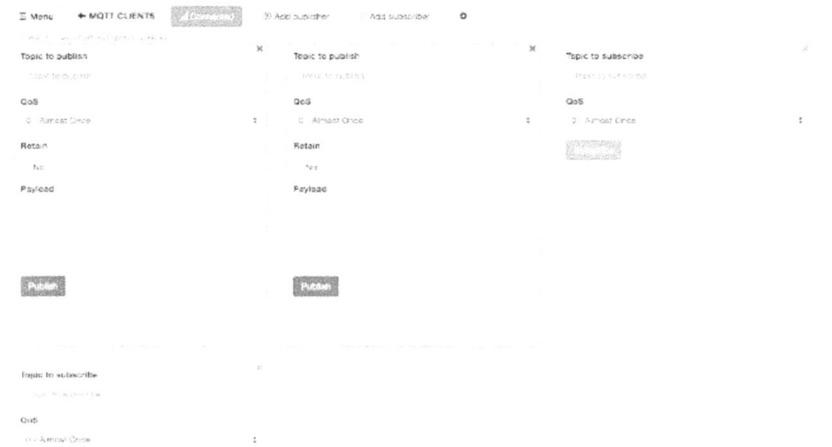

FIGURE 6.7 MQTTBox.

productivity. MQTT clients and load testing tools are integrated, and it is powerful enough to supercharge the MQTT workflow.

6.8 FLOW DIAGRAM

Figure 6.8 represents the flow diagram for the project. EEG signals from the heart rate sensor and the signal from the MEMS sensor are monitored and sent to the detection system. The occurrence of a seizure is detected using two parameters: A rise or drop in the pulse rate and fall detection. If a seizure is detected, the alert system sends a message to the caregiver or family members. If the seizure lasts for more than five minutes, the alert system automatically sends a message to a nearby hospital.

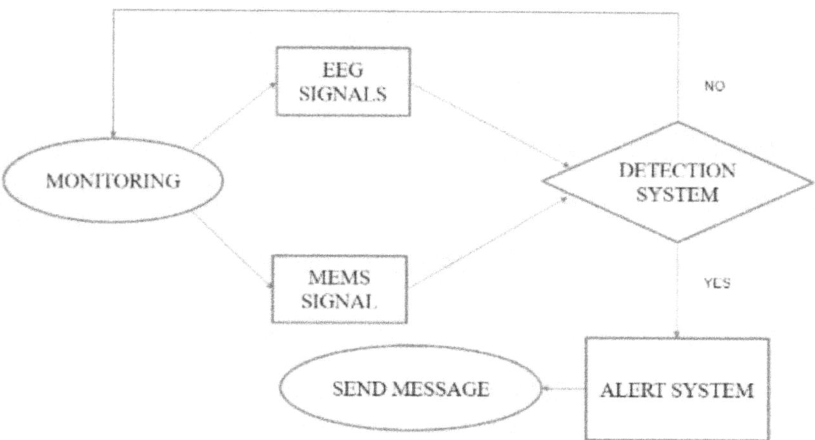

FIGURE 6.8 Flow diagram.

```
COM5
pulse: 553
X:368
Y:341
pulse: 554
X:368
Y:341
pulse: 560
X:369
Y:342
pulse: 564
X:369
Y:341
pulse: 521
X:368
Y:342
pulse: 557
```

FIGURE 6.9 Output.

6.9 EXPERIMENTAL RESULTS AND OUTPUT

The heart rate sensor and MCP3008 are connected to NodeMCU. The MCP3008 is connected to the MEMS sensor. The output from the MEMS sensor, which is an analog, is converted to digital with the help of the ADC MCP3008 and given to NodeMCU. When there is a drop or rise in the heartbeat, the MEMS sensor readings are taken to detect muscular convulsions or a fall. If detected, the MQTT protocol is activated and an alarm message is sent to the patient's family member or caregiver through the mobile application. Records of the patient's seizure and other medications are maintained in the mobile application.

6.10 PERFORMANCE ANALYSIS

Figures 6.10 and 6.11 show the performance analysis of the project. The output from the heart rate sensor and MEMS accelerometer sensor are recorded in the graph. The accuracy is high; hence, false alarm rates can be reduced.

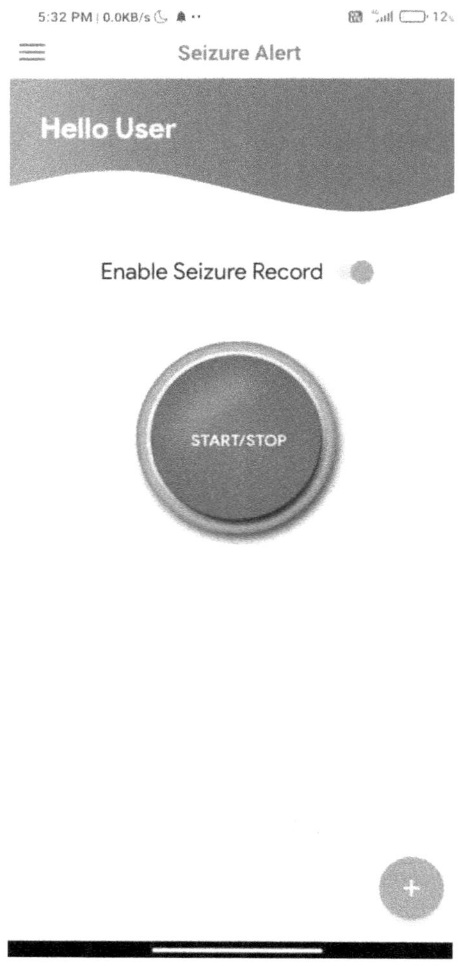

FIGURE 6.10 Screenshot of application.

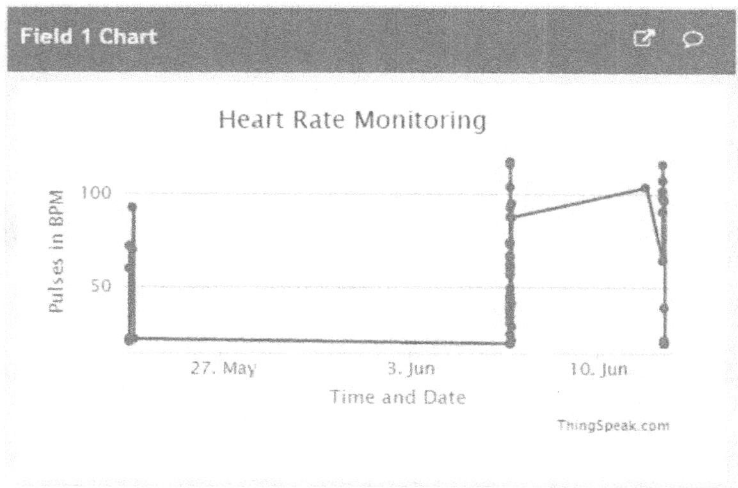

FIGURE 6.11 Performance analysis of heart rate sensor.

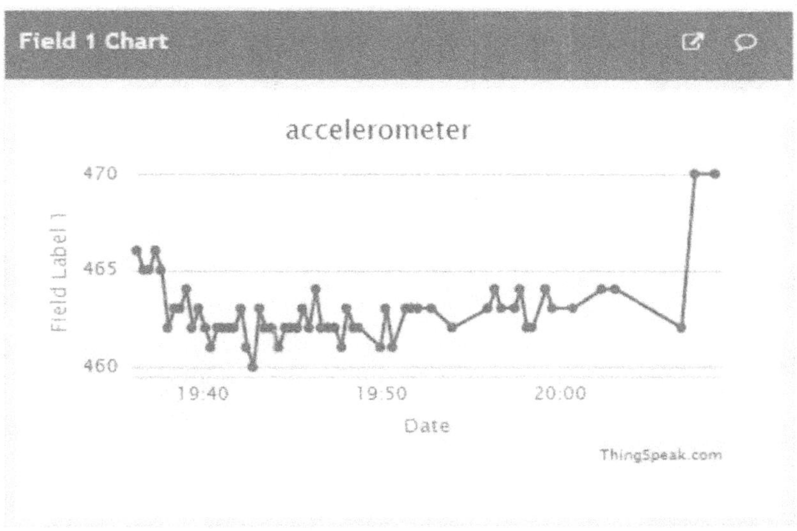

FIGURE 6.12 Performance analysis of MEMS sensor.

6.11 CONCLUSION

A lightweight, rugged, cost-effective wearable device is developed which will help millions of victims of epilepsy around the globe. With the device in their possession, a person with epilepsy can move around freely without worries.

REFERENCES

[1] M. Radman, M. Moradi, A. Chaibakhsh, M. Kordestani and M. Saif, "Multi-Feature Fusion Approach for Epileptic Seizure Detection From EEG Signals," in *IEEE Sensors Journal*, vol. 21, no. 3, pp. 3533–3543, 1 Feb 2021, doi: 10.1109/JSEN.2020.3026032.

[2] S. Sheykhivand, T. Y. Rezaii, Z. Mousavi, A. Delpak and A. Farzamnia, "Automatic Identification of Epileptic Seizures From EEG Signals Using Sparse Representation-Based Classification," in *IEEE Access*, vol. 8, pp. 138834–138845, 2020, doi: 10.1109/ACCESS.2020.3011877.

[3] Y. S. Park, G. Rees Cosgrove, J. R. Madsen, E. N. Eskandar, L. R. Hochberg, S. S. Cash and W. Truccolo, "Early Detection of Human Epileptic Seizures Based on Intracortical Microelectrode Array Signals," in *IEEE Transactions on Biomedical Engineering*, vol. 67, no. 3, pp. 817–831, March 2020, doi: 10.1109/TBME.2019.2921448.

[4] S. Kusmakar, C. K. Karmakar, B. Yan, T. J. O'Brien, R. Muthuganapathy and M. Palaniswami, "Automated Detection of Convulsive Seizures Using a Wearable Accelerometer Device," in *IEEE Transactions on Biomedical Engineering*, vol. 66, no. 2, pp. 421–432, 2019, doi: 10.1109/TBME.2018.2845865.

7 Early Diabetic Retinopathy Detection Using Augmented Continuous Particle Swarm Optimization Clustering

Bhimavarapu Usharani

CONTENTS

7.1 INTRODUCTION

Diabetes is a disorder that emerges due to malfunction of the pancreas, which retards the recovery of patients in the presence of health ailments. Diabetes affects the vital organs of the body like the eye [1], heart [2], kidney [3], nerves

DOI: 10.1201/9781003207856-7

[4], and so on. The subsequent sections provide a brief overview of diabetes and its impact on different organs of the human body.

7.1.1 Heart

Rubler et al. [5] identified the case of heart failure due to diabetes. It was elaborated on and confirmed by Kannel et al. [6]. Around 19% to 30% of diabetic patients may have heart failure [7]. The risk of heart failure in diabetic patients is higher than for nondiabetic patients. The risk of heart failure in type 1 diabetes is over 30% higher, and for type 2 diabetes, it is over 10% when compared to the risk of heart failure due to smoking or any other coronary diseases [8].

7.1.2 Kidneys

Diabetes also damages the kidneys, leading to the chronic condition called diabetic nephropathy [9]. Diabetes plays a significant role in faster progression of diabetic nephropathy. Diabetic nephropathy occurs in about 20% to 40% of diabetic patients [10]. Kidney disease occurred with type 1 diabetes for over 12.6% of patients [11], and with type 2 diabetes, it was over 2.0% [12].

7.1.3 Eyes

Diabetes affects the retina of the eye [13]. Diabetes is one of the leading causes of blindness [14], and almost 80% of blindness is due to diabetes [15]. Diabetic retinopathy is a situation where the retina of the diabetic patient is damaged due to blood leaks from the blood vessels of the retina. Around 75% of people who are suffering from diabetes will have diabetic retinopathy [16]. Diabetic retinopathy is divided into two stages: Non-proliferative diabetic retinopathy (NPDR) and proliferative diabetic retinopathy (PDR) [17]. Table 7.1 presents the severity levels of diabetic retinopathy [18–20].

TABLE 7.1
Diabetic Retinopathy (DR) Severity Levels

Severity Level	Description
No NPDR	No abnormalities
Mild NPDR	Microaneurysms only
Moderate NPDR	More microaneurysms and exudates
Severe NPDR	Intraretinal microvascular anomalies, intraretinal hemorrhage, abnormal blood vessel growth
PDR	Neovascularization, preretinal hemorrhage
Gestational DR	The newborn child has type 2 diabetes

Detection of diabetic retinopathy is essential at an early stage to prevent blindness with appropriate treatment. The first sign of diabetic retinopathy is the presence of red lesions called microaneurysms [21].

7.1.4 Color Fundus Images

In 1926, the first fundus camera provided a 20° view of the retina [22]. Fundus images are two-dimensional images of three-dimensional retina tissue, and various retina structures can be better visualized [23]. Fundus images provide a sharp, high-contrast image of the retina within the focal plane [24]. In this chapter, fundus images are pre-processed by excluding noise from the fundus image, which is further processed using enhancement techniques to highlight the details of the image.

In the present chapter, the researchers focus on the concept of detecting diabetic retinopathy in the early stage to reduce the risk of vision loss. In the pre-preprocessing phase, the image is resized to 250 × 250 pixels. Then the resized image is subjected to contrast enhancement by utilizing the contrast-limited adaptive histogram equalization algorithm to identify the lesions in the image. In the next step, we perform segmentation to extract the useful lesion information from the image. Then, feature extraction is applied to distinguish the candidate regions as microaneurysms or non-microaneurysms. In this work, we utilize a particle swarm optimization (PSO) clustering variant model applied to diabetic retinopathy databases such as MESSIDOR, DIARETDBO, and E-OPTHA. The contribution is summarized as follows:

- Early detection of non-proliferative diabetic retinopathy utilizing augmented continuous particle swarm optimization clustering for segmentation of fundus images, which improves the accuracy of diagnosis for non-proliferative diabetic retinopathy.
- Pre-processing to improve the contrast of the image by applying the contrast-limited adaptive histogram equalization algorithm.
- Augmented continuous particle swarm optimization clustering algorithms are applied in the segmentation phase.
- To distinguish the candidate regions as microaneurysms or non-microaneurysms, seven different features are extracted.
- Extensive experiments were conducted using the MESSIDOR, DIARETDBO, and E-OPTHA diabetic retinopathy datasets.

The results of the experiments on datasets that are publicly available demonstrate that the proposed technique outperforms renowned techniques in terms of high-order statistics measures. To compare clusters, we use high-order statistics such as kurtosis and skewness. These two high-order statistical measures provide a more accurate description of the shape of the cluster. The main challenge in image clustering is how to manipulate clusters based on the previous complex representations and to identify new clusters. Existing cluster algorithms used the mean, median, variance, and covariance to represent the cluster. In this work, we use kurtosis and skewness for representation of the clusters. The main advantage of using these two high-order statistics is to identify low-complexity clusters. The skewness represents the asymmetry of the cluster, whereas the kurtosis represents the concentration of the cluster. In the case where two different clusters possess similar statistical properties, then the clusters are merged. The challenging task is the detection of new clusters and merging of old and new clusters. Aggregation of clusters is by examining the entropy, kurtosis, and skewness of the clusters.

The rest of the chapter is organized as follows. Section 7.2 provides an overview of PSO clustering, fitness measures, and terminology. Section 7.3 presents a literature survey of the contributions made by several researchers in the early detection of diabetic retinopathy and microaneurysm detection. The proposed technology is discussed in Section 7.4. Finally, the chapter concludes with the conclusion section.

7.2 PRELIMINARIES

Particle swarm optimization [25] is used for continuous optimization. PSO consists of a predefined number of particles called a swarm, say, *Nd*. Each particle *pi*, $1 \le i \le Nd$, is associated with a position X_i, *d* and a velocity V_i, *d*, $1 \le d \le D$, in the *d*th dimension of the search space; the dimension *D* is same for all particles. First, all the particles must be initialized with a random position and velocity to move in the search space. At each iteration *t*, every particle finds its own best solution ($Pbest_i$) and the global best solution (*Gbest*). The formulas for the particle's updated position and velocity are given as follows.

Velocity update:

Velocity Update Formula

$$v_{i,k}(t+1) = Wv_{i,k}(t) + C_1 r_{1,k}(t)(y_{i,k}(t) - x_{i,k}(t)) + C_2 r_{2,k}(t)(y(t) - x_{i,k}(t))$$

In this equation, *W* is the inertia weight, and *C*1 and *C*2 are the global constants. Position update:

Position Update Formula

$$x_i(t+1) = x_i(t) + v_i(t+1)$$

The particle updates $Pbest_i$ as well as *Gbest* as follows:

Pbest Formula

$$Pbest_i = \begin{cases} P_i, if(Fitness(P_i) < Fitness(Pbest_i)) \\ Pbest_i, otherwise \end{cases}$$

Gbest Formula

$$Gbest = \begin{cases} Pbest_i, if(Fitness(Pbest_i) < Fitness(Gbest)) \\ Gbest, otherwise \end{cases}$$

Particle swarm optimization algorithm [25]:

1. Evaluate the fitness measure for each particle.
2. Evaluate the velocity and position updates.
3. Find the $Pbest_i$ and $Gbest$. The particle swarm optimization algorithm continues its iteration until it reaches a specified number of iterations or when the velocity value becomes zero.

7.2.1 Particle Swarm Optimization Clustering

Clustering is a technology that groups similar data points into the same group from the given dataset [26]. Some applications of clustering algorithms are image segmentation [27], pattern analysis [28], and image compression [29]. Clustering based on swarm intelligence, such as PSO, can be used for clustering analysis [30]. Particle swarm optimization-based algorithms consider datapoints as particles. The initial clusters of particles are collected from other clustering algorithms. The cluster of particles is updated continuously based on the center of the clusters and velocity and position of the cluster until the cluster center converges.

The main disadvantages of hierarchical clustering are:

1. Time complexity.
2. Works well for large datasets, but it is challenging to determine the number of clusters with dendrograms.

The main disadvantages of density-based clustering are:

1. DBSCAN does not work well for high-dimensional data.
2. DBSCAN fails for varying density clusters.
3. Does not work well for large datasets.
4. The user must give the radius and minimum number of points in the cluster's neighborhood in advance.

Particle swarm optimization clustering algorithm [30]:

1. Evaluate the fitness measure for each particle in each cluster, $\forall \times i \mathcal{E} C_j$ (Cj is a cluster j).
2. Evaluate the velocity and position updates for each particle in a cluster $\forall C_j$.

3. Replace *Pbest* with individual *i*th cluster center and *Gbest* with neighbor cluster centers.

The particle swarm optimization clustering algorithm iterates until it reaches the maximum iteration or converges. The formulas for velocity updates, position updates, *Pbest*, and *Gbest* have already been discussed.

The fitness measure used for PSO clustering is:

Fitness Measure

$$J_e = \frac{\sum_{j=1}^{N_c} \left[\frac{\sum_{\forall z_p \in C_j} d(z_p, m_j)}{|C_j|} \right]}{N_c}$$

where

$$d(z_p, m_j) = \sqrt{\sum_{k=1}^{N_b} (z_{pk} - m_{jk})^2}$$

The cluster centroids used for the particle swarm optimization image clustering algorithm [31] are:

1. $\vartheta_i(t+1) = w\vartheta_i(t) + c_1 r_1(t)\left(y_i(t) - x_i(t)\right) + c_2 r_2(t)\left(\hat{y}(t) - x_i(t)\right)$
2. $x_i(t+1) = x_i(t) + \vartheta_i(t+1)$

An advantage of particle swarm optimization clustering is that it reduces the effect of initial conditions and parallel search for optimal clustering.

7.3 REVIEW OF LITERATURE

In this work, we are using particle swarm optimization-based image clustering. In the context of PSO image clustering, each particle is a set of *n* coordinates, where each one corresponds to the dimensional position of a cluster centroid. Each particle represents a position *Nd*. Its position is then adjusted based on the particle local and global best position. Table 7.2 provides information about the fitness measures used in different projects.

7.3.1 Microaneurysm Detection

Detection of microaneurysms aids in early detection of diabetic retinopathy. Microaneurysms are the first symptom of diabetic retinopathy and cause blood

TABLE 7.2
State-of-the-Art Techniques for Fitness Measures on Particle Swarm Optimization Clustering

[32]	$\frac{1}{1+\Sigma\Sigma UD+\Sigma\Sigma(1-u)}$
[33]	$\Sigma\frac{\frac{\Sigma d(M,P)Zjr}{Zj}}{n}$
[34]	$\Sigma\Sigma\lvert x-c\rvert^2$
[35]	$\mathrm{Sqrt}(\Sigma(p-q)^2)++\Sigma(p\wedge q)$
[35]	$\Sigma\frac{\frac{\Sigma d(M,P)Z}{p}}{n}$
[36]	$\Sigma\Sigma\,(T_{ij}-T)^2$
[37]	$\frac{k}{J+J0}$

leakage to the retina. Microaneurysms are small, circular red lesions with a diameter of 50 to 125 μm.

One group [32] used the pre-processing techniques of hue, saturation, and lightness images, gamma correction, contrast-limited adaptive histogram equalization, histogram stretching, clipping, standard deviation, mean, circular Hough transform, top hat transform, and a feature extraction algorithm and used the dataset of receiver operating characteristic curve (ROC), a local dataset with accuracy of 92.7%, recall of 97.39%, and precision of 82%.

The authors [33] used the pre-processing techniques of green channel, median filter, contrast-limited adaptive histogram equalization, Gaussian filter, and normalization; the random forest classifier; and the MESSIDOR and DIARETDB2 databases. Another group [34] used the pre-processing techniques of mean filter, standard deviation, and color equalization and used a classifier support vector machine and the ROC database. One study [35] used the pre-processing techniques of resize, green channel extraction, median filter, and standard mean and deviation and used a local dataset.

Another study [36] used the pre-processing techniques of mean filter, standard deviation, mean, histogram stretching, and clipping; the support vector machine classifier; and the MESSIDOR and DIARETDB1 datasets. In one study, the authors [37] used the pre-processing techniques of green channel, grayscale, median filter, Gaussian filter, contrast-limited adaptive histogram equalization, Kirch filter, Frangi filter, local entropy, entropic thresholding classifier decision tree, 1-neural network, radial basis function (RBF) kernel support vector machine, and polynomial support vector machine.

In another study, the authors [38] used the pre-processing techniques of mean filter, contrast-limited adaptive histogram equalization, and Gaussian filter and the *k*-nearest neighbor, naive Bayes, and AdaBoost classifiers. One group [39] used the pre-processing techniques of resizing, green channel, masking, opening, and closing and a convolution neural network classifier.

Another group [40] used the pre-processing techniques of green channel, contrast-limited adaptive histogram equalization, and median filter; Frangi filter, morphology, and ACO classifiers; and the MESSIDOR and DIARETDB1 datasets. While yet another group [41] used the pre-processing techniques of resizing, green channel, and flood-filling green channel; the SoftMax classifier; and the ROC dataset. This group [42] used the pre-processing techniques of green channel, NLM filter, and contrast-limited adaptive histogram equalization and the region-growing algorithm classifier with the DIARETDB0 dataset. While this group [43] used the pre-processing techniques of green channel, Gaussian filter, and shade correction algorithm and the *k*-nearest neighbor and support vector machine classifiers with local datasets.

7.4 PROPOSED METHODOLOGY

The main aim of this research is to diagnose diabetic retinopathy in the early stage with high accuracy. This research focuses on the detection of microaneurysms. Detecting microaneurysms with particle swarm optimization continuous clustering segmentation increases the accuracy of microaneurysm detection. The proposed methodology is shown in Figure 7.1.

7.4.1 Pre-Processing

The pre-processing phase helps to improve the quality of the retina image. Spatial domain techniques operate on pixels. The advantages of spatial domain techniques are efficient computation and the need for fewer processing resources. In a pixel-based approach, the input information is the pixel itself. The image produced after applying the pixel-based approach is of high contrast, and these enhancement techniques depend on the gray levels. In this study, the pre-processing step uses histogram processing, as this technique works on pixels. The stages used in pre-processing are resizing, conversion of the RGB image to grayscale, and contrast-limited adaptive histogram equalization (CLAHE) [44]. The pre-processing phase of the retina image is shown in Figure 7.2.

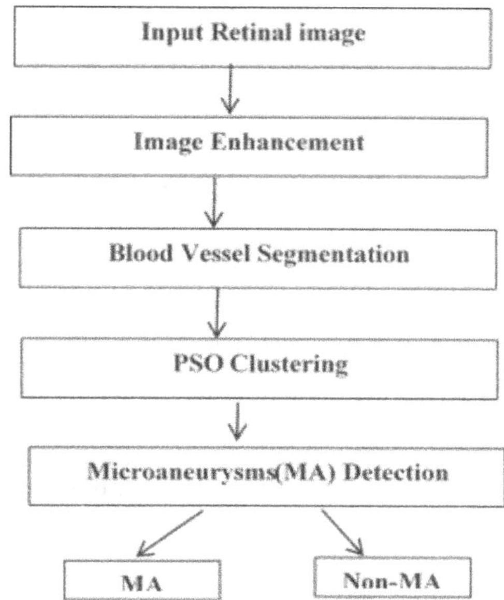

FIGURE 7.1 Proposed methodology flowchart.

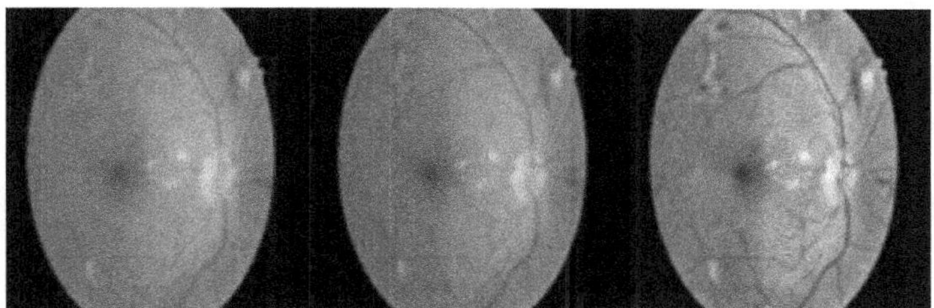

FIGURE 7.2 (Left) Resized image; (Middle) gray image; (Right) image after applying CLAHE.

7.4.2 Segmentation

The main objective of segmentation is to rearrange or change the retina image's appearance to make it more significant and easier to differentiate and extract the features of the retina image. For better segmentation and to increase the accuracy of the segmented image, optimization algorithms are used. In this work, we use PSO clustering variants to segment the pre-processed image. The segmentation phase helps in the detection of microaneurysms from the retina image. We use two different PSO continuous clustering variants, new continuous and improved continuous PSO clustering algorithms, to segment the pre-processed image.

7.4.3 Augmented Continuous Particle Swarm Optimization Clustering

Augmented continuous particle swarm optimization clustering is used to effectively segment microaneurysms.

Algorithm 1: Augmented continuous particle swarm optimization (ACPSO)
Result: *Gbest* of the whole swarm
Initialization: Generate 3 × swarm size particles

1. Generate particles based on swarm size.
2. Generate clusters using a centroid updating scheme. Evaluate fitness measures for the particles.
3. For each particle, apply the neighborhood search scheme.
4. Iterate for all particles. For each particle, update position using centroid updating and neighbor search scheme and velocity using velocity generation scheme. Evaluate the fitness measure. Update *Pbest* and *Gbest*.
5. Return *Gbest* velocity generation scheme:
   a. Generate three random numbers and normalize these numbers.
   b. Sort these numbers and use these three numbers during the velocity update scheme.

7.4.4 Fitness Measures

The fitness measure is the primary accuracy of the segmented retina image. The fitness measure measures the quality of the clusters. Each particle x_n in a cluster is represented as $x_n = (x_{n,1}, \ldots x_{n,k})$, where $x_{n,k}$ refers to the kth cluster centroid vector of the nth particle. A swarm represents several data clustering solutions. The quality of the particle in the image is measured using the fitness function. The fitness measures that are using in the previously discussed augmented continuous particle swarm optimization clustering algorithm are shown in Table 7.3.

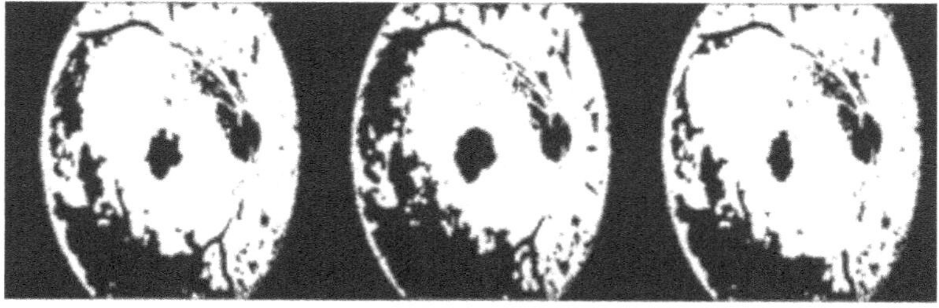

FIGURE 7.3 PSO clustering.

TABLE 7.3
Fitness Measures Used for PSO Clustering in the Proposed System

Measure	Formulae
Entropy	$\sum_{i=0}^{\infty}\sum_{j=0}^{\infty}\frac{p}{\log p}$
Kurtosis	$\frac{1/n\sum(y-\bar{y})^2}{s^4}$
Skewness	$\frac{1/n\sum(y-\bar{y})^2}{s^3}$

TABLE 7.4
List of Features

S. No.	Feature Description	Formula
f1	Entropy	$\sum_{i=0}^{\infty}\sum_{j=0}^{\infty}\frac{p}{\log p}$
f2	Max probability	$\text{Max}\{p_{ij}(x,y)\}$
f3	Energy	$\Sigma\Sigma P_{IJ}^2$
f4	Mean	$\sum_{i=0}^{\infty}\sum_{j=0}^{\infty}\frac{p}{NXM}$
f5	Variance	$\sum_{i=0}^{\infty}\sum_{j=0}^{\infty}(P(I-J)-\mu)^2$
f6	Dissimilarity	$\sum_{i=0}^{\infty}\sum_{j=0}^{\infty}P(I-J)$
f7	Contrast	$\sum_{i=0}^{\infty}\sum_{j=0}^{\infty}P(I-J)^2$

7.4.5 Feature Extraction

In the feature extraction stage of the proposed system, we extract the lesion from the segmented image. A set of features, namely area, perimeter, circularity, and diameter, is used to extract lesions. Irrelevant and redundant features should be eliminated from the segmented image to improve accuracy. The features are listed in Table 7.4. The image after feature extraction is shown in Figure 7.4. The extracted features are fed into the random forest classifier to differentiate between microaneurysms and non-microaneurysms.

7.5 RESULTS

We evaluated the performance of the microaneurysm detection technique on the publicly available datasets DIARETDB1, MESSIDOR, and E-OPTHA. The DIARETDB1 database, based on 130 images, consists of mild non-proliferative diabetic retinopathy. The retina images in the DIARETDB1 database are associated with real-world images; we evaluated the performance on these retina images. The MESSIDOR database consists of 1,200 fundus images collected from three ophthalmologic departments. The images in the MESSIDOR database are taken from three charged coupled device cameras with an angle of 45° field of view. E-OPTHA contains color-based fundus images used for diabetic retinopathy diagnosis. For experimentation, the anaconda IDE on an Intel core i5 3.4-GHz processor is used.

In the DIARETDB0 database, out of 130 images, 104 images are utilized for training, and 26 images are used for testing. To indicate the number of true and false positives, we use TP and FP; TN and FN are for true and false negatives. The metric levels are provided in Table 7.5.

Performance measures used in the proposed technique are given in Table 7.6. We compare the accuracy, sensitivity, and specificity of the present method with other research works in Table 7.7. The statistics used to measure the similarity and

TABLE 7.5
Metric Levels

Metric	Description
True positive (TP)	Count of correctly classified microaneurysm pixels
True negative (TN)	Count of correctly classified non-microaneurysm pixels
False positive (FP)	Misclassified count of non-microaneurysms treated as microaneurysms
False negative (FN)	Misclassified count of microaneurysms treated as non-microaneurysms

TABLE 7.6
Performance Metrics

Measure	Formula
Sensitivity	$\frac{TP}{(TP+FN)}$
Specificity	$\frac{TN}{(TN+FP)}$
False positive rate	$\frac{FP}{(FP+TN)}$
False negative rate	$\frac{FN}{(TP+FN)}$
Accuracy	$\frac{(TP+FN)}{(TP+FP+TN+FN)}$

TABLE 7.7
Comparison of Accuracy, Sensitivity, and Specificity with Other Techniques

Project	Dataset	Accuracy	Sensitivity	Specificity
[45]	E-OPTHA	92.28%	86.80%	92.10%
[42]	DIARETDB0	78%	87.88%	58.82%
[46]	ROC, local dataset	—	64.1%	—
35]	Local dataset	—	42.26%	—
Present work	E-OPTHA	91.15%	89.95%	87.45%
	MESSIDOR	89.93%	88.56%	85.45%
	DIARETDB1	93.84%	91.42%	90.01%

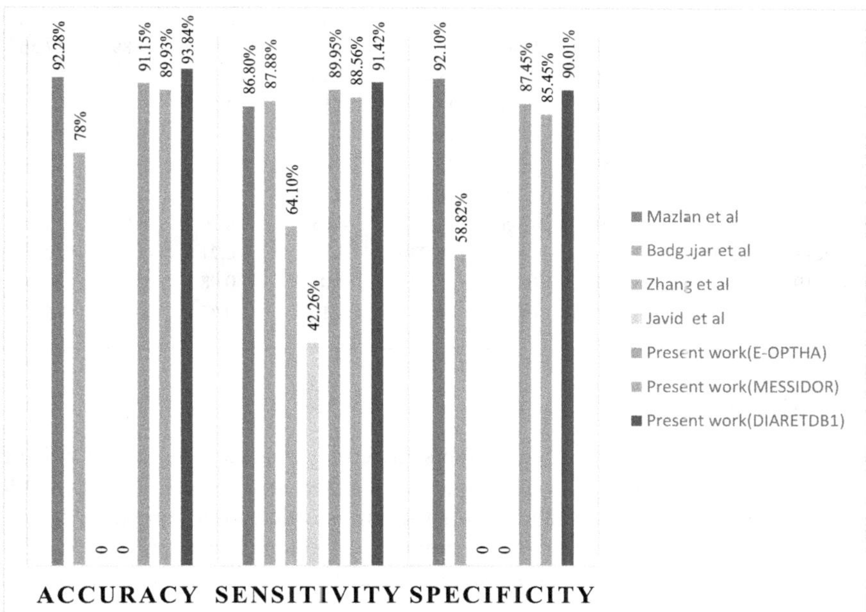

FIGURE 7.4 Performance measure comparison.

distribution of the data are kurtosis and skewness. Kurtosis confirms the symmetry of the data distribution. To identify the symmetry of the data distribution in the cluster, we use kurtosis and skewness to assess predictions about the distribution of the data in the clusters.

The present work is compared with the existing approaches, as shown in Figure 7.4. The kurtosis and skewness measures are used as the accuracy measures, and these statistical measures for the present work are compared with the existing particle swarm optimization algorithm in Table 7.8.

TABLE 7.8
Similarity Measures

	PSO				ACPSO			
Image Id	**Entropy**	**Kurtosis**	**Skew**	**Runtime**	**Entropy**	**Kurtosis**	**Skew**	**Runtime**
Image01	3.57	−0.75	−1.11	16.45	2.58	−0.83	−1.25	16.34
Image02	4.33	−1.8	0.39	19.51	4.38	−1.9	0.28	18.89
Image03	4.10	−1.94	−9.25	19.47	4.23	−1.98	−9.53	18.98
Image04	4.91	−0.87	1.06	20.64	4.99	−0.97	0.99	19.29
Image05	4.20	−1.82	0.41	18.28	4.45	−1.93	0.33	17.85
Image06	1.24	−1.46	−0.73	17.88	1.34	−1.23	0.87	16.67
Image07	4.10	−1.85	−0.38	18.19	4.28	−1.94	−0.45	17.76
Image08	3.57	−1.89	−0.34	18.30	3.87	−1.94	−0.41	17.89
Image09	4.07	−1.78	0.47	18.85	4.89	−1.11	0.59	17.85
Image10	4.78	−0.45	1.25	18.14	4.97	−0.51	1.33	17.56
Image11	4.23	−1.79	−0.46	18.25	4.51	−1.99	−0.89	17.56
Image12	3.25	0.94	−1.72	18.41	3.48	0.89	−1.87	17.85
Image13	4.52	6.13	5.28	18.08	4.89	2.23	2.87	17.67
Image14	4.01	−1.99	−0.07	18.25	3.34	0.97	0.98	16.49
Image15	4.23	−1.94	0.24	18.24	3.46	0.80	0.15	17.51
Image16	4.23	3.07	2.25	18.01	3.45	2.87	1.73	17.65
Image17	4.18	−0.89	1.05	18.53	4.08	0.96	1.03	17.45
Image18	3.15	0.73	−1.65	18.03	3.12	0.71	−1.78	17.88
Image19	4.16	−1.99	−0.10	18.08	4.08	0.98	0.89	17.68
Image20	4.28	−1.99	0.01	18.33	4.15	0.87	0.01	17.83

7.6 CONCLUSION

Automatic detection of microaneurysms in retinal images reduces the risk of vision loss. In this chapter, a technique is proposed and demonstrated through experimental outcomes, enhancing microaneurysm detection compared to the existing methods. Future work on the proposed technique can extend its scope to the diagnosis of cotton wool spots, hemorrhage, exudates, and diabetic retinopathy grading.

REFERENCES

[1] CP Wilkinson, Frederick L Ferris III, Ronald E Klein, Paul P Lee, Carl David Agardh, Matthew Davis, Diana Dills, Anselm Kampik, R Pararajasegaram, Juan T Verdaguer, et al. Proposed international clinical diabetic retinopathy and diabetic macular edema disease severity scales. Ophthalmology, 110(9):1677–1682, 2003.

[2] Sihem Boudina and Evan Dale Abel. Diabetic cardiomyopathy, causes and effects. Reviews in Endocrine and Metabolic Disorders, 11(1):31–39, 2010.

[3] AR Andersen, J Sandahl Christiansen, JK Andersen, S Kreiner, and T Deckert. Diabetic nephropathy in type 1 (insulin-dependent) diabetes: an epidemiological study. Diabetologia, 25(6):496–501, 1983.

[4] Mark J Brown and Arthur K Asbury. Diabetic neuropathy. Annals of Neurology: Official Journal of the American Neurological Association and the Child Neurology Society, 15(1):2–12, 1984.

[5] Shirley Rubler, Joel Dlugash, Yusuf Ziya Yuceoglu, Tarik Kumral, Arthur Whitley Branwood, and Arthur Grishman. New type of cardiomyopathy associated with diabetic glomerulosclerosis. American Journal of Cardiology, 30(6):595–602, 1972.

[6] William B Kannel, Marthana Hjortland, and William P Castelli. Role of diabetes in congestive heart failure: the Framingham Study. American Journal of Cardiology, 34(1):29–34, 1974.

[7] Inga S Thrainsdottir, Thor Aspelund, Gudmundur Thorgeirsson, Vilmundur Gudnason, Thordur Hardarson, Klas Malmberg, Gunnar Sigurdsson, and Lars Rydén. The association between glucose abnormalities and heart failure in the population-based Reykjavik Study. Diabetes Care, 28(3):612–616, 2005.

[8] Marcus Lind, Ioannis Bounias, Marita Olsson, Soffia Gudbjörnsdottir, AnnMarie Svensson, and Annika Rosengren. Glycaemic control and incidence of heart failure in 20 985 patients with type 1 diabetes: an observational study. The Lancet, 378(9786):140–146, 2011.

[9] American Diabetes Association et al. Nephropathy in diabetes. Diabetes Care, 27(suppl 1):s79–s83, 2004.

[10] Carl Erik Mogensen. Microalbuminuria, blood pressure and diabetic renal disease: origin and development of ideas. In The Kidney and Hypertension in Diabetes Mellitus, pages 655–706. Springer, 2000.

[11] Peter Hovind, Lise Tarnow, Peter Rossing, Malene Graae, Inge Torp, Christian Binder, and Hans-Henrik Parving. Predictors for the development of microalbuminuria and macroalbuminuria in patients with type 1 diabetes: inception cohort study. BMJ, 328(7448):1105, 2004.

[12] Amanda I Adler, Richard J Stevens, Sue E Manley, Rudy W Bilous, Carole A Cull, Rury R Holman, UKPDS Group, et al. Development and progression of nephropathy in type 2 diabetes: the United Kingdom Prospective Diabetes Study (UKPDS 64). Kidney International, 63(1):225–232, 2003.

[13] Julius Hirschberg. Uber diabetische netzhautentzündung. DMW-Deutsche Medizinische Wochenschrift, 16(51):1181–1185, 1890.

[14] George W Blankenship and Jay S Skyler. Diabetic retinopathy: a general survey. Diabetes Care, 1(2):127–137, 1978.

[15] Harry Keen. The prevalence of blindness in diabetes. Journal of the Royal College of Physicians of London, 7(1):53, 1972.

[16] Harold A Kahn and Robert F Bradley. Prevalence of diabetic retinopathy age, sex, and duration of diabetes. British Journal of Ophthalmology, 59(7):345–349, 1975.

[17] HW Larsen. Diabetic retinopathy (dissertation). Acta Ophthalmologica Supplemen ts, 60:i960, 1960.

[18] Andrew J Gay and Arthur L Rosenbaum. Retinal artery pressure in asymmetric diabetic retinopathy. Archives of Ophthalmology, 75(6):758–762, 1966.

[19] JH Dobree. Proliferative diabetic retinopathy: evolution of the retinal lesions. The British Journal of Ophthalmology, 48(12):637, 1964.

[20] Elsie R Carrinton. Pregnancy and diabetes. Annals of Internal Medicine, 59(1 Part 1):120–124, 1963.

[21] AJ Ballantyne and A Loewenstein. Retinal micro-aneurysms and punctate haemorrhages. The British Journal of Ophthalmology, 28(12):593, 1944.

[22] Amar Agarwal. Fundus Fluorescein and Indocyanine Green Angiography: A Textbook and Atlas. SLACK Incorporated, 2007.

[23] Thomas Behrendt and Eileen Slipakoff. Spectral reflectance photography. International Ophthalmology Clinics, 16(2):95–100, 1976.

[24] WH Woon, FW Fitzke, AC Bird, and J Marshall. Confocal imaging of the fundus using a scanning laser ophthalmoscope. British Journal of Ophthalmology, 76(8):470–474, 1992.

[25] James Kennedy and Russell Eberhart. Particle swarm optimization. In IEEE International of First Conference on Neural Networks, 1995.

[26] Michael R Anderberg. The broad view of cluster analysis. Cluster Analysis for Applications, pages 1–9, 1973.

[27] Siddheswar Ray and Rose H Turi. Determination of number of clusters in *k*-means clustering and application in colour image segmentation. In Proceedings of the 4th International Conference on Advances in Pattern Recognition and Digital Techniques, pages 137–143. Calcutta, India, 1999.

[28] Xiaobo Li and Zhixi Fang. Parallel clustering algorithms. Parallel Computing, 11(3):275–290, 1989.

[29] Richard CT Lee. Clustering analysis and its applications. In Advances in Information Systems Science, pages 169–292. Springer, 1981.

[30] James Kennedy. Stereotyping: Improving particle swarm performance with cluster analysis. In Proceedings of the 2000 Congress on Evolutionary Computation. CEC00 (Cat. No. 00TH8512), volume 2, pages 1507–1512. IEEE, 2000.

[31] Mahamed G Omran, Andries P Engelbrecht, and Ayed Salman. Image classification using particle swarm optimization. In Recent Advances in Simulated Evolution and Learning, pages 347–365. World Scientific, 2004.

[32] D Jeba Derwin, S Tamil Selvi, O Jeba Singh, and B Priestly Shan. A novel automated system of discriminating microaneurysms in fundus images. Biomedical Signal Processing and Control, 58:101839, 2020.

[33] MM Habib, RA Welikala, A Hoppe, CG Owen, AR Rudnicka, and SA Barman. Detection of microaneurysms in retinal images using an ensemble classifier. Informatics in Medicine Unlocked, 9:44–57, 2017.

[34] D Jeba Derwin, S Tami Selvi, and O Jeba Singh. Secondary observer system for detection of microaneurysms in fundus images using texture descriptors. Journal of Digital Imaging, 33(1):159–167, 2020.

[35] Malihe Javidi, Hamid-Reza Pourreza, and Ahad Harati. Vessel segmentation and microaneurysm detection using discriminative dictionary learning and sparse representation. Computer Methods and Programs in Biomedicine, 139:93–108, 2017.

[36] D Jeba Derwin, S Tamil Selvi, and O Jeba Singh. Discrimination of microaneurysm in color retinal images using texture descriptors. Signal, Image and Video Processing, 14(2):369–376, 2020.

[37] Sarni Suhaila Rahim, Chrisina Jayne, Vasile Palade, and James Shuttleworth. Automatic detection of microaneurysms in colour fundus images for diabetic retinopathy screening. Neural Computing and Applications, 27(5):1149–1164, 2016.

[38] Bo Wu, Weifang Zhu, Fei Shi, Shuxia Zhu, and Xinjian Chen. Automatic detection of microaneurysms in retinal fundus images. Computerized Medical Imaging and Graphics, 55:106–112, 2017.

[39] Piotr Chudzik, Somshubra Majumdar, Francesco Calivá, Bashir Al-Diri, and Andrew Hunter. Microaneurysm detection using fully convolutional neural networks. Computer Methods and Programs in Biomedicine, 158:185–192, 2018.

[40] Turab Selcuk and Ahmet Alkan. Detection of microaneurysms using ant colony algorithm in the early diagnosis of diabetic retinopathy. Medical Hypotheses, 129:109242, 2019.

[41] Rangwan Kasantikul and Worapan Kusakunniran. Improving supervised microaneurysm segmentation using autoencoder-regularized neural network. In 2018 Digital Image Computing: Techniques and Applications (DICTA), pages 1–7. IEEE, 2018.

[42] Ravindra D Badgujar and Pramod J Deore. Region growing based segmentation using Forstner corner detection theory for accurate microaneurysms detection in retinal fundus images. In 2018 Fourth International Conference on Computing Communication Control and Automation (ICCUBEA), pages 1–5. IEEE, 2018.

[43] Su Wang, Hongying Lilian Tang, Yin Hu, Saeid Sanei, George Michael Saleh, Tunde Peto, et al. Localizing microaneurysms in fundus images through singular spectrum analysis. IEEE Transactions on Biomedical Engineering, 64(5):990–1002, 2016.

[44] Karel Zuiderveld. Contrast limited adaptive histogram equalization. In Graphics Gems IV, pages 474–485. Academic Press Professional, Inc., 1994.

[45] Noratikah Mazlan, Haniza Yazid, Hamzah Arof, and Hazlita Mohd Isa. Automated microaneurysms detection and classification using multilevel thresholding and multilayer perceptron. Journal of Medical and Biological Engineering, pages 1–15, 2020.

[46] Xinpeng Zhang, Zhitao Xiao, Fang Zhang, Philip O Ogunbona, Jiangtao Xi, and Jun Tong. Shape-based filter for micro-aneurysm detection. Computers & Electrical Engineering, 84:106620, 2020.

8 Computational Fluid Dynamics of Carotid Artery Blood Flow for Low-Gravity Environments

Vishwajeet Shankhwar, Dilbag Singh, Renuka Garg, Kamleshwar Kumar Verma and K.K. Deepak

CONTENTS

8.1 INTRODUCTION

Gravity plays a major role in the development of muscular and natural skeletal structure [1]. The absence of gravity causes multisystem deconditioning, including bone demineralization, muscle degeneration, cardiovascular deconditioning, spinal elongation and back pain [2–4]. The absence of gravity, weightlessness or microgravity indicates that g-forces are not zero but are insignificant or very small [5]. Microgravity exposure causes redistribution of blood from the lower limbs of the body to the thoracic area due to a decrease in the body's gravitational hydrostatic pressure gradient [1, 6]. Efficient counter-measures are needed to prevent complaints of deconditioning in the cardiovascular system (CVS). Negative lower-body pressure is used to suppress reductions in blood flow of the lower limbs and reduce weakening of the muscular system [7]. Earth simulations are used to mimic microgravity, such as head-down bed rest, water immersion, dry floatation and parabolic flights [8, 9]. As for real microgravity, all earth

DOI: 10.1201/9781003207856-8

simulations have their own specifics, but some of the differences in human physiology brought on by simulation are similar to those experienced by astronauts [10]. It has also been studied that blood moving to the brain and face causes astronauts to have round, puffy faces from blood supplied by the carotid artery. To understand more about the blood flow in the carotid artery in earth's gravity and microgravity, the present study was designed. The main purpose of the study is to analyze variation in blood flow, areas of stress and turbulence energy in the artery during microgravity conditions via fluid simulation. Because it's very difficult to conduct space experiments on earth, it can be done through computational fluid dynamics (CFD) [11]. There has been a lot of research done in this area. Huetter et al. did modeling on coronary artery diseases and predicted outcomes [12]. CFD is a very important tool in the fluid dynamics design and simulation process. Mona et al. performed simulation on artery hyperelastic wall properties [13]. Basically, CFD can reduce the time needed for instrument design and development by removing unnecessary prototyping [14]. Generally, there are two modes of analysis, 2D and 3D. Compared to 2D, 3D is more practical and precise, but it always takes more computation time. Due to higher geometrical complexity, cardiovascular disease has often attracted little consideration from a computational perspective. CFD uses mathematical analysis and data structures to investigate and resolve the difficulties of fluid flows. Computers are used to accomplish the calculations needed to simulate the free-stream movement of the fluid and the interaction of the fluid with the outside defined by boundary conditions. Herein research has yielded software that advances the precision and speed of composite simulations such as laminar or turbulent flows. Blood flow investigation by CFD has developed significantly in the last few years. CFD can be used to examine movement, velocity, shear stress, streamlined flow and other fluid parameters. It also provides blood movement and streamlines particle flow visualization. The present research examines the blood supply to the internal carotid artery (ICA) and external carotid artery (ECA) from the common carotid artery (CCA). In the human body, the carotid arteries are the major blood capillaries that distribute blood to the head, neck and face. There are two carotid arteries, one on the right side of the body and the other on the left. Each carotid artery is bifurcated into ICA and ECA. The ICA supplies the brain with blood, while the ECA supplies the face and collar with blood. The CCA has complex geometry and requires high-resolution scanning. Therefore, a 3D computational model was created from a computed tomography scanned image, and dimensions were taken from the available literature [15].

8.2 MATERIALS AND METHODS

8.2.1 Carotid Artery Geometry

In Creo, a 3D model of the carotid artery geometry was developed, and the blood flow was analyzed in Ansys Fluent. In the model, the CCA was reported to be 5 cm proximal to the flow divider, 5 cm distal to the ICA and 3 cm distal to the

ECA. Section size (100 mm) was chosen to conform with 3D carotid geometry recreated by other authors [14, 15]. Distal divisions of the ECA were not studied due to their negligible size. After completing the geometry, the file was imported to Ansys for CFD analysis because Creo was used only to design the geometry.

8.2.2 Boundary Conditions and Mesh Sensitivity

With the geometry exported and recognized by Ansys, meshing was done and boundary conditions were given. The final meshed carotid artery for simulation after the assignment of optimized refinement at the required localized regions is illustrated in Figure 8.1.

However, to generate this final optimized and meshed volume, mesh sensitivity analysis was performed, and the subsequent results were plotted against the outlet velocity, as shown in Figure 8.2.

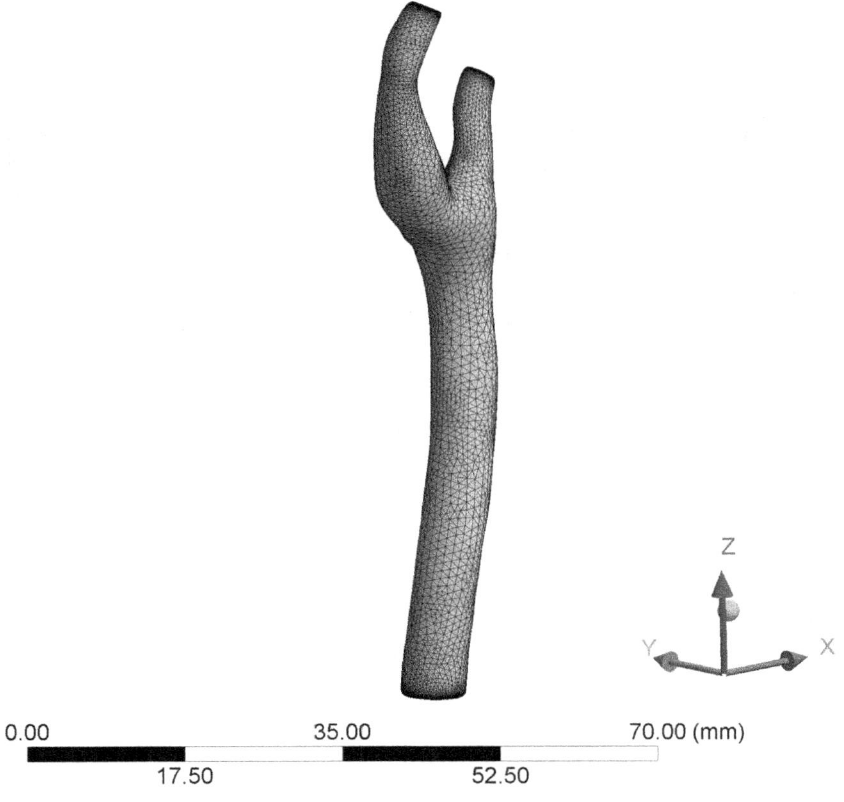

FIGURE 8.1 Human common carotid artery with its chief branches, ICA and ECA, after meshing.

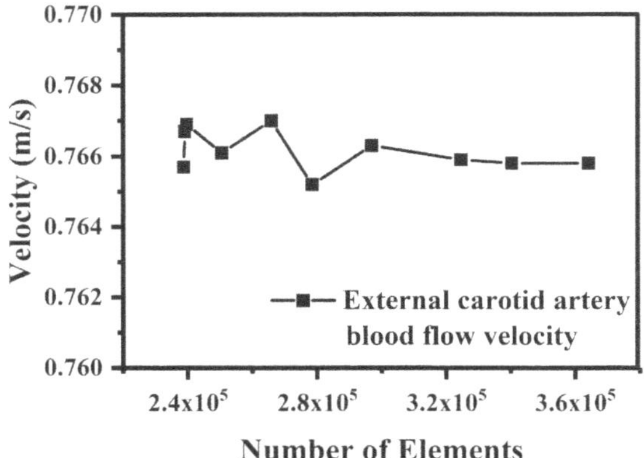

FIGURE 8.2 Mesh sensitivity graph: Number of elements used in Ansys during meshing vs. blood flow velocity in external carotid artery.

This also illustrates the convergence of the resultant velocity with the increasing elements. The subsequent optimized level of refinement was employed from the convergence data as the final mesh definition. The viscosity was taken as 0.003 kg/m-s; specific heat was taken as 3,513 J/kg-K; thermal conductivity was taken as 0.003 W/m-K; density was taken as 1,060 kg/m^3; and temperature was taken as 310 K (36.85°C), which is about the standard temperature of a human body. The velocity at the outlet depends on the inputs. The continuity equation and Navier-Stokes equation are the elementary governing equations, presented as Equations (8.1) and (8.2). The Navier-Stokes equation signifies the conservation of momentum, whereas the equation of continuity signifies the conservation of mass.

$$\frac{\partial \rho}{\partial t} + \nabla(\rho v) = 0 \tag{8.1}$$

$$\rho\left(\frac{\partial v}{\partial t} + v\nabla v\right) = -\nabla p + \mu \nabla^2 v + f \tag{8.2}$$

The viscosity coefficient is taken as μ, which is a function of shear rate, and ρ is taken as density. ∇^2 is the Laplace operator, ν is the fluid velocity vector and ρ is the fluid pressure. If the shear rate increases, the blood becomes less viscous [17]. Blood viscosity is modeled by means of the Carreau fluids model. The Carreau model is mathematically defined by Equation (8.3):

$$\mu_{\text{eff}}(\dot{\gamma}) = \mu_{\text{inf}} + (\mu_0 - \mu_{\text{inf}})\left(1 + (\lambda\dot{\gamma})^2\right)^{\frac{n-1}{2}} \tag{8.3}$$

where μ_{eff} is the effective viscosity, μ_0 is the zero shear viscosity, μ_{inf} is the infinite shear viscosity, λ is the time constant and n is the power law index.

For the case of blood [18],

$$\mu_0 = 0.056\ \text{kg.ms}^{-1},\ \mu_{inf} = 0.056\ \text{kg.ms}^{-1},\ \lambda = 3.0301\ (\text{s})\ \text{and}\ n = 0.3568$$

Further, the user-defined variable inlet velocity was used to apply the variable velocity, and a user-defined function was employed with the average values of the blood velocity at different time intervals, as shown in Figure 8.3.

Earth's gravity was taken as 9.8 m/s^2 in the negative z-axis direction, and microgravity was taken as 0.0001 m/s^2. Laminar flow was investigated for 1,000 iterations. Per the previous literature [19, 20], CCA blood flow input was reported as 0.3 m/s, and the cardiac output increased by 20% in microgravity. So, in the present analysis, these values were taken into account for simulation as boundary conditions. Herein, simulation was done to observe the results obtained in earth's gravity and microgravity conditions when the inlet blood velocity increased by 20%. Moreover, in Ansys Fluent, mesh independence analysis must be used, and not inspecting this is a very common error in CFD analysis. To make sure that the results converged and the solutions were independent of mesh resolution, the mesh independence or mesh sensitivity analysis was employed. The simulation was run several times with an increment of mesh size. As the mesh resolution changes, the solution may or may not change. If the solution does not change

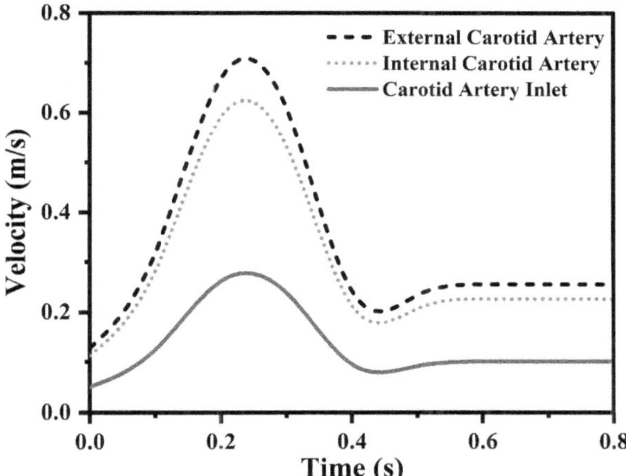

FIGURE 8.3 User-defined carotid artery inlet blood velocity and outlet blood flow velocity at the ECA and ICA branches.

because of mesh resolution, the solution is not dependent, and an acceptable mesh size has been obtained for further analysis.

8.3 RESULTS AND DISCUSSION

The total number of cells were 242,742 tetrahedral cells, 471,393 triangular interior faces and 48,026 nodes. The result was found to be converged by Ansys Fluent at the 729th iteration, but to make sure that the solution did not depend on the mesh resolution, a mesh resolution study was conducted by simulating the model multiple times with different mesh sizes. As the number of elements reached 3.45×10^5, the solution did not vary much; the variation was <5%, which means the solution was no longer dependent on mesh size.

The obtained mesh size was accepted for further analysis. The user-defined blood flow velocity was used as the inlet with a maximum velocity of 0.3 m/s, and the velocity in the ECA and ICA was found to be 0.7658 and 0.680 m/s, respectively. For incremental blood flow, the inlet was increased by 20%. In response to this, the maximum blood flow velocity for the ECA and ICA was found to be 0.909 and 0.805 m/s, respectively, under earth's gravity.

A higher velocity of 0.9151 and 0.810 m/s in blood flow was detected in microgravity conditions for ECA and ICA, respectively, as shown in Figure 8.4.

In the case of turbulence kinetic energy, it increased from 0.0815 to 0.1052 m^2/s^2, as shown in Figure 8.5.

It was also found that the maximum velocity was not in the middle but near the internal side wall of the ECA in the current simulation, while the highest velocity was in the middle and not the inner side wall of ICA. It was observed that the blood velocity increased by 19.71% in the external carotid artery and 19.11% in the internal carotid artery when calculated from baseline to microgravity, as shown in Table 8.1, whereas the increment was 18.69% and 18.38%, respectively, for earth gravity.

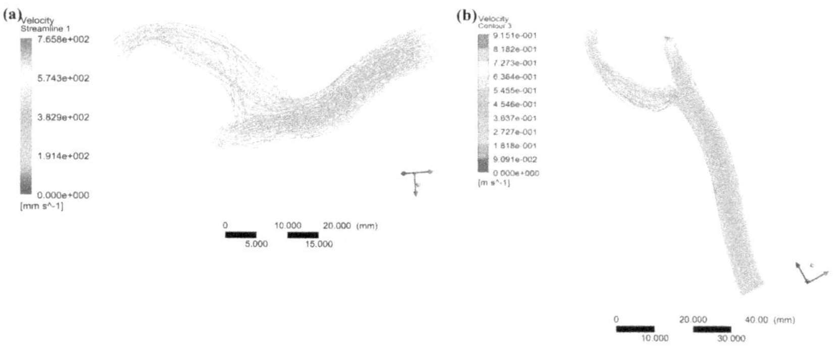

FIGURE 8.4 Blood flow velocity contour in human carotid artery: (a) for earth's gravity; (b) for microgravity.

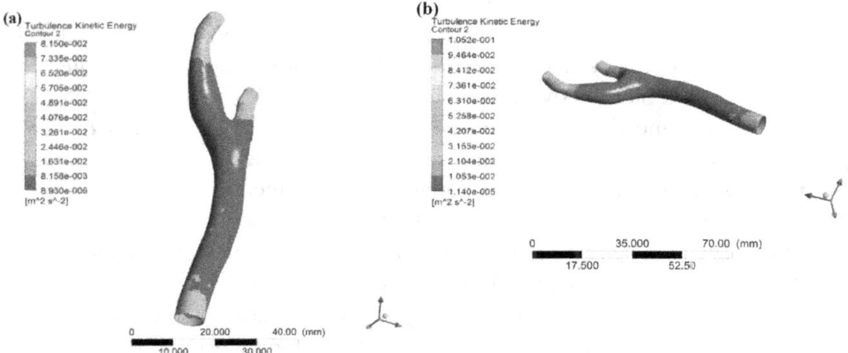

FIGURE 8.5 Turbulence kinetic energy contour for blood flow in carotid artery: (a) for earth's gravity; (b) for microgravity.

TABLE 8.1
All Blood Flow Velocity Profiles of Carotid Artery and Its Branches

		When Inlet Velocity Increased by 20%	
Region	**Baseline or Default**	**Earth Gravity**	**Microgravity**
Inlet Velocity (m/s)	0.3	0.36	0.36
ECA Velocity (m/s)	0.7658	0.909	0.915
ICA Velocity (m/s)	0.680	0.805	0.810
Turbulence Kinetic Energy (m^2/s^2)	0.0815	0.1026	0.1052

The turbulence kinetic energy was increased by 29% when compared from baseline to microgravity, whereas for earth gravity, it was 26% for the same.

It was also observed that as the increment given was less in the ICA as compared to the ECA, narrow arteries may offer higher resistance to blood flow. This could also be validated given that the inlet radius was 3.498 mm, and the ICA outlet radius was 1.807 mm. It was observed that after increasing the inlet by 20%, the ICA outlet increased by only 19.11%, which means narrow arteries have high stress and are resistive for fluid flow. It can be also inferred that the blood flow increment depends on gravity because the increments in the ECA and ICA were higher in microgravity as compared to the earth gravity condition. The validation of the current model can be done by comparing the results with the previous literature. The CFD results obtained are similar to those in previous publications [15, 16, 21].

8.4 CONCLUSION

In the current study, blood was described using a one-phase fluid model that neglected the existence of solid parts in it. This study examined the effect of microgravity on blood flow in the carotid artery. It was observed that blood starts moving more rapidly toward the thoracic cavity from the lower body under the influence of microgravity as compared to earth gravity. It can also be stated that gravity pulls down blood moving upward and decreases the blood flow velocity.

Though CFD models were created with reference to the results of three-dimensional MRI, it is debatable whether calculated outcomes, like flow velocity, are as precise as hemodynamic parameters directly measured by a catheter or echocardiography. There are some limitations to the present study. To reduce the calculation time, the fixed boundary condition was used, but wall movement with elasticity could have been included to increase correctness. However, approximation of the elastic vessel property distribution in microgravity is difficult; therefore, a typical fluid structure contact calculation cannot resolve this problem. Justification regarding the blood flow split to each branch or flow streamlines was insufficient. Future studies and simulations should be done on the basis of the fluid structure interface exhibited in terms of a precise elastic property and boundary layer turbulence blood flow simulation. Perfect boundary conditions must be used to compare the impact of microgravity. Subject-specific cardiac output and hypertension were not considered in our calculations. Therefore, there may be a discrepancy between the individually measured data and calculated data.

REFERENCES

[1] P. A. Carvil, J. Attias, S. N. Evetts, J. M. Waldie, and D. A. Green, "The effect of the gravity loading countermeasure skinsuit upon movement and strength," *J. Strength Cond. Res.*, vol. 31, no. 1, pp. 154–161, 2017.

[2] A. D. Moore, S. M. C. Lee, M. B. Stenger, and S. H. Platts, "Cardiovascular exercise in the U.S. space program: Past, present and future," *Acta Astronaut.*, vol. 66, no. 7–8, pp. 974–988, 2010.

[3] M. V. Narici and M. D. De Boer, "Disuse of the musculo-skeletal system in space and on earth," *Eur. J. Appl. Physiol.*, vol. 111, no. 3, pp. 403–420, 2011.

[4] V. Shankhwar, D. Singh, and K. K. Deepak, "Effect of novel designed bodygear on gastrocnemius and soleus muscles during stepping in human body," *Microgravity Sci. Technol.*, pp. 1–10, 2021.

[5] S. M. Schneider, "Space physiology VI: Exercise, artificial gravity, and countermeasure development for prolonged space flight," pp. 2183–2192, 2013.

[6] L. D. Montgomery, A. J. Parmet, and C. R. Booher, "Body volume changes during simulated microgravity: Auditory changes, segmental fluid redistribution, and regional hemodynamics," *Ann. Biomed. Eng.*, vol. 21, no. 4, pp. 417–433, 1993.

[7] D. E. Watenpaugh, "Human cutaneous vascular responses to whole-body tilting, Gz centrifugation, and LBNP," *J. Appl. Physiol.*, vol. 96, no. 6, pp. 2153–2160, 2004.

[8] A. Pavy-Le Traon, M. Heer, M. V. Narici, J. Rittweger, and J. Vernikos, "From space to Earth: Advances in human physiology from 20 years of bed rest studies (1986–2006)," *Eur. J. Appl. Physiol.*, vol. 101, no. 2, pp. 143–194, 2007.

[9] R. A. Stabler *et al.*, "Impact of the Mk VI Skinsuit on skin microbiota of terrestrial volunteers and an international space station-bound astronaut," *NPJ Microgravity*, vol. 3, no. 1, pp. 1–8, 2017.

[10] T. Haider *et al.*, "Effects of long-term head-down-tilt bed rest and different training regimes on the coagulation system of healthy men," *Physiol. Rep.*, vol. 1, no. 6, pp. 1–13, 2013.

[11] A. C. Benim, A. Nahavandi, A. Assmann, D. Schubert, P. Feindt, and S. H. Suh, "Simulation of blood flow in human aorta with emphasis on outlet boundary conditions," *Appl. Math. Model.*, vol. 35, no. 7, pp. 3175–3188, 2011.

[12] L. Huetter, P. H. Geoghegan, P. D. Docherty, M. Soltanipour Lazarjan, D. Clucas, and M. Jermy, "Application of a meta-analysis of aortic geometry to the generation of a compliant phantom for use in particle image velocimetry experimentation," *IFAC-PapersOnLine*, vol. 48, no. 20, pp. 407–412, 2015.

[13] M. Alimohammadi, J. M. Sherwood, M. Karimpour, O. Agu, S. Balabani, and V. Díaz-zuccarini, "Aortic dissection simulation models for clinical support: Fluid-structure interaction vs. rigid wall models," *Biomed. Eng. Online*, vol. 14, p. 34, 2015.

[14] A. Polanczyk, M. Podgorski, T. Wozniak, L. Stefanczyk, and M. Strzelecki, "Computational fluid dynamics as an engineering tool for the reconstruction of hemodynamics after carotid artery stenosis operation: A case study," *Medicina*, vol. 54, no. 3, 2018.

[15] Vishwajeet, D. Singh, and K. K. Deepak, "Modelling and simulation of carotid artery in microgravity," in *5th IEEE International Conference on Signal Processing, Computing and Control*, pp. 339–341, 2019.

[16] S. Ogoh, A. Hirasawa, S. de Abreu, P. Denise, and H. Normand, "Internal carotid, external carotid and vertebral artery blood flow responses to 3 days of head-out dry immersion," *Exp. Physiol.*, vol. 102, no. 10, pp. 1278–1287, 2017.

[17] T. Sochi, "Non-newtonian rheology in blood circulation," *arXiv.org*, pp. 1–26, 2013.

[18] M. W. Siebert and P. S. Fodor, "Newtonian and non-Newtonian blood flow over a backward-facing step—A case study," in *Excerpt from Proc. COMSOL Conf. 2009 Bost.*, p. 5, 2009.

[19] A. R. Hargens and L. Vico, "Long-duration bed rest as an analog to microgravity," *J. Appl. Physiol.*, vol. 120, no. 8, pp. 891–903, 2016.

[20] P. Norsk, A. Asmar, M. Damgaard, and N. J. Christensen, "Fluid shifts, vasodilatation and ambulatory blood pressure reduction during long duration spaceflight," *J. Physiol.*, vol. 593, pp. 573–584, 2015.

[21] H. F. Younis et al., "Hemodynamics and wall mechanics in human carotid bifurcation and its consequences for atherogenesis: Investigation of inter-individual variation," *Biomech. Model. Mechanobiol.*, vol. 3, no. 1, pp. 17–32, 2004.

9 Predictions of Loan E-Signing Based on Financial Status of Applicants Using Machine Learning

Apoorv Vats, Rashi Singh, Geetanjali Rathee and Hemraj Saini

CONTENTS

9.1 INTRODUCTION

Representing information and data in the form of graphics is called data visualization, and the tools are used to see trends, patterns and so on in data. It has been used in this chapter to better understand the financial history of loan applicants [1]. Financial history is the record of a person's current loans and their dates, amounts, and so on. Since the financial history contains data related to a person's finances, it is easy to find out whether a person has the assets with which they would be able to pay back the loan [2]. This way, we use financial history to determine e-signing of loans. There are several techniques for e-signing of loans, such as digitized loans. We can make use of the financial history to determine

DOI: 10.1201/9781003207856-9

e-signing of the loan, which leads us to the introduction of digitized loans [3]. Digitized loans are used to maintain financial transactions. Digital lending/digitized loans basically make use of web-based computing so as to originate and renew loans for speedy and efficient decisions. In digital lending, an online loan application is offered by a bank on its website, and it can be completely automated. It helps financial institutions by providing many opportunities to improve productivity with cheaper, faster automated services. As noted previously, lending companies work by analyzing the financial history of the loan applicant and then determine whether the applicant is too risky [4, 5]. For this, the applicant needs to fill out a form, which can be done physically or through a website which acts as an intermediary between the lending company and applicant. Such intermediaries receive an enormous number of applications, and therefore it is not possible to manually analyze all the applications. In this chapter, an optimized model has been developed to predict whether an applicant using a website will be risky for a loan using the e-signing process.

9.2 LITERATURE REVIEW

Patil et al. [6] worked on creating a model with an accuracy of around 64% and an algorithm that helps in predicting whether a person will be able to complete e-signing of a loan. An advantage of this model is to target those predicted not to reach the e-signing stage with customized on-boarding. The abstract and idea were taken from previously mentioned work, and in this chapter, the accuracy has been improved on a different dataset and reached 65.04% by processing the dataset using a stacking classifier.

Goyal et al. [7] evaluated predicting the financial status of an organization in the R language. The experiment was done five times on the same dataset, and the tree model for a genetic algorithm was found to be the best model for predicting customer finance. The outcome of this paper is to understand the methodology of experimenting several times with the same dataset but different algorithms.

Chen et al. [8] worked on increasing the accuracy, lowering the false positive rate, increasing the speed for software-defined networking controllers, and solving cloud-related problems like private cloud isolation of users and network flow control using XGBoost. From the previously mentioned paper, this paper has implemented the use of XGBoost and adopted some keywords, which have been used in this paper.

Prokhorenkova et al. [9] investigated the key algorithmic techniques behind CatBoost. The methods used in the paper were designed to combat predicting changes caused by a special type of target leakage present in all current applications of gradient reinforcement algorithms. The outcome of the paper was to understand the accuracy shown by the CatBoost algorithm in various situations and some keywords, which have been used in this work. Ke et al. [10] solved the problem of efficiency and scalability, which are inadequate when the feature dimension is high and the data size is large in LightGBM. To address this issue, two novel methods were proposed: Gradient-based one-sided sampling (GOSS) and exclusive feature bundling (EFB). In this paper, LightGBM's effectiveness and some keywords were established, which have been used in this work.

Daoud et al. [11] compared XGBoost, CatBoost, and LightGBM. The purpose of this research was to compare the effectiveness of the three gradient methods. New features were generated, and various techniques were used for ranking and selection of the best features. The implementation showed that LightGBM, when compared to CatBoost and XGBoost, is more accurate and faster. The findings of this paper helped in increasing the accuracy of the model in this paper by implementing all three algorithms together using a voting and stacking classifier.

Kumar et al. [12] presented a paper on breast cancer prediction with the help of a voting classifier. The aim of the study was to compare the results of supervised learning classification models and a combination of these algorithms with a voting classifier technique. The dataset was taken from the University of Wisconsin's database. This paper helped in understanding the working and usage of the voting classifier, in learning about a few keywords related to the same, and in creating a model with better accuracy than the rest of the algorithms.

Malmasi et al. [13] tested a stacking classifier on native language identification, as it was a new approach and was not previously implemented. This work presented a set of tests using three individual-based models and with multiple configurations and algorithms. The paper helped in understanding the working and usage of the stacking classifier, in learning about a few keywords related to the same, and in creating a model with the best accuracy among all the algorithms.

Although several scientists/researchers have proposed various machine learning-based e-signing methods or schemes including classifiers, the authors have not tested these on various confusion matrix parameters through voting or stacking classifiers for e-signing loan applications.

9.3 PROPOSED APPROACH

The conventional method for e-signing loan applications used by intermediaries between banks and applicants was that banks used to wait for the applicant to finish the whole process of filling out the forms and then identify if the person were a risk, but this required a lot of time and resources, as there were many applications being filed. Since the intermediaries receive an enormous number of applications, everything is slowly moving toward making use of machine-learning models where the model will itself learn and then, using the algorithm, identify whether the applicant for the e-signing of loan is risky. Classification is one of the most important decision-making techniques in many real-world problems. In this work, the main objective is to classify the data as risky or not risky, that is, whether the applicant would be completing the e-signing process and improving the classification accuracy. As discussed previously, this survey has analyzed various classification techniques. It was observed that techniques like voting and stacking classifiers suited our problem, with the stacking classifier providing the best accuracy.

9.4 SYSTEM MODEL

The proposed phenomenon is analyzed over two different classifiers—voting and stacking classifiers—against various simulation results.

9.4.1 Voting Classifier

The proposed system is analyzed through a voting classifier, as shown in Figure 9.1.

The voting classifier is a machine-learning algorithm that predicts the output by taking the results of each classifier based on majority voting. It can be seen in Figure 9.1 that for the classification models (C_1, C_2, C_3) and their predictions (P_1, P_2, P_3), which have been calculated using various algorithms, and then through majority voting, the final output P_f is predicted. Instead of creating separate models for each algorithm, this algorithm helps in creating a single model which forecasts output on the basis of the combined majority of voting for each output class. Voting classifiers are of two types, hard voting, which supports the majority, and soft voting, which supports the average.

9.4.2 Stacking Classifier

The proposed system is analyzed through a stacking classifier, as depicted in Figure 9.2. Stacking is an ensemble learning algorithm that uses a meta-classifier to combine multiple classification models. The classification models are separately

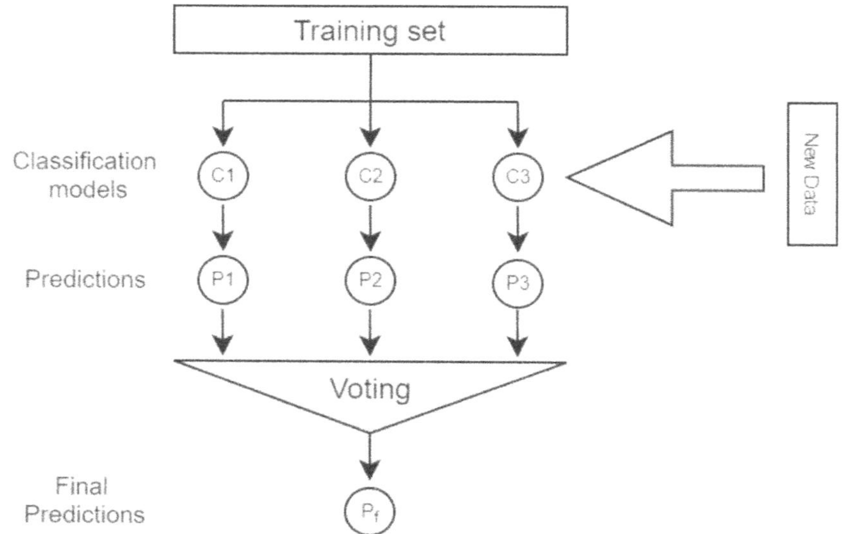

FIGURE 9.1 Voting classifier.

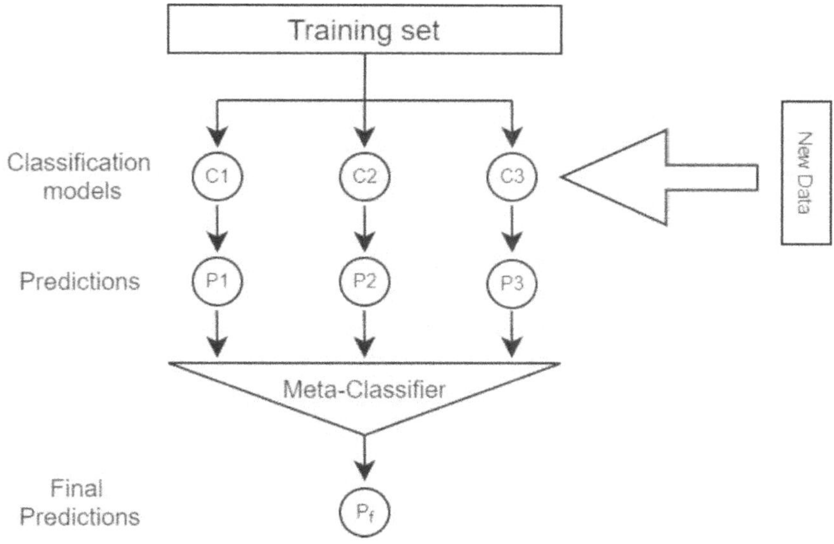

FIGURE 9.2 Stacking classifier.

trained on the basis of the complete training set, and then the meta-classifier fits on the basis of the output of the first-level classifier.

It can be seen in Figure 9.2 that the Classification models (C_1, C_2, C_3) and their predictions (P_1, P_2, P_3) have been calculated using various algorithms, and then, through the meta-classifier, the final output P_f is predicted. Stacking uses the strength of each individual estimator by using its output as input of a final estimator. In the model presented in this chapter for the voting classifier, three algorithms were used for voting: XGBoost, CatBoost, and LightGBM, with weights 1, 1, and 1, respectively, in hard voting and 1, 3, and 5, respectively, in soft voting. The reason for using these three algorithms was that after testing for various combinations of algorithms, the best accuracy was seen in these. For the stacking classifier, the three algorithms used for first-level classification were XGBoost, CatBoost, and LightGBM, and the final estimator for the meta-classifier for the model was logistic regression. To improve the accuracy, various splits were tried. The splits tried were 80–20, 70–30, and 60–40. A correlation matrix was used to visualize the relationship between two variables, and a confusion matrix was used to evaluate the model and calculate true positives and true negatives.

9.4.3 Confusion Matrix

A confusion matrix is a table used to show performance of a model in a test dataset that is known as true values. The following are a few important terms used in a confusion matrix from which the formula of accuracy, precision, and so on can be derived.

- *True positives (TPs)*: These are cases in which we predicted yes (they will sign), and they did sign.
- *True negatives (TNs)*: We predicted no, and they did not sign.
- *False positives (FPs)*: We predicted yes, but they did not actually sign (Type I error).
- *False negatives (FNs)*: We predicted no, but they did sign (Type II error).

Figures 9.3 and 9.4 show the confusion matrix for 80–20 and 70–30 splits, respectively, for the algorithms XGBoost, CatBoost, LightGBM, hard voting classifier, soft voting classifier, and stacking classifier. Figure 9.5 shows the confusion matrix for 60–40 splits for the algorithms XGBoost, CatBoost, LightGBM, hard voting classifier, soft voting classifier, and stacking classifier.

9.4.4 Dataset Used

In this study, the dataset used was downloaded from Kaggle. The dataset contains 17,908 entries and parameters of financial history, as provided in Table 9.1.

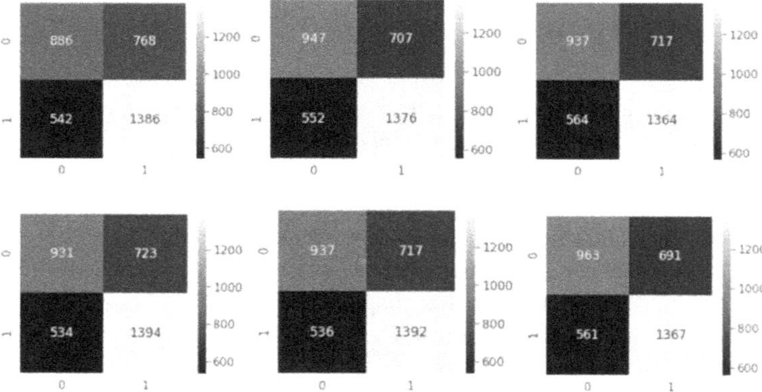

FIGURE 9.3 Confusion matrix for 80–20 splits of various algorithms.

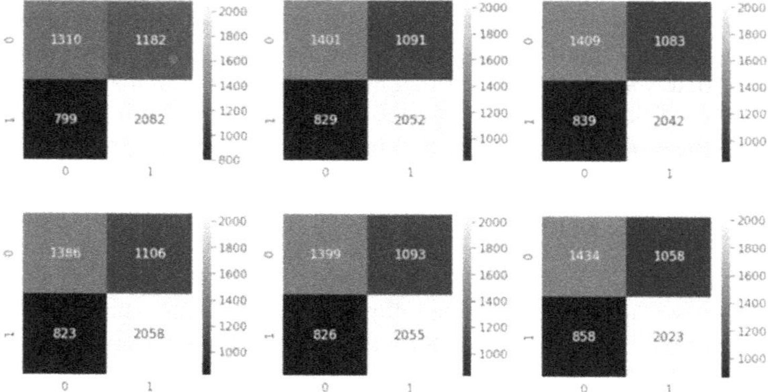

FIGURE 9.4 Confusion matrix for 70–30 splits of various algorithms.

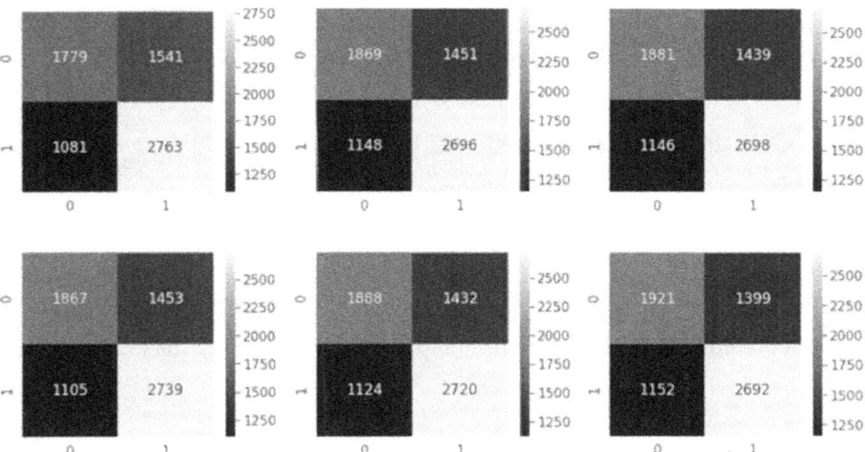

FIGURE 9.5 Confusion matrix for 60–40 splits of various algorithms.

TABLE 9.1
Features of the Dataset

S. No.	Parameters	Information
1	entry_id	Unique identity of the applicant
2	age	Age of the applicant
3	pay_schedule	How often applicant is paid
4	home_owner	Whether the applicant owns a home
5	income	Monthly income of the applicant
6	months_employed	Number of months the applicant has been employed
7	years_employed	Number of years the applicant has been employed
8	current_address_year	How many years has the applicant has been at their current address
9	personal_account_m	Number of months the applicant has had a personal account
10	personal_account_y	Number of years does the applicant has had a personal account
11	has_debt	Whether the applicant has debt
12	amount_requested	Amount the applicant has applied for
13	risk_score	Given to applicant by finance/engineering teams
14	risk_score_2	Given to applicant by finance/engineering teams
15	risk_score_3	Given to applicant by finance/engineering teams
16	risk_score_4	Given to applicant by finance/engineering teams
17	risk_score_5	Given to applicant by finance/engineering teams
18	ext_quality_score	Given to applicant by finance/engineering teams
19	ext_quality_score_2	Given to applicant by finance/engineering teams
20	inquiries_last_month	Number of inquiries made by applicant in last month
21	e_signed	E-signing completed or not

The present dataset is used for comparative analysis against various machine-learning algorithms for ensuring better precision on the e-signing of loans.

9.5 COMPARATIVE STUDY

We tried various algorithms in our model to test for the best accuracy. The algorithms are as follows:

- **Naïve Bayes**
  A machine learning algorithm based on probability, which uses Bayes' theorem given in Equation (9.1) and is used for classification tasks.

$$P(A|B) = \frac{P(B|A)P(A)}{P(B)} \tag{9.1}$$

  Naïve Bayes is mostly used for larger datasets with fewer variables.

- **Logistic Regression**
  Usually used when the dependent variable or target is categorical. Therefore, it can be said that it is a method used for problems with two class values. It makes use of the sigmoid function given in Equation (9.2) and is used to map real values (predictions) to values between 0 and 1 (probabilities).

$$p = \frac{1}{1+e^{-y}} \tag{9.2}$$

- **Artificial Neural Network**
  Similar to the human brain, with neurons interconnected to one another. An artificial neural network (ANN) is usually used in places where what has happened in the past is repeated in almost the same way.
- ***K*-Nearest Neighbor**
  Used for classification as well as regression and stores all the available cases, and the new cases are classified based on similarity.
- **Support Vector Machine Linear**
  A linear model for classification and regression problems that can be used for solving both linear and non-linear problems. In this algorithm, a hyperplane is used to separate the data into classes, and it supports both dense and sparse input.
- **Kernel Support Vector Machine**
  The kernel is a set of mathematical functions that take data as input, are used by the support vector machine (SVM), and transform it into the required form.

- **Decision Tree**
  Can be represented as a flowchart-like tree structure. In it, each internal node is a test on an attribute, each branch is a result of the test, and each leaf node holds a class label. It is used in operations research, specifically in decision analysis, to help identify a plan to reach a goal.
- **Random Forest**
  A supervised learning algorithm. Each tree in a random forest gives a class prediction, and the class with the most votes becomes our prediction. In the end, it merges them together, and a stable and accurate prediction is obtained. Both classification and regression problems make use of random forests.
- **XGBoost**
  A decision tree-based group machine learning algorithm. It is used for small to medium amounts of structured or tabular data. It pushes the limits of computing power for boosted tree algorithms, thus improving the performance and computational speed.
- **AdaBoost**
  One of the earliest boosting machine-learning algorithms to be used in solving problems. It helps to combine many weaker classification models into a single strong classifier and is used for both classification and regression problems. Its function involves putting more weight on instances that are difficult to classify and less weight on the ones that have already been handled well.
- **Gradient Boosting**
  Also used for regression and classification problems, which can produce a group of weak prediction models, generally decision trees with a fixed size as base learners.
- **CatBoost**
  An algorithm that is used for gradient boosting and on decision trees. It can work with various data types to solve many problems that businesses face today. It builds one of the most accurate models on whatever dataset it is fed with, requiring minimal data prep.
- **LightGBM**
  A gradient-boosting framework based on the concept of decision trees. It is used when the requirement is to increase the efficiency of the model, and it focuses on the accuracy of results. LightGBM makes use of two novel techniques: Exclusive feature bundling and gradient-based one-sided sampling.

9.6 PERFORMANCE ANALYSIS

To analyze the performance of models, we have used histograms, provided in Figure 9.6, as they are fantastic exploratory tools that display the distribution of continuous data.

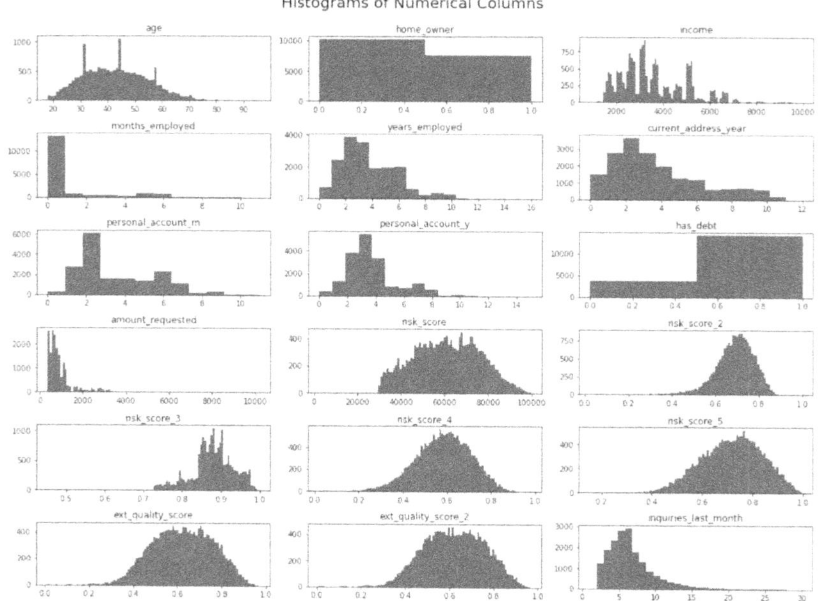

FIGURE 9.6 Histograms of numerical columns.

From the previous plots, we can conclude that the average applicant has age: 44, income: between $2,000 and $4,000, months employed: 0, years employed: 2, and personal account: 2–3.

The correlation matrix or covariance matrix, as provided in Figure 9.7, defines the correlation between two variables. It is used to briefly describe the strength and direction of the linear association between two quantitative variables and has a value between –1 (negative combination) and +1 (positive combination). If it is closer to 1 when the data points are closer to the straight line, the linear correlation is stronger, while if it is closer to 0, the direct association is weak. As discussed earlier, various algorithms have been tried to predict the e-signing of loans. The following figures show the accuracy of all the models tested and implemented on the dataset for different splits and the numerical values for the same. All the given entities in the following figures were calculated using numerical values from the confusion matrix. The formulae for the same are *Accuracy* (measure of correctness) = *(TP + TN)/Total*. *Precision* (When it predicts yes, how often is it correct?) = *TP/(TP + FP)*. *Recall* (measure of our model correctly identifying true positives) = *TP/Total*. *F1-Score* = weighted average of the true positive rate (recall) and precision.

From Figures 9.8 and 9.9, it can be seen that the stacking classifier has the maximum accuracy, 65.04%.

From Figures 9.10 and 9.11, it can be seen that the stacking classifier has the maximum accuracy, 64.34%.

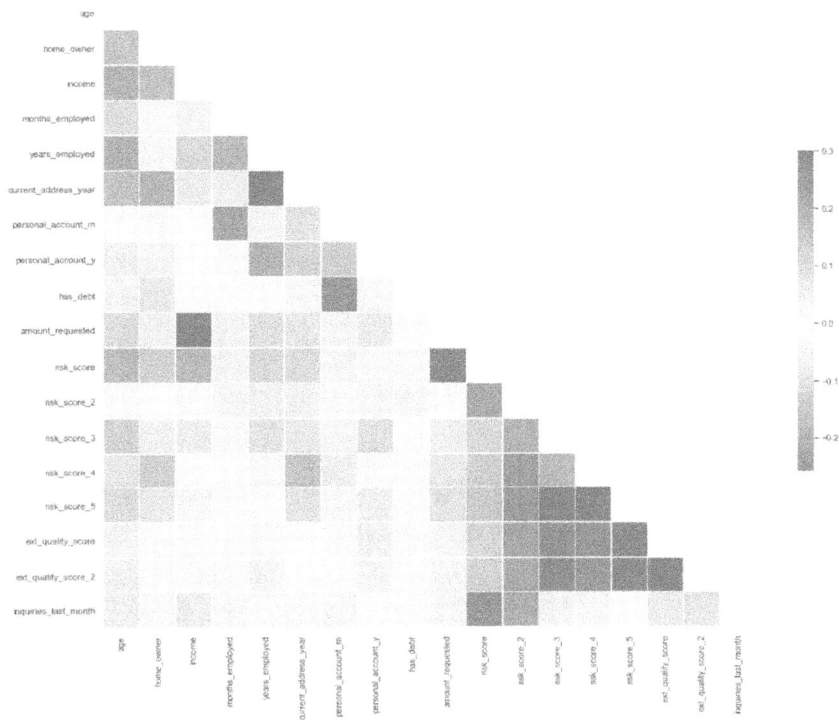

FIGURE 9.7 Correlation matrix using heatmap.

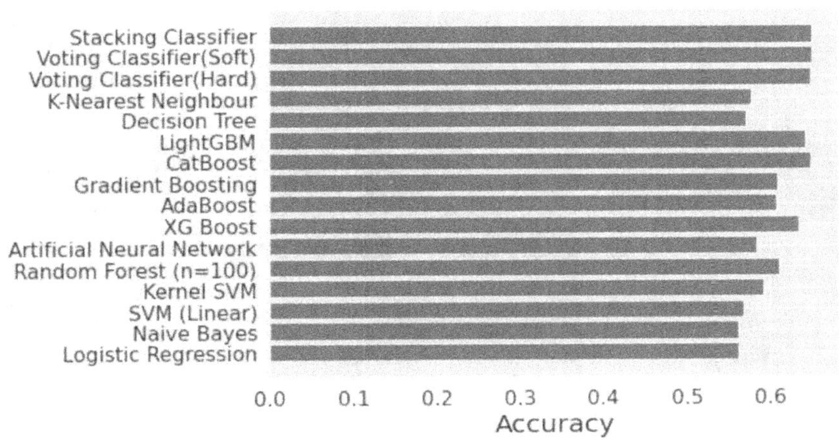

FIGURE 9.8 Accuracy graph for various algorithms for split 80–20.

Model	Accuracy	Precision	Recall	F1 Score
Logistic Regression	0.562535	0.576386	0.706432	0.634817
Naive Bayes	0.561697	0.578924	0.681017	0.625834
SVM (Linear)	0.568398	0.577769	0.735996	0.647354
Kernel SVM	0.591569	0.605730	0.690871	0.645505
Random Forest (n=100)	0.610553	0.630830	0.666494	0.648172
Artificial Neural Network	0.584590	0.621951	0.581950	0.601286
XG Boost	0.634283	0.643454	0.718880	0.679079
AdaBoost	0.608599	0.626931	0.673755	0.649500
Gradient Boosting	0.609157	0.628780	0.668568	0.648064
CatBoost	0.648520	0.660586	0.713693	0.686113
LightGBM	0.642379	0.655454	0.707469	0.680469
Decision Tree	0.571748	0.604233	0.592324	0.598219
K-Nearest Neighbour	0.577889	0.609015	0.602697	0.605839
Voting Classifier(Hard)	0.649079	0.658479	0.723029	0.689246
Voting Classifier(Soft)	0.650195	0.660028	0.721992	0.689621
Stacking Classifier	0.650475	0.664237	0.709025	0.685901

FIGURE 9.9 Numerical entities for various algorithms for split 80–20.

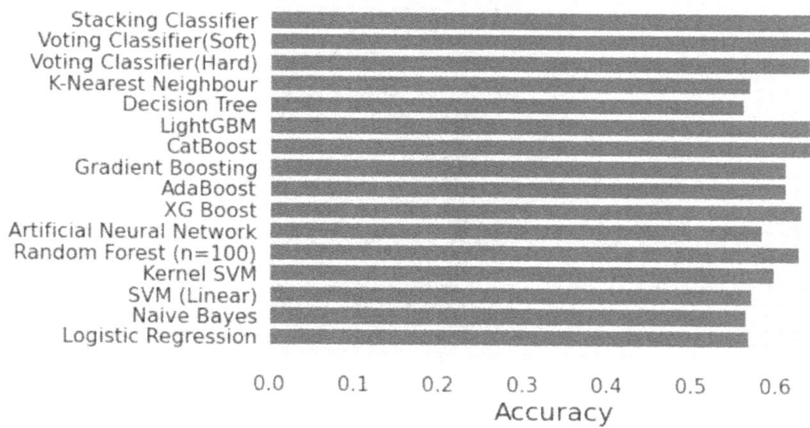

FIGURE 9.10 Accuracy graph for various algorithms for split 70–30.

From Figures 9.12 and 9.13, it can be seen that the stacking classifier has the maximum accuracy, 64.39%. The performance was tested over three different splits, and the best accuracy, precision, recall, and F1 score were for the 80–20 split: 65.04%, 66.4%, 70.9%, and 68.59%, respectively.

Model	Accuracy	Precision	Recall	F1 Score
Logistic Regression	0.567839	0.578977	0.711211	0.638318
Naive Bayes	0.565047	0.579486	0.688303	0.629224
SVM (Linear)	0.572306	0.579449	0.737938	0.649160
Kernel SVM	0.598921	0.609337	0.702187	0.652475
Random Forest (n=100)	0.627768	0.642603	0.688997	0.664992
Artificial Neural Network	0.583845	0.600750	0.667477	0.632358
XG Boost	0.631305	0.637868	0.722666	0.677624
AdaBoost	0.611949	0.629980	0.669559	0.649167
Gradient Boosting	0.611576	0.627325	0.678931	0.652109
CatBoost	0.642658	0.652879	0.712253	0.681275
LightGBM	0.642286	0.653440	0.708782	0.679987
Decision Tree	0.562814	0.591409	0.597362	0.594371
K-Nearest Neighbour	0.569700	0.598682	0.599098	0.598890
Voting Classifier(Hard)	0.640983	0.650442	0.714335	0.680893
Voting Classifier(Soft)	0.642844	0.652795	0.713294	0.681705
Stacking Classifier	0.643402	0.656605	0.702187	0.678631

FIGURE 9.11 Numerical entities for various algorithms for split 70–30.

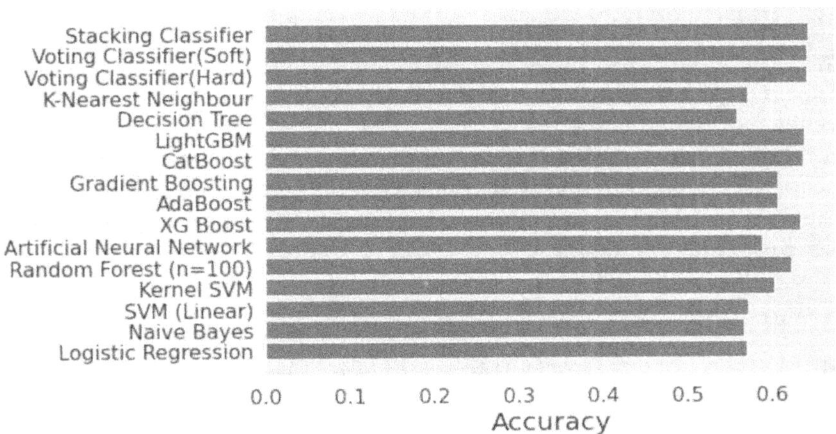

FIGURE 9.12 Accuracy graph for various algorithms for split 60–40.

Model	Accuracy	Precision	Recall	F1 Score
Logistic Regression	0.570491	0.581267	0.713580	0.640663
Naive Bayes	0.567141	0.580778	0.694849	0.632713
SVM (Linear)	0.572446	0.580366	0.733611	0.648052
Kernel SVM	0.602736	0.609095	0.724766	0.661915
Random Forest (n=100)	0.622976	0.640245	0.678720	0.658922
Artificial Neural Network	0.589754	0.592555	0.753642	0.663460
XG Boost	0.634003	0.641961	0.718783	0.678203
AdaBoost	0.607621	0.625455	0.669875	0.646904
Gradient Boosting	0.607761	0.625121	0.671956	0.647693
CatBoost	0.637214	0.650109	0.701353	0.674759
LightGBM	0.639168	0.652163	0.701873	0.676106
Decision Tree	0.559464	0.590289	0.585068	0.587667
K-Nearest Neighbour	0.572725	0.599745	0.612383	0.605998
Voting Classifier(Hard)	0.642937	0.653387	0.712539	0.681682
Voting Classifier(Soft)	0.643216	0.655106	0.707596	0.680340
Stacking Classifier	0.643914	0.658030	0.700312	0.678513

FIGURE 9.13 Numerical entities for various algorithms for split 60–40.

9.7 CONCLUSION

This chapter proposed voting and stacking classifier techniques for e-signing of loans. Both techniques were analyzed over various test splits to measure the accuracy of the proposed phenomenon. The simulated response was analyzed and showed better performance for the stacking classifier and 80–20 test split accuracy. Further, the results were compared using precision, recall, and F1 score matrices. This work could be further improved with better data pre-processing and hyper-parameter tuning.

REFERENCES

[1] Aparicio, M., & Costa, C. J. Data visualization. *Communication Design Quarterly Review*, 3(1), pp. 7–11, 2015.

[2] Kim, J. H., Iyer, V., Joshi, S. B., Volkin, D. B., & Middaugh, C. R. Improved data visualization techniques for analyzing macromolecule structural changes. *Protein Science*, 21(10), pp. 1540–1553, 2012.

[3] Markham, J. W. *A Financial History of Modern US Corporate Scandals: From Enron to Reform*. Routledge, 2015.

[4] Hoellthaler, G., Braunreuther, S., & Reinhart, G. Digital lean production: An approach to identify potentials for the migration to a digitalized production system in SMEs from a lean perspective. *Procedia Cirp*, 67, pp. 522–527, 2018.

[5] Rong, L. I. U. Thinking about interlibrary loan and document delivery service in university library [J]. *Journal of the Library Science in Jiangxi*, 2, 2008.

[6] Patil, S. B., Chougale, A. S., Chougule, R. P., Havaldar, A. A., & Belagali, S. S. Speculating the likeliness of e-validating a loan based on financial transactions. *Journal of Advances in Computational Intelligence Theory*, 2(3), 2019.

[7] Goyal, A., & Kaur, R. Accuracy prediction for loan risk using machine learning models. *International Journal of Computer Science Trends and Technology*, 4(1), pp. 52–57, 2016.

[8] Kumar, U. K., Nikhil, M. S., & Sumangali, K. Prediction of breast cancer using voting classifier technique. In *2017 IEEE International Conference on Smart Technologies and Management for Computing, Communication, Controls, Energy and Materials (ICSTM)* (pp. 108–114). IEEE, 2017.

[9] Chen, Z., Jiang, F., Cheng, Y., Gu, X., Liu, W., & Peng, J. XGBoost classifier for DDoS attack detection and analysis in SDN-based cloud. In *2018 IEEE International Conference on Big Data and Smart Computing (Bigcomp)* (pp. 251–256). IEEE, 2018.

[10] Prokhorenkova, L., Gusev, G., Vorobev, A., Dorogush, A. V., & Gulin, A. CatBoost: unbiased boosting with categorical features. *arXiv preprint arXiv:1706.09516, 2017.*

[11] Ke, G., Meng, Q., Finley, T., Wang, T., Chen, W., Ma, W., & Liu, T. Y. LightGBM: A highly efficient gradient boosting decision tree. *Advances in Neural Information Processing Systems*, 30, pp. 3146–3154, 2017.

[12] Al Daoud, E. Comparison between XGBoost, LightGBM and CatBoost using a home credit dataset. *International Journal of Computer and Information Engineering*, 13(1), pp. 6–10, 2019.

[13] Malmasi, S., & Dras, M. Native language identification with classifier stacking and ensembles. *Computational Linguistics*, 44(3), pp. 403–446, 2019.

10 Heel-End- and Toe-End-Based Gait Kinematics of Female Young Adults

Implications of Therapeutic Intervention

Kunal Kundu, Ghanshyam Shivhare, Vaidehi Patil, Jyotindra Narayan and Santosha K. Dwivedy

CONTENTS

10.1 INTRODUCTION

The assessment of human walking, known as gait analysis, has advanced the knowledge base of sports activities,[1] security establishments,[2] and neurological disorders.[3] Biomechanical gait analysis is the systematic study of lower limb-aided human motion by augmenting the body mechanics and muscle actions. Quantified in terms of a gait cycle, human walking is analyzed for the period elapsed between initial and end heel strike of a lower limb. Human gait attributes are mainly

DOI: 10.1201/9781003207856-10

categorized into two forms in the literature: Kinematics-based and kinetics-based attributes.[4] The former characterizes the walking pattern without involving the forces, that is, joint angles and derivatives of joint angles. In contrast, the latter includes the components of the force, namely ground reaction forces (GRFs), muscle-ligament dynamic interactions, and joint torques. Employing these gait attributes in medical applications, several technological developments have been instituted to detect gait abnormalities, recognize postural debilities, and address the clinical problems accordingly.[5–7] Moreover, in recent research on imaging gait analysis, positive correlations have been found for gait analysis based on an electronic walkway and fMRI-aided stepping device.[8] Gait analysis is a promising diagnostic tool to understand gait responses in different pathological conditions such as surgery, bracing, therapy, and rebuilding the healthy walking pattern. The information of heel- and toe-end kinematics is essential during neurological testing of lower extremities in case of different gait pathologies.[9–11] However, a few other factors, like personality, mood, age, and sociocultural aspects, also influence the individual's gait pattern. Considering the desirable walking pattern an essential criterion to examine the well-being of different age groups, several mathematical models have been formulated based on 2D and 3D datasets with kinematic and kinetic attributes of human locomotion.[12–14]

Researchers have explored various methods of acquiring gait data.[15–17] In general, two variants of sensor-predicated systems, namely non-wearable sensors (NWSs) and wearable sensors (WSs), are mentioned extensively for gait analysis.[17] Non-wearable sensor-predicated systems, with or without a marker, are further sub-categorized into floor sensors and image processing-based setups. Different optic augmented approaches like camera triangulation, IR thermography, structured light, and time-of-flight (ToF) are involved in image processing setups, whereas pressure-sensing mats and ground-reaction-force plates are utilized in floor sensor-based setups. Samson et al.[18] exploited ToF-based camera setups to investigate foot pressures with better resolution. Recently, Narayan et al.[19] presented a biomechanical gait analysis using a Kinect camera with structured light principles and National Instruments (NI)-LabView software interface. On the other hand, wearable sensor-predicated systems are sub-categorized as inertial motion sensors (IMUs), electromyography (EMG) sensors, ultrasonic sensors, ground reaction force plates, and goniometers. In work by Narayan et al.[20] on the gait trajectory-based control of lower-limb rehabilitation devices, IMU sensors are used to measure the reference trajectory. Wentinket al.[21] employed EMG sensors to detect the gait initiated by a prosthetic leg and found them 138 ms faster than inertial sensors. Dominguez et al.[22] introduced a digital goniometer to compute the knee joint's angular position during walking.

Moreover, many NWSs combine to establish a walkway-based setup for clinical gait analysis, such as CONTEMPLAS[23] and commercial gait quantification systems such as BTS GaitLab[24] and Tekscan: Pressure Mapping.[25] Similarly, several WSs are conjugated to establish commercial setups for gait analysis, such as a motion sensor- and force plate-based M3D gait analysis system[26] and an inertial tracker-based 'Moven' (later named as Xsens MVN).[27] The revolutionary layout of NWS-predicated hardware in the laboratory makes these systems more expensive than WS. However, the RGB depth sensor embedded Kinect camera has recently been found as an affordable NWS-predicated method for gait identification in 2D and 3D, exploiting the structured light principle to track human joint forms of motion.[28] Microsoft Kinect has justified its worth in analyzing standing balance, posture control, and biomechanical gait compared with marked-predicated setups.[29–31]

After exploring the kinematics and kinetic attributes of human gait, researchers have designed and developed many humanoid robots, lower-limb rehabilitation devices, and dummies for surgical applications.[32–35] In this work, the literature is limited to such applications of lower-body kinematics. In general, kinematics offers a relationship between the definite space and the end effector of the system to generate and control joint trajectories using actuators.[36] Stolle et al.[37] proposed a seven-bar linkage-based rehabilitation device for each foot to imitate the kinematic attributes of walking during gait therapy. The syncing of the left-right side is carried out by a chain-sprocket arrangement and motor speed control. In a study by Pongpipatpaiboon et al.,[38] kinematic gait analysis for hemiparetic subjects is performed to investigate the beneficial effects of an ankle-foot orthotic (AFO) device on toe clearance. To imitate the human foot using an ankle rehabilitation robot, Syrseloudis et al.[39] presented a novel 2-DOF serial-parallel platform with features of good rigidity, improved stiffness, low redundancy, and low cost. Li et al.[40] presented a five-link bipedal model of a lower-limb rehabilitation device and formulated the kinematics using Denavit-Hartenberg (DH) parameters through the waist to toe-end. Zakaria et al.[41] presented the DH-convention- and geometric-based kinematics of a 3-DOF lower-limb exoskeleton robot. They considered the length of the foot from heel to toe-end. In a recent work on a robotic-based lower-limb rehabilitation system, Wang et al.[42] proposed a 4-DOF mechanism to assist the 2-DOF at the hip, 1-DOF at the knee, and 1-DOF at the ankle. In the kinematics, DH parameters at the ankle joint are framed by considering the vertical distance to the foot sole. Workspace analysis and trajectory planning are also presented for the designed rehabilitation robot.

While designing lower-limb rehabilitation devices with ground clearances, the consideration of ankle-to-heel and ankle-to-toe distances is significant in lower-body kinematics. Therefore, there is an emergent need to study and analyze the heel-end and toe-end kinematics of lower extremities during human gait. To the authors' knowledge, very limited demonstrations are available in the literature where heel-end- and toe-end-based kinematic gait analysis for Indian female adolescents has been carried out. The main contributions of the current work are as follows:

- The lower-limb joint angles of female adolescents (21.8 ± 2.14 years) are estimated in the gait sagittal plane using MS Kinect-NI LabView experimental setup. Thereafter, the joint angular velocities and joint angular accelerations are evaluated over a gait cycle.

- The forward kinematics and inverse kinematics of the heel-based lower extremity are formulated using DH conventions. The velocity and acceleration kinematics are thereafter derived using Jacobian relations.
- Including the horizontal foot length from heel to toe and the tibio-talar ankle angle, the complete kinematics of the toe-based lower extremity is formulated using DH conventions and Jacobian relations.
- The simulation result for heel-end and toe-end kinematics is carried out using anthropometric parameters of female adolescents and compared over a gait cycle.

The rest of the work is organized as follows. In Section 10.2, the basic terminologies related to healthy human walking are illustrated. The Kinect-LabView experimental setup and details are provided in Section 10.3. Sections 10.4 and 10.5 present the formulation of kinematic relations for heel-end and toe-end, respectively. Results and discussion are given in Section 10.6. Concluding remarks are presented in Section 10.7.

10.2 BASIC TERMINOLOGIES OF HUMAN GAIT

To understand the related work, experimental setup, and results of the current work, there is a need to review the gait cycle's basic terminologies. The time passed between two matched instances performed by a leg during an ordinary walk is characterized as a gait cycle. Five pivotal events followed by each foot through a gait cycle are first heel contact (FHC), heel up (HU), toe-up (TU), feet parallel (FP), and last heel contact (LHC). Both FHC and LHC denote a foot's matched states at the time interval of one gait cycle.

The total gait cycle is divided into four periods: Mid-stance, terminal stance, initial swing, and terminal swing. The mid-stance and terminal stance configure a stance phase where a portion of the foot is in ground contact, while the initial and terminal swings constitute a swing phase where the foot always stays in the air. The entire stance period encompasses nearly 60% of the period over a gait cycle. A schematic representation of human walking with pivotal events and periods is shown in Figure 10.1.[43] In addition to events and periods, the significant attributes of human walking are described by stride length and cycle time. The distance covered and time elapsed between FHC and LHC are defined as stride length and cycle time.

10.3 EXPERIMENTAL SETUP AND RELATED WORK

First, in the experimental setup, MS Kinect was installed due to its efficient depth detection quality even in dim light settings and its promising ability to deal with the borderline uncertainties in a human pose. As shown in Figures 10.2a and 10.2b, the MS Kinect comprises an RGB camera, an infrared (IR) emitter, an infrared depth sensor, a tilt motor, a three-axis accelerometer, and an array of four microphones.

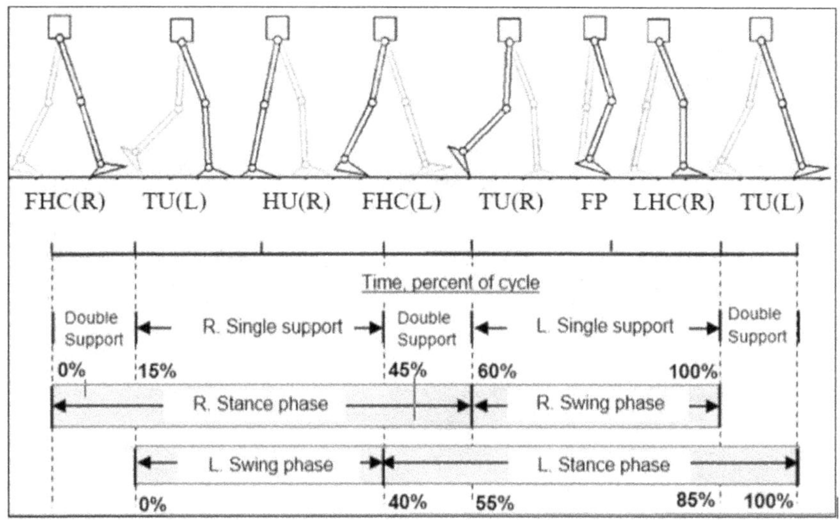

FIGURE 10.1 Gait cycle of a healthy human.

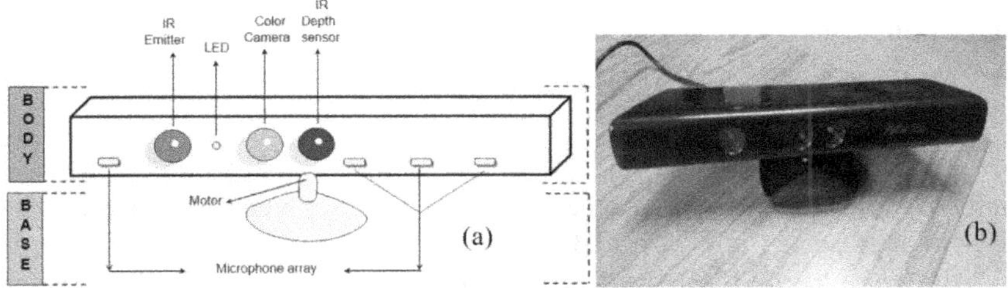

FIGURE 10.2 Illustration of (a) schematic diagram of MS Kinect; and (b) MS Kinect camera used in the experiment.

The detailed specifications of different features for the selected Kinect camera are provided in Narayan et al.[19]. The range of view (ROV) is configured at 57° horizontal and 43° vertical directions with a vertical tilt of ±27°. Kinect-SDK's hardware setup is connected with a 64-bit Windows 10 i7 processor and 8 GB DDR memory. The Kinect and SDK can access 20 joints of the human body even in a sitting position. After constructing the MS-Kinect setup, NI-LabView was installed to read the skeleton data using the Kinesthesia toolkit. Graphical algorithms were formed inside the toolkit to analyze the joint triples of a human subject. After capturing the coordinate information related to the joint triples, the joint angles were estimated using vector algebra and cosine formulations. Thereafter, the joint angles were stored in the angle evaluation block and displayed

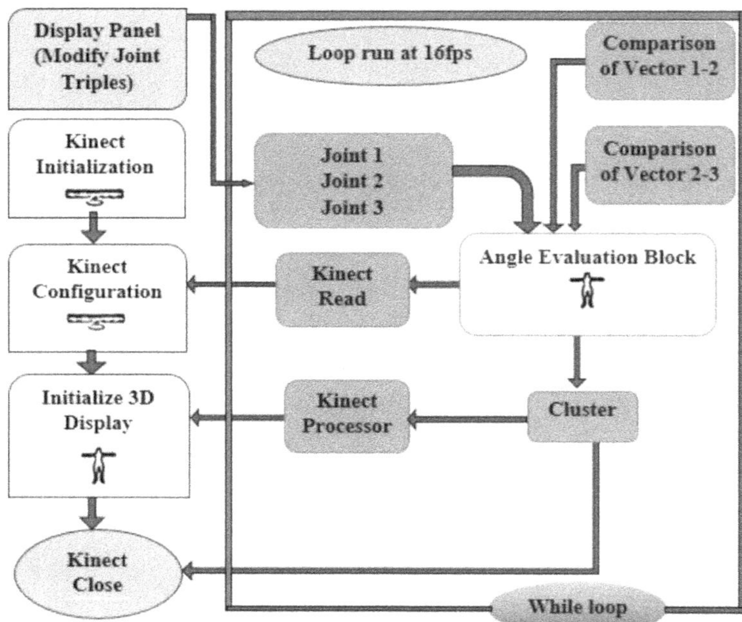

FIGURE 10.3 Flowchart for the evaluation of joint angles.

on the LabView interface. The schematic flowchart of the complete procedure is given by represented in Figure 10.3.

After configuring the Kinect-LabView setup and placing it at 0.8 m height over the ground, five healthy female adolescents (19 to 25 years, 21.8 ± 2.14 years) were asked to track a path after taking consent from them. Figure 10.4a shows all the relevant distance specifications which were exploited during the experiment recordings. The participants were suggested to cover the marked path and stop at the exit of the Kinect's ROV. Figure 10.4b illustrates the skeleton data of a young female participant as an instance. The recording of the joint angles for each participant was carried out for 1.6–2.0 seconds. In this experimental work, the term 'healthy' is defined as a participant who is free from any neurological disorders, severe wounds in the lower extremities, trauma, and consumption of nonsteroidal anti-inflammatory drugs (NSAIDs). The other crucial parameters of the healthy participants are as follows: Body height: 158 ± 2.28 cm, body mass: 52.4 ± 3.26 kg, stride length: 1.09 ± 0.04 cm, cycle time: 0.89 ± 0.04 sec.

After estimating joint angles, the joint angular velocities and acceleration are computed using first- and second-order differences over time. Figure 10.5a,b,c

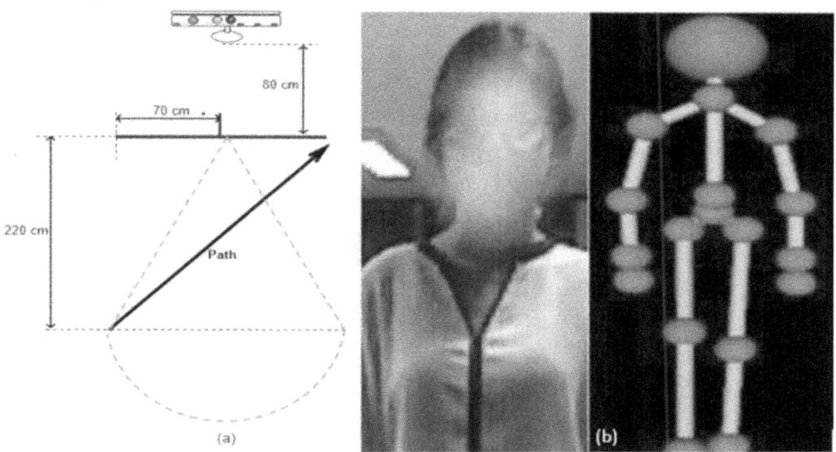

FIGURE 10.4 (a) Path configuration in the experimental setup; (b) female participant with tracked body joints.

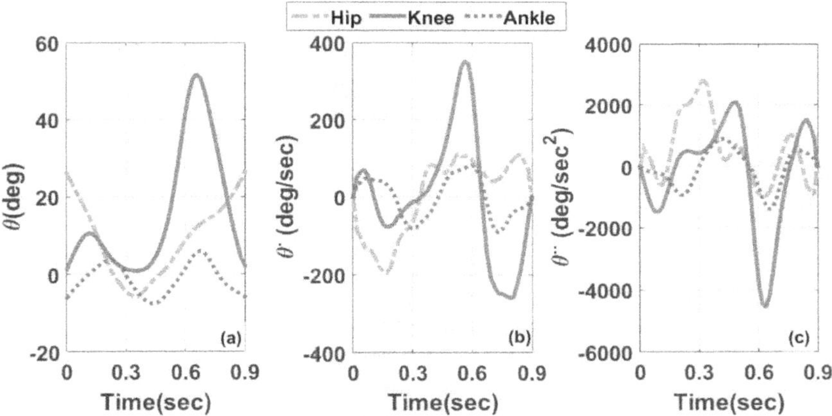

FIGURE 10.5 Hip, knee, and ankle: (a) joint angles; (b) angular velocity; (c) angular acceleration.

presents the mean angular position, mean angular velocities, and mean angular accelerations for lower-limb joints in the sagittal plane, respectively.

The mean range of movements (ROM) for hip (maximum flexion/minimum extension), knee (maximum flexion/minimum extension), and ankle joint (maximum dorsiflexion/minimum plantarflexion) are 26.36°/–5.8°, 51.87°/0.84°, and 5.92°/–6.12°, respectively. The details of the mean range of joint angles (θ), angular velocities $(\dot{\theta})$, and angular accelerations $(\ddot{\theta})$ are presented in Table 10.1, along with the respective tie over a gait cycle.

TABLE 10.1
Range of Joint Angular Movements, Angular Velocity, and Angular Acceleration in the Sagittal Plane

Parameters	Maximum	Time (sec)	Minimum	Time (sec)
θ_{hip} (deg)	26.36	0.9	–5.81	0.34
θ_{knee} (deg)	51.87	0.66	0.84	0.34
θ_{ankle} (deg)	5.92	0.68	–6.12	0
$\dot{\theta}_{hip}$ (deg/s)	111.65	0.53	–194.89	0.17
$\dot{\theta}_{knee}$ (deg/s)	352.94	0.56	–260.00	0.81
$\dot{\theta}_{ankle}$ (deg/s)	83.18	0.60	–92.03	0.73
$\ddot{\theta}_{hip}$ (deg/s^2)	2820.99	0.32	–963.44	0.64
$\ddot{\theta}_{knee}$ (deg/s^2)	2099.28	0.49	–4135.59	0.64
$\ddot{\theta}_{ankle}$ (deg/s^2)	900.22	0.43	–1397.16	0.66

10.4 HIP-KNEE-ANKLE-HEEL-BASED KINEMATICS

For realizing kinematics of heel-based lower limb of female adults, a 3-DOF linkage configuration is considered to represent the hip-knee-ankle-heel anatomical structure, as shown in Figure 10.6. The hip, knee, and ankle joint angles, denoted by θ_1, θ_2, and θ_3, perform flexion/extension movements in the sagittal plane. The three respective segments, thigh, calf, and vertical-foot, are denoted by l_1, l_2, and l_3. The center of mass distances for the three segments are denoted by l_{c1}, l_{c2}, and l_{c3}. Considering the hip joint as the reference point, the kinematics is described to plan heel contact motion using lower-limb joint parameters and vice versa. The downward y-direction and right x-direction at each lower-limb joint are considered negative and positive sign conventions. The kinematic modeling is classified into two types: Forward kinematic and inverse kinematics, as explained further.

10.4.1 Forward Kinematics

In the forward kinematic analysis, the end-effector (heel) coordinates are computed using link parameters (lower limb segments) and the joint variables (lower limb joints) for a specified reference frame. The kinematic configuration of the lower limb can be easily defined employing Denavit-Hartenberg parameters,[44] as shown in Table 10.2.

The forward kinematics is carried out by transforming the initial coordinate frame at the hip joint to the final coordinate frame at the heel-end using DH

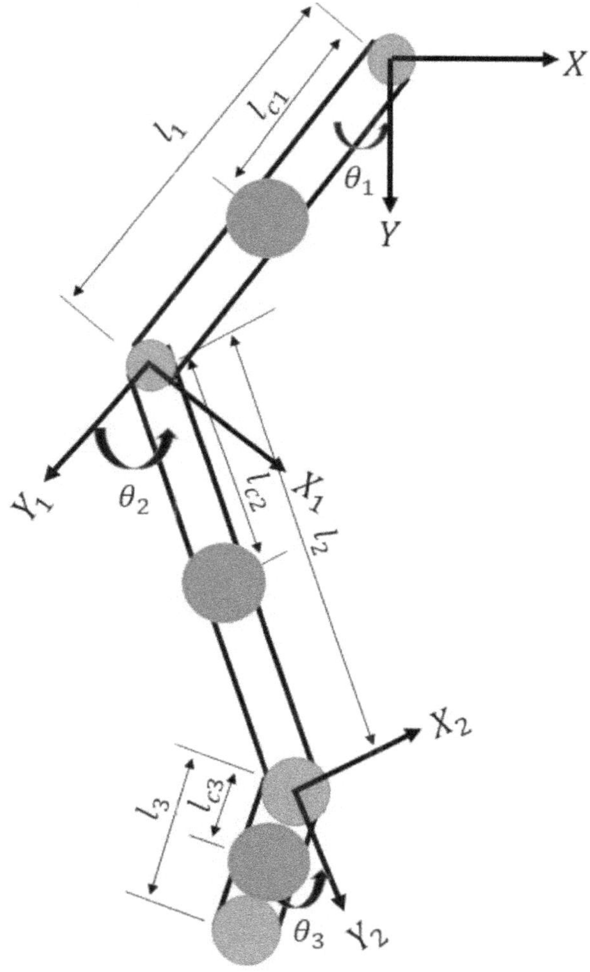

FIGURE 10.6 Three-DOF structure representation of lower limb w:th the heel end.

TABLE 10.2
DH Parameters for the Hip-Knee-Ankle-Heel Structure

S. No.	Link Length, a_j (mm)	Link Twist, a_j (deg)	Joint Distance, d_j (mm)	Joint Angle, θ_j (deg)
1.	l_1	0	0	$90° - \theta_1$
2.	l_2	0	0	$-\theta_2$
3.	l_3	0	0	$-\theta_3$

parameters. The transformation matrix between two consecutive lower-limb joints $(j-1 \text{ to } j)$ can be formulated as:

$$T_j^{j-1} = \begin{bmatrix} C\theta_j & -S\theta_j C\alpha_j & S\theta_j S\alpha_j & a_j C\theta_j \\ S\theta_j & C\theta_j C\alpha_j & -C\theta_j S\alpha_j & a_j S\theta_j \\ 0 & S\alpha_j & C\alpha_j & d_j \\ 0 & 0 & 0 & 1 \end{bmatrix} \tag{10.1}$$

After multiplying the transformation matrices $\left(T_{Hip}^{Knee} \bullet T_{Knee}^{Ankle} \bullet T_{Ankle}^{Heel}\right)$, one can get the final transformation matrix as:

$$T_{Hip}^{Heel} = T_{Hip}^{Knee} \bullet T_{Knee}^{Ankle} \bullet T_{Ankle}^{Heel} = \begin{bmatrix} S\theta_{123} & -C\theta_{123} & 0 & l_1 S\theta_1 + l_2 S\theta_{12} + l_3 S\theta_{123} \\ C\theta_{123} & S\theta_{123} & 0 & -l_1 C\theta_1 - l_2 C\theta_{12} - l_3 C\theta_{123} \\ 0 & 0 & 1 & 0 \\ 0 & 0 & 0 & 1 \end{bmatrix} \tag{10.2}$$

where

$S\theta_j = \sin\left(\theta_j\right)$, $C\theta_j = \cos\left(\theta_j\right)$, $S\theta_{jk} = \sin\left(\theta_j + \theta_k\right)$, $C\theta_{jk} = \cos\left(\theta_j + \theta_k\right)$, $S\theta_{jkl} = \sin\left(\theta_j + \theta_k + \theta_l\right)$, $C\theta_{jkl} = \cos\left(\theta_j + \theta_k + \theta_l\right)$; $j = 1, k = 2, l = 3$.

10.4.2 Inverse Kinematics

Inverse kinematics is defined as the estimation of joint variables (hip, knee, and ankle joint angles) in terms of given end-effector (heel-end) coordinates and link parameters (lower limb segments). The geometric-based analytical method is used in this work to establish the inverse kinematic relations. Exploiting the known values of heel-end position coordinates (x_3, y_3) and ankle-heel length (l_3), one can find the following relation for ankle joint coordinates (x_2, y_2) in terms of lower-limb joint angles $(\theta_1, \theta_2, \theta_3)$:

$$\begin{cases} x_2 = x_3 - l_3 \cos\varphi \\ y_2 = y_3 - l_3 \sin\varphi \end{cases} \tag{10.3}$$

where

$$\varphi = 90° - \left(\theta_1 + \theta_2 + \theta_3\right) \tag{10.4}$$

Now, use the cosine formula for the knee joint as follows:

$$\cos\theta_2 = \frac{\left(x_2^2 + y_2^2 - l_1^2 - l_2^2\right)}{\left(2 \times l_1 \times l_2\right)} \tag{10.5}$$

Therefore, the knee joint angle (θ_2) can be estimated as:

$$\theta_2 = \cos^{-1}\left\{\frac{\left[\left(x_2^2 + y_2^2 - l_1^2 - l_2^2\right)\right]}{\left(2 \times l_1 \times l_2\right)}\right\} \tag{10.6}$$

Moreover, the ankle joint coordinates (x_2, y_2) can also be expressed as:

$$\begin{cases} x_2 = l_1 \sin\theta_1 + l_2 \sin(\theta_1 + \theta_2) = \cos\theta_1 (l_2 \sin\theta_2) + \sin\theta_1 (l_1 + l_2 \cos\theta_2) \\ y_2 = -l_1 \cos\theta_1 - l_2 \cos(\theta_1 + \theta_2) = -\cos\theta_1 (l_1 + l_2 \cos\theta_2) + \sin\theta_1 (l_2 \sin\theta_2) \end{cases} \tag{10.7}$$

The following relations can be formed for the hip joint using Equation (10.7):

$$\begin{cases} \cos\theta_1 = \dfrac{\left[x_2 \times l_2 \sin\theta_2 - y_2 (l_1 + l_2 \cos\theta_2)\right]}{\left(x_2^2 + y_2^2\right)} \\ \sin\theta_1 = \dfrac{\left[y_2 \times l_2 \sin\theta_2 + x_2 (l_1 + l_2 \cos\theta_2)\right]}{\left(x_2^2 + y_2^2\right)} \end{cases} \tag{10.8}$$

Therefore, solving for the previous sine and cosine relations, one can get the expression of the hip joint (θ_1) as follows:

$$\theta_1 = \tan^{-1}\left\{\frac{\left[\left[y_2 \times l_2 \sin\theta_2 + x_2 (l_1 + l_2 \cos\theta_2)\right]\right]}{\left[\left[x_2 \times l_2 \sin\theta_2 - y_2 (l_1 + l_2 \cos\theta_2)\right]\right]}\right\} \tag{10.9}$$

Now, one can obtain the ankle joint angle (θ_3) by substituting the hip joint angle (θ_1) and knee joint angle (θ_2) into Equation (10.4):

$$\theta_3 = 90° - \varphi - \theta_1 - \theta_2 \tag{10.10}$$

10.4.3 Velocity and Acceleration Kinematics

Employing the Jacobian matrix, the velocity kinematics offers heel-end motion analysis over a gait cycle. Thereafter, the mathematical relations of acceleration kinematics can be established by differentiating the velocity components. The Jacobian matrix can be computed by performing first-order partial differentiation of the heel-end position with every lower-limb joint angle.[44] The linear velocity of the heel-end (v_3^0) can be expressed in terms of joint angular velocity $(\dot{\theta})$ using link Jacobian (J_v) as follows:

$$v_3^0 = J_v \dot{\theta} \tag{10.11}$$

where

$$J_v = \begin{bmatrix} J_{v1} & J_{v2} & J_{v3} \end{bmatrix}, v_3^0 = \begin{bmatrix} v_{3_x}^0 \\ v_{3_y}^0 \end{bmatrix}, \qquad \dot{\theta} = \begin{bmatrix} \dot{\theta}_1 \\ \dot{\theta}_2 \\ \dot{\theta}_3 \end{bmatrix},$$

The expression for J_v for the hip-knee-ankle-heel-based lower limb is evaluated as follows:

$$\begin{cases} J_{v_1} = \begin{bmatrix} l_1 C\theta_1 + l_2 C\theta_{12} + l_3 C\theta_{123} \\ l_1 S\theta_1 + l_2 S\theta_{12} + l_3 S\theta_{123} \end{bmatrix} \\ J_{v_2} = \begin{bmatrix} l_2 C\theta_{12} + l_3 C\theta_{123} \\ l_2 S\theta_{12} + l_3 S\theta_{123} \end{bmatrix} \\ J_{v_3} = \begin{bmatrix} l_3 C\theta_{123} \\ l_3 S\theta_{123} \end{bmatrix} \end{cases} \tag{10.12}$$

Expanding Equation (10.11) using Equation (10.12), one can get the components of linear velocity $\left(v_{3_x}^0, v_{3_y}^0\right)$ as:

$$\begin{aligned} v_{3_x}^0 &= l_1 \cos\theta_1 \times \dot{\theta}_1 + l_2 \cos(\theta_1 + \theta_2) \times \left(\dot{\theta}_1 + \dot{\theta}_2\right) + l_3 \cos(\theta_1 + \theta_2 + \theta_3) \times \left(\dot{\theta}_1 + \dot{\theta}_2 + \dot{\theta}_3\right) \\ v_{3_y}^0 &= l_1 \sin\theta_1 \times \dot{\theta}_1 + l_2 \sin(\theta_1 + \theta_2) \times \left(\dot{\theta}_1 + \dot{\theta}_2\right) + l_3 \sin(\theta_1 + \theta_2 + \theta_3) \times \left(\dot{\theta}_1 + \dot{\theta}_2 + \dot{\theta}_3\right) \end{aligned} \tag{10.13}$$

Furthermore, the components of linear acceleration $\left(a_{3_x}^0, a_{3_y}^0\right)$ for the heel end could be derived as:

$$\begin{aligned} a_{3_x}^0 = &-l_1 \sin\theta_1 \times \dot{\theta}_1 - l_2 \sin(\theta_1 + \theta_2) \times \left(\dot{\theta}_1 + \dot{\theta}_2\right) - l_3 \sin(\theta_1 + \theta_2 + \theta_3) \\ &\times \left(\dot{\theta}_1 + \dot{\theta}_2 + \dot{\theta}_3\right) + l_1 \cos\theta_1 \times \ddot{\theta}_1 + l_2 \cos(\theta_1 + \theta_2) \times \left(\ddot{\theta}_1 + \ddot{\theta}_2\right) \\ &+ l_3 \cos(\theta_1 + \theta_2 + \theta_3) \times \left(\ddot{\theta}_1 + \ddot{\theta}_2 + \ddot{\theta}_3\right) \\ a_{3_y}^0 = &\; l_1 \cos\theta_1 \times \dot{\theta}_1 + l_2 \cos(\theta_1 + \theta_2) \times \left(\dot{\theta}_1 + \dot{\theta}_2\right) + l_3 \cos(\theta_1 + \theta_2 + \theta_3) \\ &\times \left(\dot{\theta}_1 + \dot{\theta}_2 + \dot{\theta}_3\right) + l_1 \sin\theta_1 \times \ddot{\theta}_1 + l_2 \sin(\theta_1 + \theta_2) \times \left(\ddot{\theta}_1 + \ddot{\theta}_2\right) \\ &+ l_3 \sin(\theta_1 + \theta_2 + \theta_3) \times \left(\ddot{\theta}_1 + \ddot{\theta}_2 + \ddot{\theta}_3\right) \end{aligned} \tag{10.14}$$

10.5 HIP-KNEE-ANKLE-TOE-BASED KINEMATICS

Extending the kinematics for the heel-based lower limb, as shown in Figure 10.7, a similar kind of analysis is carried out for the hip-knee-ankle-toe-based lower limb using the horizontal length between heel and toe. Moreover, the toe-end

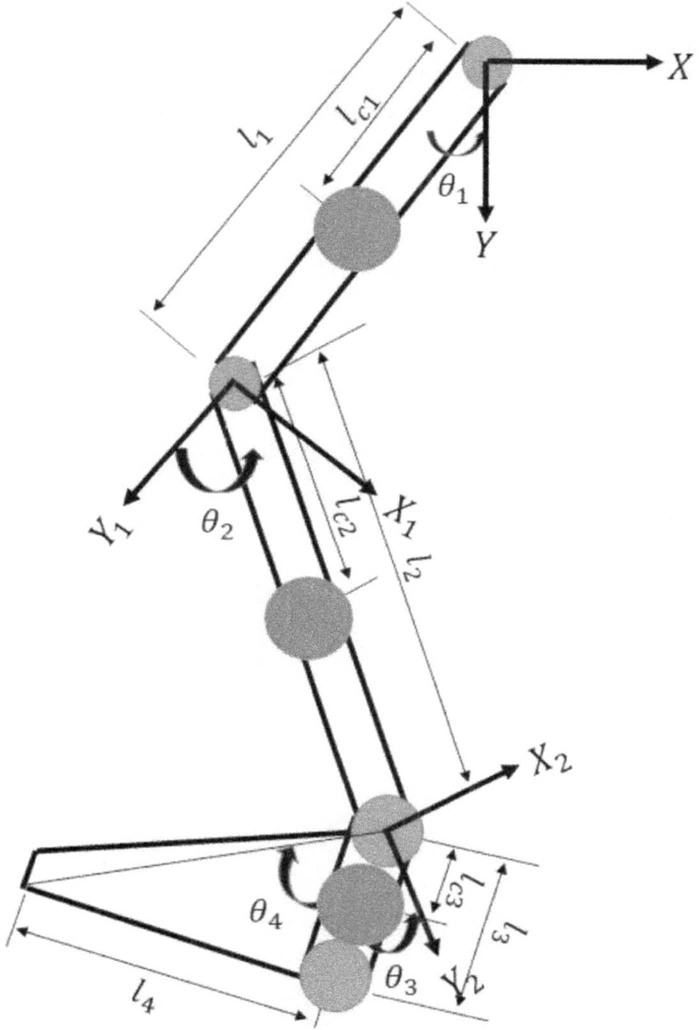

FIGURE 10.7 Three-DOF structure representation of lower limb with toe-end.

position coordinate is now denoted by (x_3, y_3). The relation for the tibio-talar angle (θ_4) using vertical ankle-heel length (l_3) and horizontal heel-toe length (l_4) can be expressed as

$$\theta_4 = -\tan^{-1}\left(\frac{l_4}{l_3}\right) \tag{10.15}$$

TABLE 10.3
DH Parameters for the Hip-Knee-Ankle-Toe Structure

S. No.	Link Length, a_j (mm)	Link Twist, α_j (deg.)	Joint Distance, d_j (mm)	Joint Angle, θ_j (deg.)
1.	l_1	0	0	$90° - \theta_1$
2.	l_2	0	0	$-\theta_2$
3.	$\left(l_3^2 + l_4^2\right)^{1/2}$	0	0	$-\theta_3 + \theta_4$

10.5.1 Forward Kinematics

Similar to the forward kinematic analysis in Section 10.4, the Denavit-Hartenberg parameters for the hip-knee-ankle-toe-based lower limb are shown in Table 10.3. The third link length and joint angle have the effect of the additional horizontal heel-toe segment.

Now, one can get the final transformation matrix $\left(T_{Hip}^{Toe}\right)$ by employing the frame transformation matrix [Equation (10.1)] for consecutive lower-limb joints as:

$$T_{Hip}^{Toe} = T_{Hip}^{Knee}.T_{Knee}^{Ankle}.T_{Ankle}^{Toe} = \begin{bmatrix} S\theta_{123} & -C\theta_{123} & 0 & l_1 S\theta_1 + l_2 S\theta_{12} + \left(l_3^2 + l_4^2\right)^{1/2}\left(S\theta_{1234}\right) \\ C\theta_{123} & S\theta_{123} & 0 & -l_1 C\theta_1 - l_2 C\theta_{12} - \left(l_3^2 + l_4^2\right)^{1/2}\left(C\theta_{1234}\right) \\ 0 & 0 & 1 & 0 \\ 0 & 0 & 0 & 1 \end{bmatrix} \tag{10.16}$$

where
$S\theta_j = \sin\left(\theta_j\right)$, $C\theta_j = \cos\left(\theta_j\right)$, $S\theta_{jk} = \sin\left(\theta_j + \theta_k\right)$, $C\theta_{jk} = \cos\left(\theta_j + \theta_k\right)$, $S\theta_{jkl} = \sin\left(\theta_j + \theta_k + \theta_l\right)$, $C\theta_{jkl} = \cos\left(\theta_j + \theta_k + \theta_l\right)$, $S\theta_{jklm} = \sin\left(\theta_j + \theta_k + \theta_l + \theta_m\right)$, $C\theta_{jklm} = \cos\left(\theta_j + \theta_k + \theta_l + \theta_m\right)$; $j = 1, k = 2, l = 3, m = 4$.

10.5.2 Inverse Kinematics

Following the geometric-based analytical approach, one can obtain similar inverse kinematic relations as those computed in Section 10.4. The only difference is noted regarding the evaluation of ankle joint coordinates $\left(x_2, y_2\right)$, which utilizes the given toe-end position coordinates $\left(x_3, y_3\right)$, ankle-heel length $\left(l_3\right)$, and heel-toe length $\left(l_4\right)$ in terms of lower-limb joint angles $\left(\theta_1, \theta_2, \theta_3, \theta_4\right)$ as follows:

$$\begin{cases} x_2 = x_3 - \left(l_3^2 + l_4^2\right)^{1/2}\left(\cos\varphi\right) \\ y_2 = y_3 - \left(l_3^2 + l_4^2\right)^{1/2}\left(\sin\varphi\right) \end{cases} \tag{10.17}$$

where

$$\varphi = 90^\circ - (\theta_1 + \theta_2 + \theta_3 - \theta_4) \tag{10.18}$$

Thereafter, the hip, knee, and ankle joint angles $(\theta_1, \theta_2, \theta_3)$ can be computed using similar formulations to those provided in Section 10.4. To avoid repetition, those formulations are omitted here.

10.5.3 Velocity and Acceleration Kinematics

Exploiting the concept of link Jacobian as mentioned in Section 10.4, the elements of J_v for the hip-knee-ankle-toe-based lower limb are computed as follows:

$$\begin{cases} J_{v_1} = \begin{bmatrix} l_1 C\theta_1 + l_2 C\theta_{12} + \left(l_3^2 + l_4^2\right)^{1/2} \left(C\theta_{1234}\right) \\ l_1 S\theta_1 + l_2 S\theta_{12} + \left(l_3^2 + l_4^2\right)^{1/2} \left(S\theta_{1234}\right) \end{bmatrix} \\ J_{v_2} = \begin{bmatrix} l_2 C\theta_{12} + \left(l_3^2 + l_4^2\right)^{1/2} \left(C\theta_{1234}\right) \\ l_2 S\theta_{12} + \left(l_3^2 + l_4^2\right)^{1/2} \left(S\theta_{1234}\right) \end{bmatrix} \\ J_{v_3} = \begin{bmatrix} \left(l_3^2 + l_4^2\right)^{1/2} \left(C\theta_{1234}\right) \\ \left(l_3^2 + l_4^2\right)^{1/2} \left(C\theta_{1234}\right) \end{bmatrix} \end{cases} \tag{10.19}$$

Thereafter, one can obtain the components of linear velocity $\left(v_{3_x}^0, v_{3_y}^0\right)$ for the toe-end lower limb as follows:

$$\begin{aligned} v_{3_x}^0 &= l_1 \cos\theta_1 \times \dot{\theta}_1 + l_2 \cos(\theta_1 + \theta_2) \times (\dot{\theta}_1 + \dot{\theta}_2) \\ &\quad + \left(l_3^2 + l_4^2\right)^{1/2} \left(\cos(\theta_1 + \theta_2 + \theta_3 + \theta_4)\right) \times (\dot{\theta}_1 + \dot{\theta}_2 + \dot{\theta}_3) \\ v_{3_y}^0 &= l_1 \sin\theta_1 \times \dot{\theta}_1 + l_2 \sin(\theta_1 + \theta_2) \times (\dot{\theta}_1 + \dot{\theta}_2) \\ &\quad + \left(l_3^2 + l_4^2\right)^{1/2} \left(\sin(\theta_1 + \theta_2 + \theta_3 + \theta_4) \times (\dot{\theta}_1 + \dot{\theta}_2 + \dot{\theta}_3)\right) \end{aligned} \tag{10.20}$$

Utilizing the expressions of linear velocity from Equation (10.20), the components of linear acceleration $\left(a_{3_x}^0, a_{3_y}^0\right)$ for the toe-end could be formulated as:

$$\begin{aligned} a_{3_x}^0 &= -l_1 \sin\theta_1 \times \dot{\theta}_1 - l_2 \sin(\theta_1 + \theta_2) \times (\dot{\theta}_1 + \dot{\theta}_2) \\ &\quad - \left(l_3^2 + l_4^2\right)^{1/2} \left(\sin(\theta_1 + \theta_2 + \theta_3 + \theta_4) \times (\dot{\theta}_1 + \dot{\theta}_2 + \dot{\theta}_3)\right) \\ &\quad + l_1 \cos\theta_1 \times \ddot{\theta}_1 + l_2 \cos(\theta_1 + \theta_2) \times (\ddot{\theta}_1 + \ddot{\theta}_2) \\ &\quad + \left(l_3^2 + l_4^2\right)^{1/2} \left(\cos(\theta_1 + \theta_2 + \theta_3 + \theta_4)\right) \times (\ddot{\theta}_1 + \ddot{\theta}_2 + \ddot{\theta}_3) \end{aligned}$$

$$
\begin{aligned}
a_{3_y}^0 &= l_1 \cos\theta_1 \times \dot{\theta}_1 + l_2 \cos(\theta_1 + \theta_2) \times (\dot{\theta}_1 + \dot{\theta}_2) \\
&+ (l_3^2 + l_4^2)^{1/2} \left(\cos(\theta_1 + \theta_2 + \theta_3 + \theta_4) \times (\dot{\theta}_1 + \dot{\theta}_2 + \dot{\theta}_3)\right) \\
&+ l_1 \sin\theta_1 \times \ddot{\theta}_1 + l_2 \sin(\theta_1 + \theta_2) \times (\ddot{\theta}_1 + \ddot{\theta}_2) \\
&+ (l_3^2 + l_4^2)^{1/2} \left(\sin(\theta_1 + \theta_2 + \theta_3 + \theta_4)\right) \times (\ddot{\theta}_1 + \ddot{\theta}_2 + \ddot{\theta}_3)
\end{aligned} \tag{10.21}
$$

10.6 RESULTS AND DISCUSSION

Taking mean values of lower-limb segments (thigh link: $l_1 = 42.1$ cm, calf link: $l_2 = 40.8$ cm, ankle-heel link: $l_3 = 6.05$ cm, and foot link: $l_4 = 13.7$ cm), joint angles, joint angular velocities, and joint angular acceleration, the kinematic formulations are applied to compute the position, velocity, and acceleration of the heel-end and toe-end in Cartesian coordinates. Figure 10.8a presents the toe-end (dash-dotted) and heel-end (line) trajectory over a gait cycle. The positional differences, that is, $((d_x = x_{TE} - x_{HE}), (d_y = y_{TE} - y_{HE}))$ between both trajectories in the *x*- and *y*-directions are shown in Figures 10.8b and 10.8c.

The maximum and minimum values of d_x are 13.95 cm at 52.22% (0.47 s) and 3.95 cm at 73.33% (0.66 s) of the gait cycle. Starting with the first heel contact, d_x is almost constant up to TU and decreases rapidly to attain its minima near FP. Thereafter, it starts increasing at a similar rate until the event of last heel contact arrives. On the other hand, the maximum and minimum value of d_y is 13.38 cm at 73.33% (0.66 s) and –2.07 cm at 42.22% (0.38 s) of the gait cycle. Initiating with the first heel contact, d_y increases marginally to attain the local maxima in early midstance. Thereafter, it decreases sharply to reach the global minima in late terminal stance and increases further to arrive at the global maxima near FP event. Finally, the difference starts falling up to LHC. The position difference at five major events of the gait cycle is shown in Table 10.4.

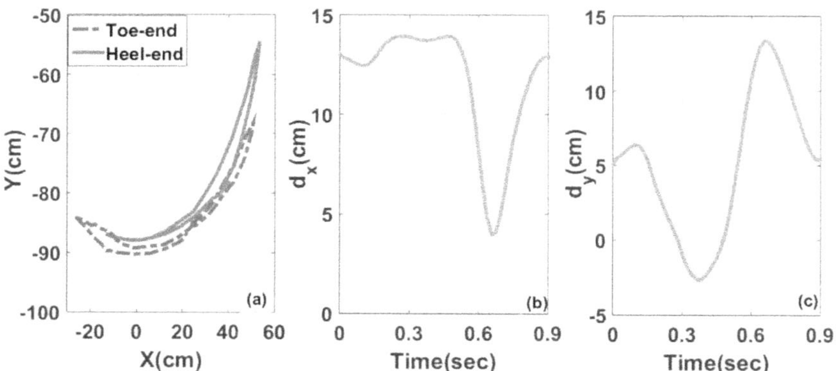

FIGURE 10.8 (a) Trajectories for heel-end and toe-end; (b) trajectory difference in the *x*-direction; (c) trajectory difference in the *y*-direction.

TABLE 10.4
Difference between Toe-End and Heel-End Position, Velocity, and Acceleration at Different Events

Events	d_x (cm)	d_y (cm)	d_{v_x} (cm/s)	d_{v_y} (cm/s)	d_{a_x} (cm/s²)	d_{a_y} (cm/s²)
FHC	13.05	5.08	0	0	0	0
HU	13.99	0.62	84.21	−1902.14	3531.01	8390.56
TU	12.86	5.54	−2780.06	5646.23	2055.69	26261.71
FP	2.80	13.72	168.26	−34.35	78950.09	−20705.46
LHC	12.91	5.41	0	0	0	0

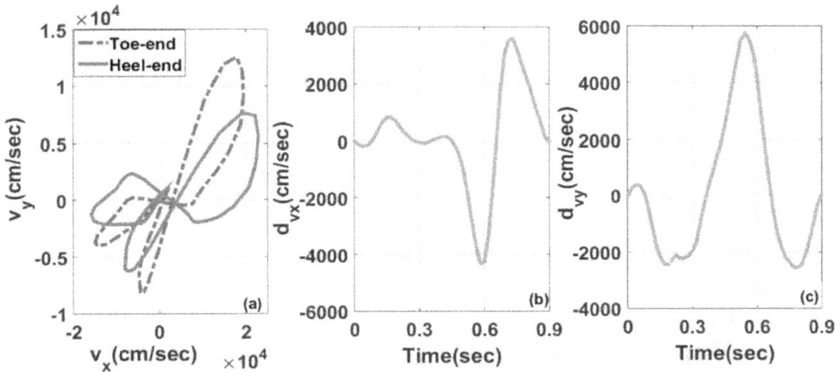

FIGURE 10.9 (a) Velocity trajectories for heel-end and toe-end; (b) velocity difference in the *x*-direction; (c) velocity difference in the *y*-direction.

Figure 10.9a presents the toe-end (dash-dotted) and heel-end (line) velocity over a gait cycle. The velocity differences, that is, $\left(\left(d_{vx} = v_{x_{TE}} - v_{x_{HE}}\right), \left(d_{vy} = v_{y_{TE}} - v_{y_{HE}}\right)\right)$ in the *x*- and *y*-directions are shown in Figures 10.9b and 10.9c. The maximum and minimum values of d_{vx} are 3,615 cm/s at 81.11% (0.73 s) and –4,325 cm/s at 64.44% (0.58 s) of the gait cycle.

Initiating from FHC, d_{vx} is marginally varying up to the terminal stance phase. As the gait cycle advances, it reduces to attain the global minima in the pre-swing phase, further reaches upwards to its global maxima near FP, and finally drops until the end of the gait cycle. On the other hand, the maximum and minimum values of d_{vy} are 5,753 cm/s at 60% (0.54 s) and –2,553 cm/s at 87.7% (0.79 s) of the gait cycle. A continuous increasing-decreasing function is observed for d_{vy}, which attains its minima near the HU and FP events of the gait cycle. The global maximum is achieved at the toe-up event of the gait cycle. The velocity difference at five major events of the gait cycle is shown in Table 10.4.

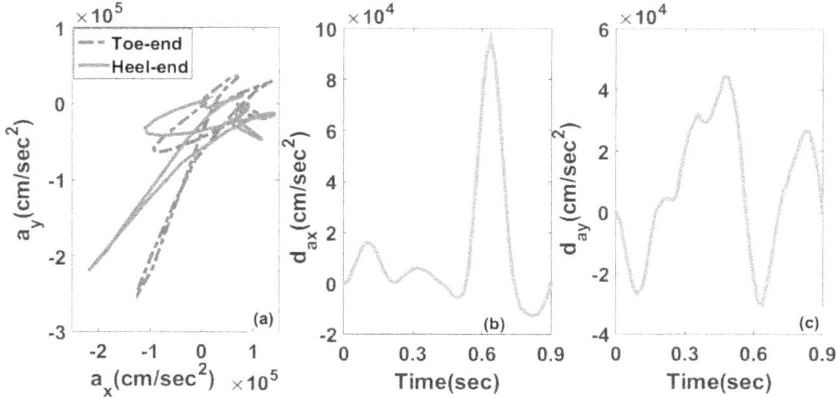

FIGURE 10.10 (a) Acceleration trajectories for heel-end and toe-end; (b) acceleration difference in x-direction; (c) acceleration difference in the y-direction.

Figure 10.10a presents the acceleration plots for toe-end (dash-dotted) and heel-end (line) over a gait cycle. The respective differences in the x- and y-directions $\left(\left(d_{ax} = a_{x_{TE}} - a_{x_{TE}}\right), \left(d_{ay} = a_{y_{TE}} - a_{y_{HE}}\right)\right)$ are shown in Figures 10.10b and 10.10c.

The acceleration difference in the x-direction, d_{ax}, attains the maximum and minimum values as 96,150 cm/s^2 at 71.11% (0.64 s) and –12,540 cm/s^2 at 92.22% (0.83 s) of the gait cycle. Originating from FHC, d_{ax} is marginally low up to the TU event. Thereafter, it increases to achieve the global maximum near the FP event and further falls to reach global minimum near the end of the gait cycle. Furthermore, the maximum and minimum values of d_{ay} are found to be 44,380 cm/s^2 at 52.22% (0.47 s) and –30,540 cm/s^2 at 71.11% (00.64 s) of the gait cycle. The acceleration difference in the y-direction d_{ay} attains its minima at the start of the mid-stance and pre-swing phase, whereas it touches the maxima near the late stance and late swing phase of the gait cycle. The acceleration difference at five major events of the gait cycle is shown in Table 10.4.

The results mentioned previously show that both lower-limb configurations follow a similar pattern, with axial and angular differences based on foot parameters. Although the toe-end configuration poses more natural human walking characteristics, the heel-end configuration provides desired gait characteristics with less computational cost. Additionally, this work can be interpreted as a helpful resource to analyze the ground clearances between the heel and toe over a gait cycle. Additionally, the complete work presents a knowledge base of lower-limb biomechanical joint movements while developing gait rehabilitation devices.

10.7 CONCLUSIONS

In this work, gait kinematics was presented for young female adults in the sagittal plane. The foot configurations, namely heel-end and toe-end, were considered to derive forward, inverse, velocity, and acceleration kinematics of the lower extremity. The toe-end configuration was formed by including the horizontal foot length, vertical length, and tibio-talar angle. Initially, biomechanical joint angles of five healthy subjects were recorded using a Microsoft Kinect-NI LabView experimental setup. The first- and second-order derivatives were computed as joint angular velocities and joint angular accelerations. Thereafter, utilizing the joint and anthropometric parameters, the trajectory, velocity, and acceleration plots were presented for both foot configurations of the lower limb. The differences between both configurations were discussed at major events of a gait cycle. This work can provide extensive information on gait kinematics during the design of effective lower-limb rehabilitation devices. Moreover, it will serve as a comprehensive source to understand the ground clearances between heel-end and toe-end foot configurations during therapeutic exercises. In the future, machine-learning algorithms will be explored to predict joint motion for different age and gender groups.

ACKNOWLEDGMENTS

The authors acknowledge the Department of Scientific and Industrial Research, India, for establishing the PRISM (Promoting Innovations in Individuals, Start-ups, and MSMEs) scheme under which this project work was carried out.

REFERENCES

[1] Mok, K.M., Bahr, R. and Krosshaug, T., 2018. Reliability of lower limb biomechanics in two sport-specific sidestep cutting tasks. *Sports Biomechanics, 17*(2), pp. 157–167.

[2] Singh, J.P., Jain, S., Arora, S. and Singh, U.P., 2018. Vision-based gait recognition: a survey. *IEEE Access, 6*, pp. 70497–70527.

[3] Nonnekes, J., Goselink, R.J., Růžička, E., Fasano, A., Nutt, J.G. and Bloem, B.R., 2018. Neurological disorders of gait, balance and posture: a sign-based approach. *Nature Reviews Neurology, 14*(3), p. 183.

[4] Koldenhoven, R.M., Hart, J., Saliba, S., Abel, M.F. and Hertel, J., 2019. Gait kinematics & kinetics at three walking speeds in individuals with chronic ankle instability and ankle sprain copers. *Gait & Posture, 74*, pp. 169–175.

[5] Zhou, J., Butler, E.E. and Rose, J., 2017. Neurologic correlates of gait abnormalities in cerebral palsy: implications for treatment. *Frontiers in Human Neuroscience, 11*, p. 103.

[6] Raccagni, C., Nonnekes, J., Bloem, B.R., Peball, M., Boehme, C., Seppi, K. and Wenning, G.K., 2019. Gait and postural disorders in parkinsonism: a clinical approach. *Journal of Neurology*, pp. 1–8.

[7] Reinhardt, J., Rus-Oswald, O.G., Bürki, C.N., Bridenbaugh, S.A., Krumm, S., Michels, L., Stippich, C., Kressig, R.W. and Blatow, M., 2020. Neural correlates of stepping in healthy elderly: parietal and prefrontal cortex activation reflects cognitive-motor interference effects. *Frontiers in Human Neuroscience, 14*.

[8] Sun, J., Wu, P., Shen, Y., Yang, Z., Li, H., Liu, Y., Zhu, T., Li, L., Zhang, K. and Chen, M., 2018, December. Relationship between personality and gait: predicting personality with gait features. In *2018 IEEE International Conference on Bioinformatics and Biomedicine (BIBM)* (pp. 1227–1231). IEEE.

[9] Toe/Heel Walking. Available online: https://ecampusontario.pressbooks.pub/clinicalexamination/chapter/toe-heel-walking/ (accessed on 19 February 2021).

[10] Lower Limb Neurological Examination. Available online: www.ambonsall.com/pdf/LowLimbExam.pdf (accessed on 19 February 2021).

[11] Khanfar, A., Al Qaroot, B., Alsousi, A., Zughoul, B., Al Elaumi, A., Hamdan, M. and Safi, R., 2019. A novel method in assessing lower limb motor function. *Journal of Orthopaedic Surgery*, *27*(2), p. 2309499019849956.

[12] McGrath, M., Howard, D. and Baker, R., 2017. A Lagrange-based generalised formulation for the equations of motion of simple walking models. *Journal of Biomechanics*, *55*, pp. 139–143.

[13] Moreira, L., Pinheiro, C., Lopes, J.M., Sanz-Merodio, D., Figueiredo, J., Santos, C.P. and Garcia, E., 2019, February. Study of gait cycle using a five-link inverted pendulum model: first developments. In *2019 IEEE 6th Portuguese Meeting on Bioengineering (ENBENG)* (pp. 1–4). IEEE.

[14] Chereshnev, R. and Kertész-Farkas, A., 2017, July. Hugadb: human gait database for activity recognition from wearable inertial sensor networks. In *International Conference on Analysis of Images, Social Networks and Texts* (pp. 131–141). Springer, Cham.

[15] Phinyomark, A., Petri, G., Ibáñez-Marcelo, E., Osis, S.T. and Ferber, R., 2018. Analysis of big data in gait biomechanics: current trends and future directions. *Journal of Medical and Biological Engineering*, *38*(2), pp. 244–260.

[16] Zou, Q., Ni, L., Wang, Q., Li, Q. and Wang, S., 2017. Robust gait recognition by integrating inertial and RGBD sensors. *IEEE Transactions on Cybernetics*, *48*(4), pp. 1136–1150.

[17] Muro-De-La-Herran, A., Garcia-Zapirain, B. and Mendez-Zorrilla, A., 2014. Gait analysis methods: an overview of wearable and non-wearable systems, highlighting clinical applications. *Sensors*, *14*(2), pp. 3362–3394.

[18] Samson, W., Van Hamme, A., Sanchez, S., Chèze, L., Van Sint Jan, S. and Feipel, V., 2012. Dynamic footprint analysis by time-of-flight camera. *Computer Methods in Biomechanics and Biomedical Engineering*, *15*(sup 1), pp. 180–182.

[19] Narayan, J., Pardasani, A. and Dwivedy, S.K., 2020, July. Comparative gait analysis of healthy young male and female adults using Kinect-Labview setup. In *2020 International Conference on Computational Performance Evaluation (ComPE)* (pp. 688–693). IEEE.

[20] Narayan, J., Kalani, A. and Dwivedy, S.K., 2019, October. Reference trajectory based Jacobian transpose control of a novel lower limb exoskeleton system for children. In *2019 5th International Conference on Signal Processing, Computing and Control (ISPCC)* (pp. 102–107). IEEE.

[21] Wentink, E.C., Schut, V.G.H., Prinsen, E.C., Rietman, J.S. and Veltink, P.H., 2014. Detection of the onset of gait initiation using kinematic sensors and EMG in transfemoral amputees. *Gait & Posture*, *39*(1), pp. 391–396.

[22] Domínguez, G., Cardiel, E., Arias, S. and Rogeli, P., 2013, August. A digital goniometer based on encoders for measuring knee-joint position in an orthosis. In *2013 World Congress on Nature and Biologically Inspired Computing* (pp. 1–4). IEEE.

[23] Templo Clinical Gait Analysis. Available online: www.contemplas.com/clinical_gait_analysis_walkway.aspx (accessed on 28 March 2021).

[24] BTS Bioengineering. Available online: www.btsbioengineering.com/products/integrated-solutions/bts-gaitlab/ (accessed on 28 March 2021).

[25] Arafsha, F., Hanna, C., Aboualmagd, A., Fraser, S. and El Saddik, A., 2018. Instrumented wireless smart insole system for mobile gait analysis: a validation pilot study with tekscanstrideway. *Journal of Sensor and Actuator Networks*, *7*(3), p. 36.

[26] Tec Gihan Co., Ltd. Available online: www.tecgihan.co.jp/en/products/force-plate/small-for-shoes/m3d-force-plate-wired/ (accessed on 25 January 2021).

[27] Zhang, J.T., Novak, A.C., Brouwer, B. and Li, Q., 2013. Concurrent validation of Xsens MVN measurement of lower limb joint angular kinematics. *Physiological Measurement*, *34*(8), p. N63.

[28] Clark, R.A., Pua, Y.H., Bryant, A.L. and Hunt, M.A., 2013. Validity of the Microsoft Kinect for providing lateral trunk lean feedback during gait retraining. *Gait & Posture*, *38*(4), pp. 1064–1066.

[29] Ma, Y., Mithraratne, K., Wilson, N.C., Wang, X., Ma, Y. and Zhang, Y., 2019. The validity and reliability of a Kinect v2-based gait analysis system for children with cerebral palsy. *Sensors*, *19*(7), p. 1660.

[30] Napoli, A., Glass, S., Ward, C., Tucker, C. and Obeid, I., 2017. Performance analysis of a generalized motion capture system using Microsoft Kinect 2.0. *Biomedical Signal Processing and Control*, *38*, pp. 265–280.

[31] Otte, K., Kayser, B., Mansow-Model, S., Verrel, J., Paul, F., Brandt, A.U. and Schmitz-Hübsch, T., 2016. Accuracy and reliability of the Kinect version 2 for clinical measurement of motor function. *PLoS ONE*, *11*(11), p.e0166532.

[32] Hooi, T.K. and Mahyuddin, M.N., 2017, October. A study of walking gait stability and gait efficiency of a cost-effective small humanoid bipedal robot: analysis, simulation and implementation. In *2017 IEEE International Symposium on Robotics and Intelligent Sensors (IRIS)* (pp. 125–129). IEEE.

[33] Narayan, J. and Kumar Dwivedy, S., 2021. Preliminary design and development of a low-cost lower-limb exoskeleton system for paediatric rehabilitation. *Proceedings of the Institution of Mechanical Engineers, Part H: Journal of Engineering in Medicine*, p. 0954411921994940.

[34] Abel, E.W., Unger, A., Fletcher, R. and Jain, A.S., 2002, October. Development of clinical measurement of the axes of rotation of the ankle and subtalar joints. In *Proceedings of the Second Joint 24th Annual Conference and the Annual Fall Meeting of the Biomedical Engineering Society][Engineering in Medicine and Biology]* (Vol. 3, pp. 2455–2456). IEEE.

[35] Narayan, J. and Dwivedy, S.K., 2020. Towards neuro-fuzzy compensated PID control of lower extremity exoskeleton system for passive gait rehabilitation. *IETE Journal of Research*, pp. 1–18.

[36] Waldron, K.J. and Schmiedeler, J., 2016. Kinematics. In *Springer Handbook of Robotics* (pp. 11–36). Springer, Cham.

[37] Stolle, C.J., Nelson, C.A., Burnfield, J.M. and Buster, T.W., 2016, July. Improved design of a gait rehabilitation robot. In *International Workshop on Medical and Service Robots* (pp. 31–44). Springer, Cham.

[38] Pongpipatpaiboon, K., Mukaino, M., Matsuda, F., Ohtsuka, K., Tanikawa, H., Yamada, J., Tsuchiyama, K. and Saitoh, E., 2018. The impact of ankle–foot orthoses on toe clearance strategy in hemiparetic gait: a cross-sectional study. *Journal of Neuroengineering and Rehabilitation*, *15*(1), pp. 1–12.

[39] Syrseloudis, C.E., Emiris, I.Z., Lilas, T. and Maglara, A., 2011. Design of a simple and modular 2-DOF ankle physiotherapy device relying on a hybrid serial-parallel robotic architecture. *Applied Bionics and Biomechanics*, *8*(1), pp. 101–114.

[40] Li, Y., Yan, L., Qian, H., Wu, J., Men, S. and Li, N., 2014. Dynamics and kinematics analysis and simulation of lower extremity power-assisted exoskeleton. *Journal of Vibroengineering*, *16*(2), pp. 781–791.

[41] Zakaria, M.A., Majeed, A.A., Khairuddin, I.M. and Taha, Z., 2016, September. Kinematics analysis of a 3DoF lower limb exoskeleton for gait rehabilitation: a preliminary investigation. In *International Conference on Movement, Health and Exercise* (pp. 168–172). Springer, Singapore.

[42] Wang, H., Lin, M., Jin, Z., Yan, H., Liu, G., Liu, S. and Hu, X., 2020. A 4-DOF workspace lower limb rehabilitation robot: mechanism design, human joint analysis and trajectory planning. *Applied Sciences*, *10*(13), p. 4542.

[43] Kalita, B., Narayan, J. and Dwivedy, S.K., 2020. Development of active lower limb robotic-based orthosis and exoskeleton devices: a systematic review. *International Journal of Social Robotics*, pp. 1–19.

[44] Schilling, R.J., 1996. *Fundamentals of Robotics: Analysis and Control*. Simon & Schuster Trade.

11 Blockchain-Based Electronic Health Record System Enforced by Ensemble Multi-Contract Approach

J. Antony Prince, N. Hemapriya and V. Muthulakshmi

CONTENTS

11.1 INTRODUCTION

The Indian healthcare sector has struggled with a number of issues, including making healthcare more accessible, ensuring adequate healthcare services and providing a better patient experience. Patients will benefit from faster and more accurate diagnosis as well as more successful therapies if information is shared seamlessly between healthcare providers. This would also improve providers' collective capacity to make service delivery more cost effective and improve the customer experience [12] focuses on creating a visual computational model of a

DOI: 10.1201/9781003207856-11

medical app that uses blockchain technology to handle both patient and doctor databases during surgery. The platform was created to fill in the gaps left by previous iterations, which mostly used blockchain in the banking and finance industries. For the penetration of blockchain into the healthcare ecosystem of India, it's essential to start by creating a nationwide electronic health record (EHR) exchange system. Since the feasibility and long-term efficacy of each use case are currently being researched and developed, the realization of distributed ledger technology by the Indian healthcare industry will take time. Blockchain is a new platform that has the ability to reshape the system for knowledge generation and sharing in a number of sectors, including healthcare. It has the power to improve some of the most important aspects of healthcare by improving interoperability and workflow optimization while protecting overall data protection and privacy by increasing stakeholder confidence. To improve patients' data ownership, the contemporary disjoint ecosystem of healthcare providers that retains localized power over patient data would need to be decentralized using blockchain [13]. Faced with possible privacy concerns and flaws in existing personal medical data storage and sharing systems, as well as the idea of self-autonomous data ownership, a revolutionary consumer-centric medical information sharing approach using a decentralized and permissioned blockchain to protect the privacy of electronic healthcare management system has been suggested in our proposed system.

11.2 LITERATURE SURVEY

Healthcare is one of the most popular applications where blockchain is expected to have a significant effect. Kumar et al. [2] focused on the future implementations of blockchain technologies in modern healthcare systems, as well as the critical criteria for such systems, such as trustless and open healthcare systems. McGhin et al. [1] suggested that due to stringent regulatory standards, such as the Health Insurance Portability and Accountability Act (HIPAA) of 1996, blockchain implementations in the healthcare industry typically need more stringent security, interoperability, and record-sharing requirements. Researchers in academia and industry have begun to study solutions targeted toward healthcare use and focused on existing blockchain technology. Pirtle and Ehrenfeld [3] defined the aim of this technology, which is to "maintain a single record of their certifications and approvals," which will "simplify interstate licensure, bolster trust, and encourage organizations and individuals to authenticate professional qualifications." Ismail, Materwala, and Zeadally [4] suggested blockchain's replication function, as well as its privacy and protection capabilities, have a bright future in healthcare, as they will fix some of the system's inherent problems. Zhang et al. [5] proposed the creation of smart contracts that are designed on top of a blockchain to enable decentralized apps (DApps) to communicate with the blockchain programmatically and to facilitate on-chain storage. In the healthcare industry, programmable blockchains have sparked concern as a possible response to key issues, including a lack of coordination, inadequate clinical report distribution, and incomplete health records. Kassab et al. [6] presented the findings of a systematic literature review undertaken to classify, extract, analyze, and synthesize studies on the symbiosis of blockchain in healthcare and summarize and categorize current difficulties in integrating blockchain in the healthcare context. Agbo, Mahmoud, and Eklund [7] conducted a study outlining the current state of blockchain technology implementation for healthcare. More research is needed to better identify, define, and assess the usefulness of blockchain in healthcare, according to the findings. Tandon et al. [8] suggested that blockchain is being used to create new and advanced interventions to enhance the current methods of handling, exchanging, and accessing patient data and personal health information. Hathaliya et al. [9] proposed a permissioned blockchain-based healthcare architecture to strengthen the protection and privacy of patient data. Ramani et al. [10] conducted a study which suggested a safe and effective data accessibility process for patients and doctors in a healthcare system based on blockchain technology. The suggested system is therefore capable of protecting patients' privacy. The scheme's security review reveals that it can withstand well-known threats while retaining system integrity. Abdellatif et al. [11] outlined a modern, smart, and safe healthcare system (ssHealth) that uses developments in edge computing and blockchain technology to allow disease identification, remote surveillance, and rapid emergency response. The proposed framework acts as a one-stop solution for efficient healthcare management which also enables safe medical data sharing across local healthcare entities, enabling numerous national and foreign entities to be incorporated.

11.3 EVOLUTION OF BLOCKCHAIN TECHNOLOGY

One of the first contemporary propositions that progressed into blockchain as a technology was envisioned by Haber and Stornetta [17], who explored the development of a cryptographically secured chain of blocks that is resistant to tampering. They further augmented the system architecture by involving the Merkle tree to allow for storing multiple documents in a single block. Blockchain gained relevance in 2008 when Nakamoto [18] detailed an electronic peer-to-peer system that utilized digital currency to overcome the drawbacks faced in the economic crisis. His proposal was the stepping stone in building the first-ever successful decentralized digital currency, Bitcoin. Bitcoin utilized the proof-of-work consensus to overcome the Byzantine general problem where transactions are stored in the block and added to the blockchain after validation. Bitcoin miners who are part of the network validate the block by solving a cryptographic mathematics puzzle and gain Bitcoin as a reward if they succeed.

The next breakthrough in the blockchain was when Buterin [19] developed a new blockchain platform called Ethereum to fully leverage the capabilities of the blockchain system. The major addition in Ethereum that turned out to be pivotal was the ability to execute contracts in the blockchain. Ethereum comprises the Ethereum virtual machine (EVM), which is a Turing complete machine, to execute smart contracts. Ethereum uses Ether as a cryptocurrency for rewards and transactions, with the focus oriented toward easier adoption of the platform

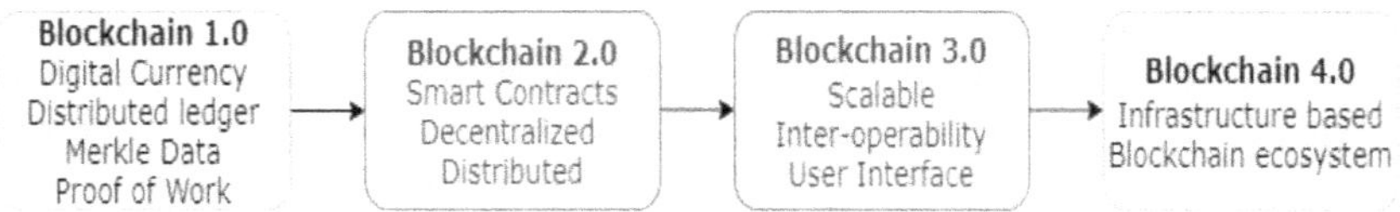

FIGURE 11.1 Evolution of blockchain technology over the years.

by developers. The contracts can be developed using Solidity or vyper and can be called using an external account or via the contract itself. Subsequently, Hyperledger was conceived as an open-source blockchain spearheaded by the Linux Foundation with a focus on developing a comprehensive set of stable frameworks, tools, and libraries for enterprise-grade blockchain deployments. Figure 11.1 indicates the evolution of blockchain technology.

Blockchain is a decentralized, distributed ledger that stores the details of a digital asset where it does not allow a single person or a governing body to control the network. Each of the blocks comprises numerous transactions with a link created among different blocks using a hash function to form a chain. When an asset is created, it is verified across the distributed network of nodes and added to a block, which is linked to the previous block, leading to a chain of blocks or blockchain. The data stored in the blockchain is immutable [20]; that is, the data cannot be altered once added to the blockchain, which is further made consistent by cryptographically linking the data by their hash value and asymmetric public-key cryptography. The general workflow of blockchain is: The request of the transaction is broadcast to a peer-to-peer network. Validation of the transaction is done by the network of nodes. The verified transaction constitutes smart contract execution logs, records, or any other information. Verified transactions are grouped together to be added to a block. The block of verified transactions is added to the blockchain by means of a consensus protocol like proof of work or proof of authority. The transaction is then added to the blockchain successfully.

The block in the blockchain combines its own hash, data, and the hash of its previous block, essentially functioning analogously to a linked list. The first block of the blockchain is known as the genesis block. Each of the blocks in the blockchain can verify multiple transactions by implementing a Merkle tree and storing the root hash. Also, tampering with data in a block will change its hash, breaking its link with the adjacent blocks and invalidating its immutability property and tamper-proof approach. Consensus is the decision-making process for selecting a leader among a group of nodes for adding a new block. Both Bitcoin and Ethereum follow the proof of work, although Ethereum has shifted from proof of work to proof of stake. New consensus approaches are an active area of research to achieve better scalability and efficiency of the blockchain.

Proof of authority (POA) is a consensus approach where the block addition rights are decided by means of the identity, which is already authenticated in a permissioned blockchain network. POA offers better performance and fault tolerance.

An interplanetary file system (IPFS) is essentially a shared file that is decentralized and follows a peer-to-peer architecture to function as a hypermedia protocol designed to store and share data. For each file uploaded to IPFS, a unique hash value is computed and stored in interested nodes along with metadata of what other node is storing it. IPFS removes duplication across the network. It is an approach toward offering secure peer-to-peer content delivery. IPFS [21] allows for addressing large amounts of data and computing immutable links in transactions along with timestamping to secure content without having to put the data themselves on-chain. It is aimed at making the web faster, safer, and more open. Ethereum is a blockchain computing platform that triggered the advent of smart contract development by including a Turing complete machine. Ethereum uses Ether for the transactions and computation costs and rewards. Ether is peer-to-peer cryptocurrency. For any transaction to be undertaken in the public Ethereum blockchain, a certain amount of Ether known as Gas is incurred to fuel the transaction execution. Ethereum allowed for the widespread adoption and consideration of blockchain in many new cases in domains spanning agriculture to finance.

The EVM is a runtime compiler in the Ethereum blockchain which acts as a Turing complete machine to execute smart contracts. It allows for compilation, verification, and deployment of smart contracts developed using Solidity or vyper. The EVM converts the smart contract into bytecode, which is then deployed to the network. Smart contracts [22] are autonomous executing codes that execute based on some condition or event. Ethereum introduced smart contracts and utilizes the Ethereum virtual machine to run and compile the contract. Smart contracts are generally coded using special languages like Solidity, vyper (Ethereum), Golang, JavaScript, Java, and C++, which can be also used for contract development on other blockchain platforms. Smart contracts are known as chaincode in the hyperledger. The general workflow of smart contract execution is: Smart contract development is carried out using supported languages. Code is uploaded to the Ethereum virtual machine. A copy of the contract is broadcast to the entire network. Contract execution is triggered due to an event or condition satisfaction. The nodes of the network validate and evaluate the code execution. The result is submitted to Ethereum for verification and validation.

Even though blockchain has seen an exponential increase in relevance, and new use cases are being proposed, blockchain does possess certain limitations which prevent it from fully reaching its potential. One primary concern is the scalability issue posed by blockchain, as the question of efficiency transactions is raised when the network starts to grow. Blockchain also raises concerns over high energy utilization. For instance, the advent of Bitcoin led to the growth of miners throughout the globe where high computational capacity and electricity are being used to achieve the proof of work consensus and earn Bitcoin. It is also considered a nascent technology that is not yet mature to replace legacy systems or be integrated with them. Yet the future of blockchain is glimmering with the hope of achieving true decentralization and security owing to extensive research.

11.4 PROPOSED FRAMEWORK

Conventionally existing healthcare institutes use paper records for patient records. This practice is generally ill advised owing to the susceptibility of the format to tampering, data loss, or destruction. Paper records also are not easy to track, lack provenance, and are susceptible to being damaged. With the advent of technological penetration, most healthcare institutes have transitioned toward a digital mode of record management. Electronic health records hold much prominence and provide multiple benefits like provenance, traceability, and security. Yet the existing digital solutions are centralized and fail when it comes to interoperability,; that is, different hospitals follow different protocols for handling medical records. This difference in mechanisms makes the patient struggle when shifting from one hospital to another. Blockchain as a technology holds much promise in modeling the future of electronic health records in the era of transition toward smart cities. Cloud-based storage or big data-based paradigms to handle EHRs have been explored in the past, but the procedures do not provide a secure accessibility mechanism and are susceptible to tampering. Blockchain provides a zero-proof knowledge-based trust system for handling electronic health records. Decentralization of the network restricts any hostile threat aimed toward the blockchain network.

The healthcare system is a vast ecosystem with a plethora of stakeholders who are involved in multitudes of interactions for the efficient functioning of the medical community. Patients generally interact with doctors, pharmacists, clinicians, and insurance providers. From the perspective of a healthcare institute, the interaction involves that of government regulators and researchers as well. The majority of the stakeholders are heavily dependent upon the patient's record to gain insights or a verification process. General record access strategies are typically time consuming and ineffective for the required quantity of records to be propagated. Another major concern is maintaining the privacy and security of the records and preventing access by any malicious entities. A robust and secure system that can optimize the record access paradigm could enable the betterment of the healthcare domain operating procedure. Figure 11.2 represents the architecture of the proposed blockchain-based EHR framework.

An Ethereum-based permissioned network with proof-of-authority consensus is to be configured and orchestrated. A permissioned network, unlike a public network, allows only authenticated users to be part of the network. The stakeholders in healthcare are broadly classified into patients, doctors, administrators, and healthcare institutes. For evaluation purposes, the Kovan testnet with proof-of-authority consensus is chosen. Testnets are networks used to test protocols and smart contracts in production-level environments. Figure 11.3 includes the primary stakeholders involved in the proposed system. The patient/user is one of the key stakeholders who becomes a part of the network by creating an identity mapping of credentials such as unique health identification number (UHID) to map with their records.

The patient holds access to their data record, and the control for others to access their record lies with the patient as well. Doctors can perform the task of record creation by joining the network, upon which a doctor ID is created via

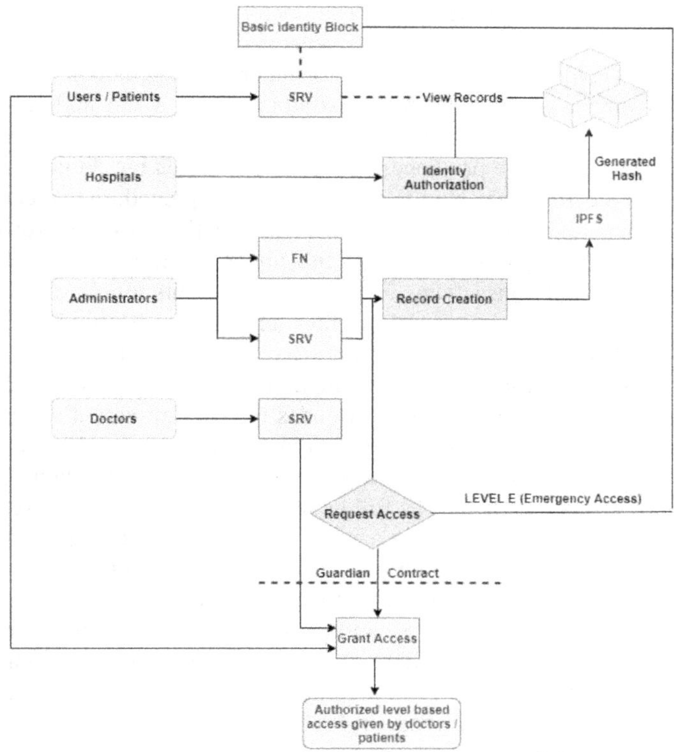

FIGURE 11.2 Workflow of the proposed EHR framework.

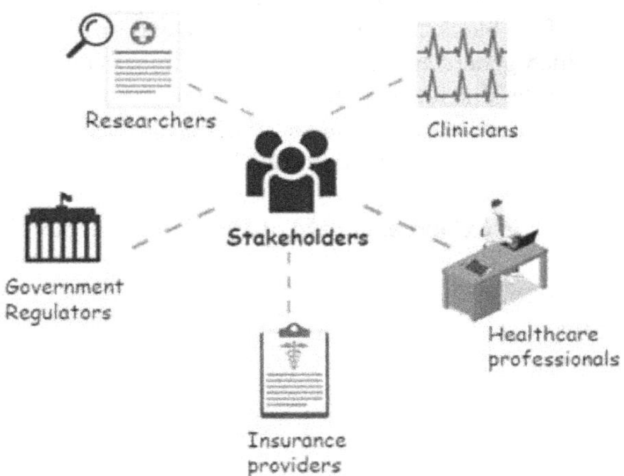

FIGURE 11.3 Primary stakeholders involved in the proposed framework.

the smart contract to map their data. The doctor can upload the data record to the IPFS network and add the file hash generated as a new record to the blockchain. Doctors hold access privileges for the record and can handle record access requests for other stakeholders. Administrators can be a full node or a partial node. This comprises researchers, clinicians, government regulators, and insurance firms. They hold the privilege to add health records but do not have direct access to data records. They have to follow the access procedure to create a level-oriented request and gain access to the records contingent on approval by the patient or doctor. Hospitals function as full nodes in the network and validate block generation and transactions. For doctors or patients to join, registration of hospitals in the network is mandatory, as they form the peer-to-peer decentralized system. As full nodes, they run their very own blockchain node and hold a copy of the blockchain which allows them to maintain the integrity of the network.

Proof of authority selects a group of nodes for the transaction validation and block addition. Out of all stakeholders in our implementation, healthcare institutes like hospitals are considered the validator nodes to stake their identity to the network. They would act as the full nodes that run their own blockchain peer copy. The tasks of network block creation, transaction validation, and network management fall under the purview of the full nodes. The administrators include but are not limited to clinicians, researchers, government agencies, and insurance providers. The administrators can function as either a full node or a simple record verification (SRV) node. SRVs analogous to the simple payment verification (SPV) node are not required to run the full blockchain node but can be part of the blockchain by means of accessing the block headers alone.

Doctors and patients can function as an SRV node with access to the transaction access and generation procedure. Doctors are tasked with adding health records to the blockchain for patients. Patients can generally access their records and manage access requests. An identity block contract deals with the creation and management of network users. The patient, doctors, and administrators can register to be part of the blockchain after verification and validation to the identity smart contract, which generates a unique identity number (UID) to represent the user based on their role. The identity smart contract is to be developed in Solidity, with mappings for doctors, patients, and administrators. Each mapping holds the UID and other membership details required to be part of the blockchain network.

<Algorithm 1: Smart Contract for Identity Management>

```
Define struct Identity
Define struct IDatum
Define mapping Identities public
Define mapping IData public
function Create Identity(roleName, accountId){
        objectIdentity = new Identity(roleName,accountId)
        mapping Identities[accountId] = objectIdentity
}
```

```
function Create IDatum(accountID, variables for essential health data){
        objectIDatum = new IDatum(function arguments)
        Mapping IData[accountID] = objectIDatum
}
function ID verify(accountID, requestedRole) return bool{
        if Identities[accountID].role matches requestedRole{
              return True
        }
        else{
              return False
        }
}
function IData call(accountID) return string{
        require accountID mapped in IData
        return IData[accountID].data
}
</>
```

Doctors and administrators with verified access in the identity contract have the privilege to create records. The health record is uploaded to the decentralized web, that is, the IPFS. The IPFS returns a unique file hash for the record uploaded, which is to be stored as a record in the blockchain. A record contract is created using Solidity to store the patient ID, adder ID, timestamp, record hash (generated from IPFS), and metadata as encapsulation with methods defined for adding, fetching, and deleting the record. For every record added, a record UID is generated by which the particular record can be queried. The patient UID allows for querying the entire record history of the patient stored in the blockchain. Solidity has events that allow for better traceability of logs and transactions. When a record is created, an event is registered in the Ethereum network mapping the patient record and patient UID. Figure 11.4 depicts the record storage mechanism of the proposed system.

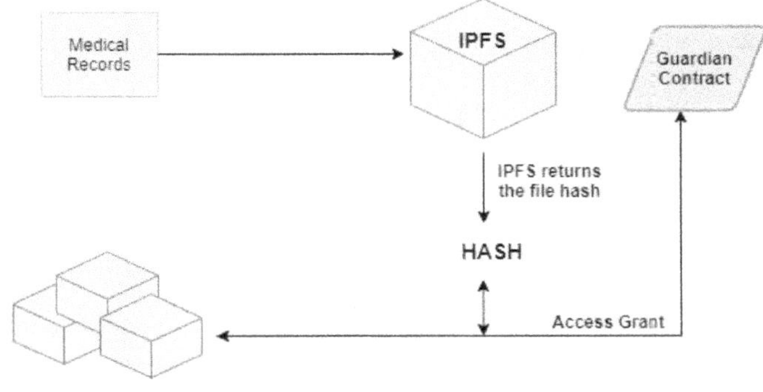

FIGURE 11.4 Health record management using IPFS and permissioned blockchain.

<Algorithm 2: Smart Contract for Record Management>

```
Define struct Record
Define mapping Records public
function Create Record(accountId, patientID,variables for record data){
  require accountID.role in doctor/admin in Identity Contract
  Record = new Record(accountId,patientID,variables for record data)
  mapping Records[concat(patientID,recordID)] = Record
  emit CREATE _ RECORD event
}
function Query Record(accountID,recordID) return value{
  require account.role matches doctor or LEVEL R access clearance
  emit RECORD _ QUERY event
  return Records[recordID].data
}
function Query Patient(accountID,patientID) return value{
  require account.role matches doctor or LEVEL P access clearance
  emit PATIENT _ QUERY event
  return Records that has patientID pattern in recordID
}
function DeleteRecord(accountID,recordID) return bool{
  require account.role matches doctor or LEVEL R access clearance
  emit RECORD _ DELETE event
  set Records[recordID].active = False
  return True
}
function concat(value a, value b) returns value{
  new value ab
  for i in a : add to ab
  for i in b : add to ab
  return ab
}
function slice(value a, length) returns (value,value){
  new value p,q
  for i in length : add to p
  for j=length to a.length : add to q
  return p,q
}
</>
```

The need for blockchain is highly validated by the secure access control it provides, augmented by cryptographic protocols. The records stored in the blockchain are highly privileged and confidential information. Patients can access their records using the patient UID, and doctors can access their records using the record UID or patient UID. The administrator access control follows a three-level

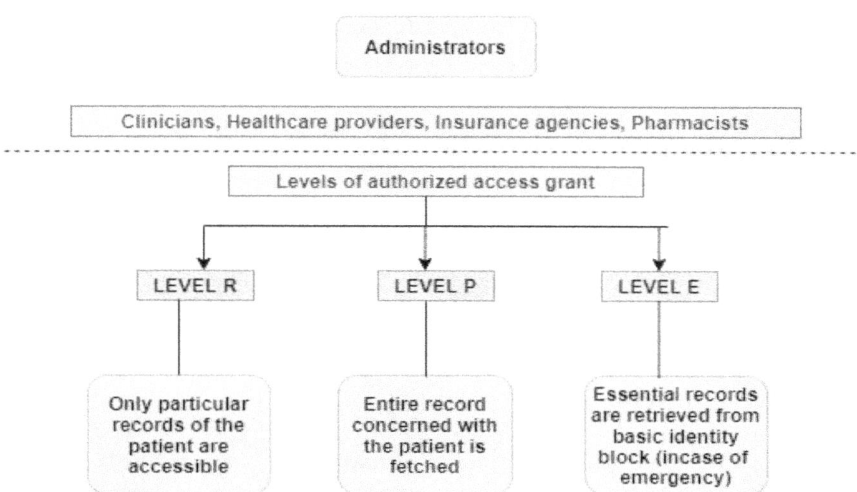

FIGURE 11.5 Various levels of authorized access grant provided to the administrators.

approach to prevent the record from reaching malicious entities. The three levels of requests are depicted in Figure 11.5.

- LEVEL R (Record)
  Access to the particular record of a patient
- LEVEL P (Patient)
  Access to the entire medical transactional records stored in the blockchain
- LEVEL E (Emergency/Essentials)
  Access to details stored in the block in the identity contract

Each of the requests is added to the guardian contract to be authorized by the patient or doctor. This granular approach to record access privileges allows for a safe and secure record access procedure. The guardian contract developed using Solidity maps the requests to level, status, and authorized notary UIDs. Events are used to generate an access log for the medical records.

<Algorithm 3: Smart Contract for Guardian Management>

```
Define struct Guard
Define mapping Guardian public
function Create Guard(accountId, Level, variables){
  require accountID.role in doctor/admin in Identity Contract

  if Level is R{
```

```
requestGuard = new Guard(accountID,Level,recordID,clearance=False)
  Guardian[guardID] = requestGuard;
  emit RECORD _ REQUEST event
  }
  else if Level is P{
requestGuard = new Guard(accountID,Level,patientID,clearance=False)
  Guardian[guardID] = requestGuard;
  emit PATIENT _ QUERY event
}
  else{
requestGuard = new Guard(accountID,Level,patientID,clearance=False)
  Guardian[guardID] = requestGuard;
  emit ESSENTIAL _ QUERY event
}
function Allow Guard(accountID,guardID) return bool{
  require account.role matches doctor or patient in GuardRequest
  Guardian[guardID] .clearance = True;
  emit REQUEST _ SUCCESS event
  return True;
  }
function Revoke Guard(accountID,guardID) return bool{
  require account.role matches doctor or patient in GuardRequest
  Guardian[guardID] .clearance = False;
  emit REQUEST _ REVOKE event
  return True;
}
</>
```

11.5 PERFORMANCE AND EVALUATION

For testing the proposed framework, the test environment has the following configuration:

- Intel Core i5–8265U CPU @ 1.60GHz–1.80 GHz
- 8.00 GB of memory with Windows 64-bit OS (version 10)

Smart contracts are developed with the Solidity programming language in the Remix IDE, and the blockchain network is the Kovan testnet, which is a proof-of-authority consensus network. Web3.py and Python are used for making remote procedure calls (RPCs) to the blockchain. The deployment is done using the MetaMask client with test Ether from the Kovan faucet.

This segment discusses what kind of data is used to test the proposed framework's efficiency. This section further goes through the metrics that are used to describe the outcomes of the current performance assessment. To determine the performance of the proposed framework, the transaction deployment time and completion time are taken into consideration. The time taken to deploy the Ethereum smart contract is referred to as the transaction deployment time. The time interval between when the transaction is completed and validated to be added to the Ethereum blockchain is termed the transaction completion time. The metrics taken into account for better evaluation of the model include execution time, transaction assessment, throughput, and latency.

Execution time: It is essentially the time interval between the transaction validation and the execution of the transaction in the blockchain network. Table 11.1 indicates the average execution time for several transactions in a block.

If the number of transactions grows, the execution time grows as well. These transactions are performed in such a way as to satisfy the functions in the smart contract. Figure 11.6 indicates the time taken by different functions/transactions such as block creation, adding of records, querying, and viewing records. This time taken would considerably increase when the number of users rise.

Throughput refers to the amount of data that could be transferred from one location to another in a unit amount of time. The delay that occurs while a system component waits for another system component to react to an action is known as

TABLE 11.1
Execution Time for Different Transactions in a Block

Transaction	Execution Time
Block creation	2 min 23 sec
Add patient records	1 min 52 sec
View patient records	48 sec
Query records	52 sec

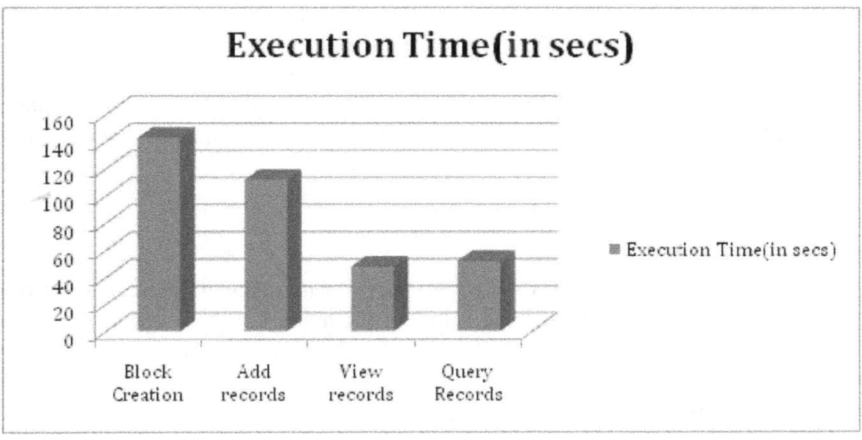

FIGURE 11.6 Average execution time taken for essential transactions.

TABLE 11.2
Transaction Fee and Data Payload Size for Various Functions

Transaction	Size (bytes)	Block Reward
$TxF_{block\_creation}$	560	0.0020
TxF_{add_block}	550	0.0140
TxF_{create_record}	240	0.0078
TxF_{view_record}	122	0.0003
TxF_{update_record}	420	0.0060

latency. In terms of the time factor, it is the difference between the time it takes to deploy a transaction and the time it takes to complete it. The assessment of transactions is done using a data payload field that is present in any Ethereum transaction. The transaction contains a data payload that is used to invoke smart contract functions. We will measure the transaction sizes of different functions of our proposed system using the data payload. The transaction sizes in bytes for these functions are shown in Table 11.2.

The table indicates the Gas reward offered in ETH (Ethers). The transaction fees for Ethereum are measured in "ETH," which is the Ethereum currency, which has wei and gwei as the units. The method for calculating the charge for Ethereum transactions is also suggested here. The product of Gas used and Gas price is the purchase fee for a transaction. It may be articulated in the following way:

$$Transaction\ Fee = gasPrice \times gasConsumed$$

11.6 RESULTS AND DISCUSSION

There are two major approaches to reimagining health knowledge exchange: One emphasizes the importance of stable enabling infrastructure, while the other emphasizes the importance of standardization in the healthcare sector. The proposed framework would enable improvement in providers' collective capability to make healthcare service delivery more cost effective and enhance the customer experience. The key parameters achieved in our proposed framework are:

11.6.1 Scalability

Scalability is the capacity of a system to perform its tasks effectively when the storage of the system fluctuates and is one of the major concerns associated with blockchain. The proof-of-work consensus protocol is computationally heavy and raises the question of scalability. Taking this into consideration, the proposal opts for proof-of-authority consensus. Also, the proposal makes use of off-chain storage to reduce the data load in the blockchain, with an access control layer making it considerably scalable.

11.6.2 Role-Based Access Mechanism

The proposed system ensures that all of the stakeholders or entities of the system are given a unique role. Any unauthorized third-party entity will not be able to intrude into the system. This parameter guarantees that the confidentiality of the healthcare records of the patient will not be jeopardized and that only registered users have access to the system. It also follows an identity at stake mechanism for maintaining integrity.

11.6.3 Security

Data in the blockchain are immutable due to hashing and cryptographic linking augmented by asymmetric public-key cryptography. The proposal introduces a guardian contract, which is an exclusive smart contract designed to map the access control privileges using a three-level clearance approach. The guardian contract deals with emergency scenarios with Level E, aggregated record access with Level P, and specificity by means of Level R.

11.6.4 Event Traceability

Events are an inheritable entity in an Ethereum contract. The Ethereum block consists of logs to represent occurrences or events. An event can be emitted from a smart contract along with arguments. Arguments can be split into indexable and non-indexable. Indexable arguments allow for filtering the entire event history in the blockchain. This allows for tracing events like record creation or access.

11.6.5 Off-Chain Storage

The off-chain storage system is implemented using the IPFS in the proposed framework which stores the patient data in the blockchain by including the patient identifier as well as the IPFS hash. IPFS uses a cryptographic hash to store the contents in a decentralized and distributed peer-to-peer (P2P) network, which guarantees that the system's security is not jeopardized when the scalability problem is addressed. Table 11.3 performs a constructive comparison between the proposed framework and other related work

TABLE 11.3
Feature Comparison Based on Performance Metrics

Parameters	[14]	[15]	[16]	Proposed Framework
Scalability	Yes	No	Yes	Yes
Role-based access	No	Yes	Yes	Yes
Off-chain storage (IPFS)	No	No	Yes	Yes
Event traceability	No	No	No	Yes
Security	Yes	Yes	Yes	Yes

11.7 CONCLUSION

We have addressed how blockchain technology could help the healthcare industry. Despite advancements in the healthcare industry and technical innovation in EHR programs, they also face concerns that could be tackled by blockchain technology. Our suggested system blends safe data management with monitored access controls for medical records. It provides a system that is simpler to use and understand for patients and other stakeholders. Since IPFS's off-chain storage mechanism is used, the architecture recommends steps to ensure that the system address the issue of data storage. The system benefits from role-based access because patient records are only open to trustworthy and connected persons. This also addresses the EHR system's knowledge asymmetry problem. Both services and the healthcare community would benefit from a permissioned patient-accessible blockchain-based solution to transforming clinical treatment, and data confidence would be preserved. The proposed blockchain system would act as an interface for a physician to update and track a patient's profile directly in a secure and approved manner. The updated hospitalization log will take into account the patient's personal records, as well as other health-related facts and insurance plans. The streamlined incorporation of medical knowledge sharing and claim and payment data would improve the patient experience.

11.8 FUTURE WORK

Blockchain is touted as playing a crucial role in the future of the healthcare system. The potential of implementing a unified interoperable permissioned blockchain for medical information sharing is immense. The payment module could be integrated into the current system. The key takeaways for consideration would be the payment made by the patient for a doctor's appointment in this blockchain-based decentralized framework to build a smooth network of patient knowledge flow and data sharing and communicate with third-party networks such as hospitals. The healthcare company that embraces this system should have a well-developed solution environment with a range of vendors from which to select. Since a consensus on the standard practice for a common blockchain-based healthcare management adoption scheme is required, multiple parties must work together. To assist the creation of the envisioned decentralized network and thus ensure the authenticity of the data being generated, processed, and shared, the stakeholders of the medical industry should invest in a unified permissioned blockchain spanning healthcare providers, payers, and other regulators involved in the healthcare field. For the promise of blockchain to be fully fulfilled, the formulation of regulatory standards by the bureaucracy and active involvement from the stakeholders in constructing an interdisciplinary trust-based nexus throughout the healthcare ecosystem is required.

REFERENCES

[1] T. McGhin, K.-K. R. Choo, C. Z. Liu and D. He, "Blockchain in healthcare applications: Research challenges and opportunities," Journal of Network and Computer Applications, vol. 135, 2019.

[2] T. Kumar, V. Ramani, I. Ahmad, A. Braeken, E. Harjula and M. Ylianttila, "Blockchain utilization in healthcare: Key requirements and challenges," 2018 IEEE 20th International Conference on e-Health Networking, Applications and Services (Healthcom), Ostrava, Czech Republic, 2018.

[3] C. Pirtle and J. Ehrenfeld, "Blockchain for healthcare: The next generation of medical records," Journal of Medical Systems, vol. 42, p. 172, 2018.

[4] L. Ismail, H. Materwala and S. Zeadally, "Lightweight blockchain for healthcare," IEEE Access, vol. 7, pp. 149935–149951, 2019.

[5] P. Zhang, M. A. Walker, J. White, D. C. Schmidt and G. Lenz, "Metrics for assessing blockchain-based healthcare decentralized apps," 2017 IEEE 19th International Conference on e-Health Networking, Applications and Services (Healthcom), Dalian, China, 2017.

[6] M. H. Kassab, J. DeFranco, T. Malas, P. Laplante, G. Destefanis and V. V. Graciano Neto, "Exploring research in blockchain for healthcare and a roadmap for the future," IEEE Transactions on Emerging Topics in Computing, 2019.

[7] C. C. Agbo, Q. H. Mahmoud and J. M. Eklund, "Blockchain technology in healthcare: A systematic review," Healthcare, 2019.

[8] A. Tandon, A. Dhir, A. K. M. Najmul Islam and M. Mäntymäki, "Blockchain in healthcare: A systematic literature review, synthesizing framework and future research agenda," Computers in Industry, vol. 122, 2020.

[9] J. Hathaliya, P. Sharma, S. Tanwar and R. Gupta, "Blockchain-based remote patient monitoring in healthcare 4.0," 2019 IEEE 9th International Conference on Advanced Computing (IACC), 2019.

[10] V. Ramani, T. Kumar, A. Bracken, M. Liyanage and M. Ylianttila, "Secure and efficient data accessibility in blockchain based healthcare systems," 2018 IEEE Global Communications Conference (GLOBECOM), Abu Dhabi, United Arab Emirates, 2018.

[11] A. A. Abdellatif, A. Z. Al-Marridi, A. Mohamed, A. Erbad, C. F. Chiasserini and A. Refaey, "ssHealth: Toward secure, blockchain-enabled healthcare systems," IEEE Network, vol. 34, no. 4, pp. 312–319, July/August 2020.

[12] T. Le Nguyen, "Blockchain in healthcare: A new technology benefit for both patients and doctors," 2018 Portland International Conference on Management of Engineering and Technology (PICMET), Honolulu, HI, USA, 2018.

[13] X. Liang, J. Zhao, S. Shetty, J. Liu and D. Li, "Integrating blockchain for data sharing and collaboration in mobile healthcare applications," 2017 IEEE 28th Annual International Symposium on Personal, Indoor, and Mobile Radio Communications (PIMRC), Montreal, QC, Canada, 2017.

[14] P. Zhang, J. White, D. C. Schmidt, G. Lenz and S. T. Rosenbloom, "FHIRChain: Applying blockchain to securely and scalably share clinical data," Computational and Structural Biotechnology Journal, vol. 16, pp. 267–278, 2018.

[15] M. G. Kim, A. R. Lee, H. J. Kwon, J. W. Kim and I. K. Kim, "Sharing medical questionnaires based on blockchain," Proceedings of 2018 IEEE International Conf erence on Bioinformatics and Biomedicine (BIBM 2018), pp. 2767–2769, 2019.

[16] A. Shahnaz, U. Qamar and A. Khalid, "Using blockchain for electronic health records," IEEE Access, vol. 7, pp. 147782–147795, 2019, doi: 10.1109/ACCESS.2019.2946373.
[17] S. Haber and W. S. Stornetta, "How to time-stamp a digital document," Journal of Cryptology, vol. 3, pp. 99–111, 1991.
[18] S. Nakamoto, "Bitcoin: A peer-to-peer electronic cash system," Cryptography Mailing List, 2009, https://metzdowd.com.
[19] V. Buterin, "A next-generation smart contract and decentralized application platform," Ethereum, pp. 1–36, January 2014.
[20] E. Politou, F. Casino, E. Alepis and C. Patsakis, "Blockchain mutability: Challenges and proposed solutions," IEEE, 2014.
[21] J. Benet, "IPFS—Content addressed, Versioned, P2P File System," ArXiv abs/1407.3561, 2014.
[22] M. Alharby and A. van Moorse, "Blockchain-based smart contracts: A systematic mapping study," ArXiv abs/1710.06372, 2017.

12 EMG Features as an Indicator of Muscle Strength for the Assessment of Non-Specific Low Back Pain

S. Saranya, S. Poonguzhali, N. Madhu Baala and S. Karunakaran

CONTENTS

12.1 INTRODUCTION

Core trunk muscles contribute to the stabilization of the trunk and facilitate movement of the arms, legs and spine [1]. Postural variations or disuse of these muscles may lead to progressive weakness. The manifestation of this muscle weakness in the form of 'non-specific' low back pain affects the overall quality of life of an individual. Treatment for back pain usually begins with a strength assessment of

DOI: 10.1201/9781003207856-12

TABLE 12.1
MRC Grading—MMT

MMT Grade	Muscle Function—Description
0	No contraction
1	Flicker or trace contraction
2	Active movement—gravity eliminated
3	Active movement against gravity
4–	Active movement against gravity and slight resistance
4	Active movement against gravity and moderate resistance
4+	Active movement against gravity and strong resistance
5	Normal power

these muscles followed by exercises to strengthen weak muscles [2, 3]. Strength testing usually involves manual muscle testing (MMT) by the examiner, who assigns grades defining muscle strength. Table 12.1 shows the Medical Research Council (MRC) 0–5-point muscle strength grading scale [4], with subdivisions for grade 4.

Though MMT is a relatively easy and common method to assess muscles, difficulty arises in grading individual muscles since musculoskeletal movement usually involves the coordination of more than one muscle. Moreover, patient position and strength, examiner strength and severity of pain are factors that affect evaluation [5]. The method is also subjective, with noticeable intra-rater variations in grading strength. Methods like dynamometry have been proposed as an alternative to MMT that quantitatively measures force in terms of strength. Use of dynamometry has proved effective in the measurement of limb muscle strength, but practical difficulties arise in fitting dynamometers to the contours of the back for trunk assessments. They also provide a gross value of strength and often present a weak methodology with varying protocols [6, 7].

The limitations can be overcome by using a more quantitative method for grading muscle strength that can aid/confirm MMT evaluation by physicians. This chapter hypothesizes that electromyogram (EMG) features, when carefully selected, can be used to quantitatively represent the strength of individual muscles that contribute to a movement and the use of EMG features can quantify the inherent strength of the muscle facilitating movement. EMG measures the electrical activity of the muscles, and studies have reported the use of EMG for successful examination of back pain [8, 9]. EMG is also used to evaluate the effects of strength training exercises during rehabilitation [10].

This chapter uses EMG features to assign strength grades based on the MRC scale of 4–, 4, 4+ and 5 for patients with chronic non-specific low back pain. Three bilateral core muscles of the low back, namely the erector spinae group (longissimus thoracis [LT]), iliocostalis lumborum (IL) and multifidus (MF), are evaluated during prone trunk extension, and the grades are compared with manual grades given by the examiner.

12.2 PARTICIPANTS AND DATA COLLECTION

Surface EMG signals were recorded from 88 participants presenting a condition of mild to moderate non-specific low back pain based on a 11-point numerical pain rating scale (NPRS), as seen in Table 12.2. The muscle strength score was in the range of 4–5 on an MMT-MRC grading scale assessed by an experienced physiotherapist. All procedures performed for this chapter involving human participants were in accordance with the ethical standards of the Institutional Ethics Committee and with the 1964 Helsinki declaration and its later amendments or comparable ethical standards. Informed consent was obtained from all individual participants included in the study. Patients with spinal deformities/injuries or surgical interventions at the back were excluded from the study.

Surface EMG signals were recorded from six electrodes placed bilaterally on the left (LT_L, IL_L, MF_L) and right (LT_R, IL_R, MF_R) sides of the trunk [Figure 12.1a]. These muscles are crucial for spine stability and mobility of the

TABLE 12.2
Anthropometric Details and Pain Characteristics

Characteristics	Values
Age (years)	32.6 ± 3.43
Weight (kg)	63.5 ± 10.3
Height (cm)	159.5 ± 8.1
BMI	23.7 ± 3.2
NPRS (0–10)	3 ± 3

Abbreviations: BMI, Body Mass Index; NPRS, Numerical Pain Rating Scale.
Data are presented as mean ± SD.

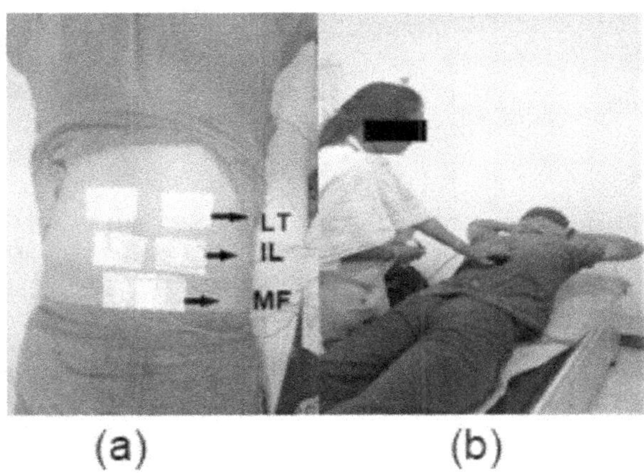

FIGURE 12.1 Data acquisition. (a) Bilateral electrode placement; (b) prone trunk extension protocol.

thoraco-lumbar region [11]. Electrodes for the MF were placed at the level of L5, 2 cm lateral to the lumbo-sacral junction. For the LT, electrodes were placed 2 cm lateral between the L1 and L2 spinal processes. IL electrodes were placed 4 cm lateral to the L3 spinal processes, and the reference was placed at the ulnar styloid process according to SENIAM recommendations and after proper skin preparation.

The protocol involves prone trunk extension until the possible end range of motion (ROM) with hands placed behind the head, as shown in Figure 12.1b. Prone trunk extension was specifically chosen because it is relatively easy to perform even in the case of severe back pain and also activates all three muscles of interest. Physicians also prefer trunk lifts in prone position as one of the initial strengthening exercises in the course of treatment [12]. The participants were verbally encouraged to sustain the position at end ROM for 5 sec against the resistance offered by the examiner. For grades 4–, 4 and 4+, the resistance varied from mild, moderate to strong relative to the examiner's maximum strength. Grade 5 involved the participant overpowering the examiner's maximal resistance. EMG was acquired using Biometrics Ltd, eight-channel wireless DataLOG (MWX8) sampled at 1000 Hz as the examiner performed MMT.

12.3 FEATURE SELECTION AND CLUSTERING

Muscle strength refers to the maximum tension that a muscle builds isometrically (static) against a resistive load. Non-redundant features with unique information on strength to demarcate muscle grades accurately are necessary [14]. As seen from Table 12.3, four features that quantify muscle strength have been identified

TABLE 12.3
Correlation between Selected EMG Features and Muscle Strength

EMG Features	Formula	Description	Muscle Strength Index
Integral EMG	$IEMG = \sum_{j=1}^{J-1} \lvert x_j \rvert$	Integral of rectified EMG signal	Natural muscle fiber recruitment and the strength of contraction [9, 13]
Root Mean Square EMG	$RMS = \sqrt{\frac{1}{J}\sum_{j=1}^{J} x_j^2}$	Root mean square value of the EMG segment under consideration	Force of isometric contraction [10]
Waveform Length	$WL = \sum_{j=1}^{J-1} \lvert x_{j+1} - x_j \rvert$	Cumulative length of the waveform within the given EMG time segment	Signal complexity [10, 15]
Willison's Amplitude	$WAMP = \sum_{j=1}^{J-1} f\left(\lvert x_{j+1} - x_j \rvert\right)$	Number of times that the difference between two adjacent amplitude values exceeds a predefined threshold	Indirect indicator of motor unit firing rate [10]

based on previous studies: integrated EMG (IEMG), root mean square (RMS), waveform length (WL) and Willison's amplitude (WAMP).

Since EMG follows a fairly Gaussian distribution for isometric contraction, a Gaussian mixture model (GMM) method that clusters data based on multivariate normal distribution is used in this chapter [17]. The model parameters mean and covariance are selected by iteratively applying an expectation maximum algorithm that converges to a maximum likelihood estimate [16]. GMM $\mathcal{P}_g$ has the following form,

$$\mathcal{P}_g(x_i;\mu_g,\Sigma_g)=\frac{e^{\frac{-1}{2}(x_i-\mu_g)^T\Sigma_g^{-1}(x_i-\mu_g)}}{\sqrt{(2\pi)^d\Sigma_g}} \tag{12.1}$$

where mean vector μ_g and covariance Σ_g determine the geometric characteristics of cluster g, and d is the dimension is the dataset. Since the desirable number of clusters is already known, and is based on the MMT grades assigned by the physician, Bayesian information criterion (BIC) is used to choose the model parameters that offer the lowest penalty for four clusters representing the four strength grades. BIC is computed based on the maximum log-likelihood resulting in combining the fit and complexity for each GMM model. The smaller the negative log-likelihood, the better the fit [18].

For unsupervised clustering, separability of clusters can be quantified using silhouette scores (Sc) and the Davis Bouldin index (Db). The similarity between the sample and its associated cluster is found, and Sc is the averaged Sc of all samples within the cluster. The Db index measures the average similarity between each cluster C_n and its most similar cluster C_m. Generally, Sc varies between –1 (incorrect clustering) and 1 (highly dense clustering), where a value close to 0 indicates overlapping clusters, and scores less than 0.5 are generally undesirable for good clustering. A lower DB index close to 0 indicates better separation between clusters.

12.4 RESULTS

12.4.1 Muscle Strength Classification

The model mixtures that had low BIC scores for the four clusters representative of the four strength grades for each muscle are in Table 12.4. Sc and Db indices with the total number of misclassifications (MCs) for each muscle are also listed. On average, the Sc index of all the muscles (~0.7) is close to 1 and DB (~0.4) less than 0.5, indicating good separability between the clustered strength grades. While no misclassifications are noted for bilateral LT and MF left muscles, two or three MCs for bilateral IL and MF right were observed, which is insignificant when considering the total number of observations (n = 88).

TABLE 12.4
GMM Model Parameters and Cluster Evaluation Metrics for the Selected Muscles

	Model Selection		Cluster Evaluation		
Muscles	**Covariance Type**	**BIC Score**	**Sc**	**Db**	**MC**
LT_L	Full unshared	–290	0.801	0.38	—
LT_R	Diagonal unshared	–396	0.71	0.48	—
IL_L	Diagonal unshared	–486	0.74	0.41	2
IL_R	Diagonal unshared	–360	0.73	0.39	3
M_L	Full shared	–447	0.82	0.46	—
M_R	Full shared	–221	0.72	0.46	2

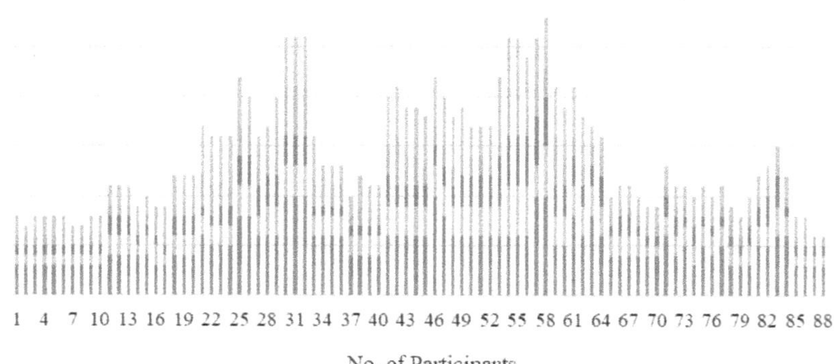

FIGURE 12.2 Comparison between muscle strength grades of each participant (n = 88) across all six muscles.

12.4.2 Individual Strength Grades

Participant (P)-wise strength grades of all the muscles under consideration is compared in Figure 12.2. The muscles are represented in different colors, and the height of each color bar is indicative of the strength scores, the lowest being 4–, and other grades have increasing heights. Most of the participants have higher strength for MF_R, the least being IL_L. Also, the strength variation between muscles is almost uniform for each case. On comparing P1 and P31, it can be observed that the strength scores of P1 varies between 4 and 4 for all muscles, while the scores for P31 lie between 4+ and 5. This indicates that strength or weakness is uniform over all the core muscles of the trunk.

12.4.3 Bilateral Symmetry of Trunk Muscles

Bilateral symmetry between the left and right side was calculated for each feature using the formula $BSI = [(L - R)/L + R)]$, where the BSI values ranged from 0 (symmetric) to 0.5 (asymmetric) [19]. In Table 12.5, a positive value indicates dominant left-side activity, and a negative value signifies a dominant right side. The BSIs of LT and IL show a slightly higher degree of activity on the left side, while MF is predominantly active on the right side. There was no significant difference in symmetry between the left and right sides for IL and MF, evident from the four features (mean $t = 0.46$ and $p < .65$). For LT, the RMS feature did not reveal any asymmetry ($t = 0.858$ and $p <.391$), but IEMG and WL indicated mild asymmetry between sides at a 99% confidence interval ($t = 1.6$ and $p < .01$) and WAMP at a 99.99% confidence interval ($t = 3.29$ and $p <.001$).

12.4.4 Comparison between Manual and Estimated Scores

Agreement between the manual and estimated MMT scores based on Cohen's kappa coefficient revealed a score of 0.48, suggesting moderate agreement. A significant difference in grading was observed for strength levels 4 and 4+ in agreement with a previous study [20] where good inter- and intra-rater agreement was reported for other grades compared to the grading of 4 and 4–5 on the modified MRC scale. As these grades represent fine deviations in strength, it poses greater difficulty for the examiner to accurately grade them. The current work based on EMG-based grading reduces this ambiguity and aids the examiner in selecting grades, making it more reliable.

12.4.5 Muscle-Wise Distribution of Grades

The distribution of strength grades in bilateral LT, IL and MF are shown in Figure 12.3a,b,c. About 50% of the participants exhibited medium strength grades (4 to 4+) for LT (left, $n = 44$ and right, $n = 47$) while IL (left, $n = 57$ and right, $n = 63$)

TABLE 12.5
Correlation between EMG Features and Bilateral Symmetry in Each Muscle Pair (Left and Right)

	Muscles								
	LT			IL			MF		
Features	*BSI*	*t*	*p*	*BSI*	*t*	*P*	*BSI*	*t*	*p*
RMS	0.018 (0.01)	0.858	.391	0.023 (0.19)	0.137	.890	–0.020 (0.19)	–0.282	.777
IEMG	0.062 (0.12)**	1.662	.098	0.021 (0.19)	0.086	.930	–0.020 (0.18)	–0.271	.786
WL	0.065 (0.13)**	1.660	.098	–0.115 (0.26)	0.567	.571	–0.013 (0.15)	–0.053	.957
WAMP	0.044 (0.12)*	3.291	.001	0.023 (0.07)	1.089	.277	0.003 (0.09)	–0.129	.896

*Significant at level $p < .01$.
**Significant at level $p < .1$.

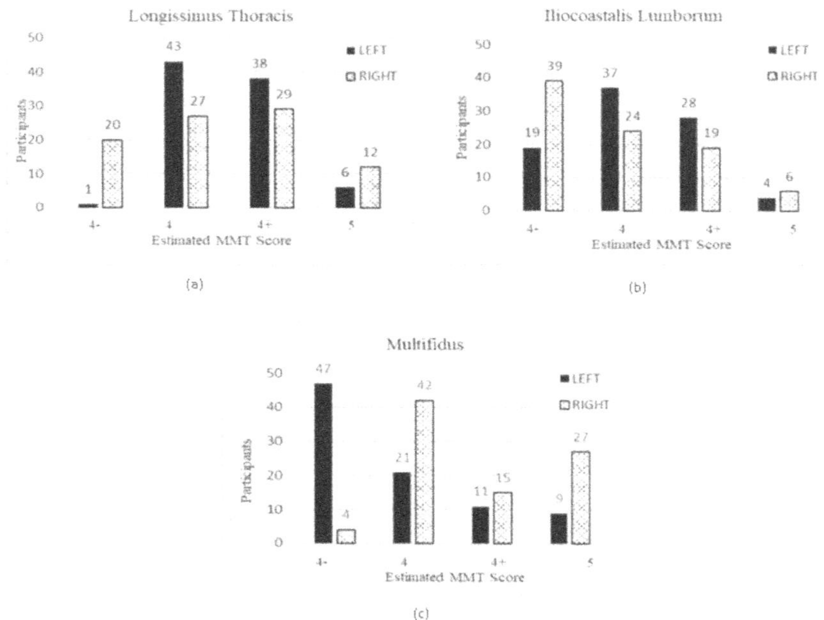

FIGURE 12.3 Estimated MMT grades (a) longissimus thoracis; (b) iliocostalis lumborum; and (c) multifidus.

strength was the lowest (4–to 4). MF showcased a significant difference between the left and right sides, where M_L had good numbers (*n* = 47) for strength level 4–, and M_R (*n* = 42) had the maximum numbers for strength level 4.

12.5 DISCUSSION

12.5.1 Current Limitations and Main Findings

The MMT procedure to grade individual muscles of the limb is quite established, but trunk muscles cannot be individually graded owing to the difficulty of manually locating the differences in strength of individual muscles. The use of dynamometry and myometry also has practical implications owing to the bulkiness of the back muscles, and any attempts require special arrangements for fitting the instruments onto the contours of the back [21]. The measurement can only give a gross score representing all the core muscles. While MMT requires an experienced and trained examiner to correctly predict strength grades [22], dynamometers need a huge age, gender and muscle/muscle group-wise normative database to compare the obtained force values [23]. Though a number of studies have reported a normative database for upper and lower extremity strengths [24, 25] and a few for cervical strength addressing neck pain [26], no recent studies have been reported for normative values of trunk muscle strength. The present chapter was able to identify individual muscle strengths of LT, IL and MF based on EMG features, quantifying them into finer grades of 4–, 4, 4+ and 5.

12.5.2 Contribution of EMG Features in Grading Muscles

Trichopterans explored the possible use of EMG features to grade strength levels of low back muscles of persons suffering from back pain. The relationship between RMS and strength grades has been well established in previous studies [27, 28], while IEMG and muscle tension have been identified in some [29]. The role of WL and WAMP has not been sufficiently explored, though they give details on the motor unit level. A combination of these four features for assessing strength grades has not been attempted in any study, though a similar study has used RMS alone for grading strength levels of tibialis muscles of hemiplegic patients [30].

12.5.3 Individual Variations in Muscle Strength

A comparison of strength levels between participants and their individual strengths has also been reported to see muscle activity trends during back pain. Very few participants had grade 5 strength levels for some muscles, a condition acceptable for back pain subjects. An overall decrease in IL strength, both left and right, is evident from Figure 12.2 across all participants and seen to be weaker when compared to the LT, whose strength scores were moderate. With respect to sides, the left side was weak when compared to the right, which can be attributed to the fact that all participants were right dominant, and postural adjustments toward the dominant side could have influenced the results.

12.5.4 Changes in Bilateral Symmetry

Mild changes in symmetry in the bilateral muscles were observed from IEMG, WL and WAMP features for the LT. WAMP showed significant changes in the LT ($p < .01$), providing an opportunity to investigate motor unit level changes in firing on both sides due to back pain. This can be attributed to the fact that, the LT being the important muscle that holds the lumbar and thoracic regions erect [21], asymmetry could have been caused by incorrect posture, a major reason for back pain. The distribution of strength grades of the MF was not uniform between the right and left sides, with the right being stronger compared to the left in a majority of the participants, but it did not show feature-level differences in symmetry, as seen in LT. Atrophy of the MF is an important factor associated with chronic back pain, and strengthening programs that increase MF muscle mass, as suggested in previous literature [31], are further recommended from the present chapter. Since the majority of the participants exhibited a weaker MF on the left side, exercises that specifically target the weaker side can be suggested. The MF has long been associated with major structural changes in patients with back pain; this chapter also confirms its intricate nature, requiring further insight.

12.5.5 Advantages and Limitations of Present Chapter

The major advantage of using EMG for muscle strength is the ease with which individual muscle strength can be graded irrespective of location when compared to dynamometers and myometers, which are difficult to use in regions other than limbs. EMG, as a measurement that involves a small cross-sectional area of the muscle underlying the electrodes, eliminates the need for gender-based demarcation in strength, as muscle strength per cm^2 is the same irrespective of gender [32]. This fact has brought EMG-based strength testing and MMT onto common ground, where the latter also does not take gender differences in consideration. The only issue in EMG-based measurements is the need for proper placement of electrodes at the muscle belly, as mild deviations can result in significant changes in feature values and can grossly affect strength measurements. Furthermore, studies involving deep-seated muscles cannot take advantage of this technique, as surface EMG can be picked up only from superficial muscles that can be palpated. Even with some limitations, there is still much scope for the proposed technique, as major muscles involving the trunk and limbs that have clinical significance can still be faithfully represented by EMG.

12.6 CONCLUSION

The present chapter emphasizes the use of selective EMG features for muscle strength grading, and the results are quite promising. The proposed method circumvents the major issues faced in current strength testing techniques (MMT and dynamometers) while also providing an opportunity to investigate intuitive changes associated with muscle physiology as a result of disease, injury and disuse. This dual benefits of EMG-based strength testing can be used in a routine clinical setup owing to the ease and minimal preparations with which the test can be successfully performed.

REFERENCES

[1] Hibbs AE, Thompson KG, French D, Wrigley A, Spears I. Optimizing performance by improving core stability and core strength. Sport Med. 2008;38:995–1008.
[2] Ripamonti M, Colin D, Rahmani A. Maximal power of trunk flexor and extensor muscles as a quantitative factor of low back pain. Isokinet Exerc Sci. 2011;19(2):83–89.
[3] Crowther A, McGregor AH, Strutton PH. Testing isometric fatigue in the trunk muscles. Isokinet Exerc Sci. 2007;15(2):91–97.
[4] Medical Research Council of the United Kingdom. Aids to the Examination of the Peripheral Nervous System. London: The White Rose Press; 1976.
[5] Fisher MI, Harrington S. Research round-up: manual muscle testing. Phys Ther Fac Publ Pap. 2015;47:1–2.

[6] Wikholm JB, Bohannon RW. Hand-held dynamometer measurements: tester strength makes a difference. J Orthop Sport Phys Ther. 2013;13:191–198.

[7] Ferrada RW, Rios CL, Perea RA, Mayorga JD, Rios CI. Isokinetic trunk strength in acute low back pain patients compared to healthy subjects: a systematic review. Int J Environ Res Public Health. 2021;18(5):2576.

[8] Ekstrom RA, Osborn RW, Hauer PL. Surface electromyographic analysis of the low back muscles during rehabilitation exercises. J Orthop Sport Phys Ther. 2008;38:736–745. doi: 10.2519/jospt.2008.2865.

[9] Ansari B, Bhati P, Singla D, Nazish N, Hussain ME. Lumbar muscle activation pattern during forward and backward walking in participants with and without chronic low back pain: an electromyographic study. J Chiropr Med. 2018;17:217–225.

[10] Oliver GD, Stone AJ, Plummer H. Electromyographic examination of selected muscle activation during isometric core exercises. Clin J Sport Med. 2010;20: 452–457.

[11] Donatelli RA. The anatomy and pathophysiology of the core. In: Sports-Specific Rehabilitation. Missouri: Churchill Livingstone, Elsevier Inc.; 2007.

[12] Ansari B, Bhati P, Singla D, Nazish N, Hussain ME. Lumbar muscle activation pattern during forward and backward walking in participants with and without chronic low back pain: an Electromyographic study. J Chiropr Med. 2018 17:217–222.

[13] Metral S, Cassar G. Relationship between force and integrated EMG activity during voluntary isometric anisotonic contraction. Eur J Appl Physiol. 1981;46:185–198.

[14] Phinyomark A, Phukpattaranont P, Limsakul C. Feature reduction and selection for EMG signal classification. Expert Syst Appl. 2012;39:7420–7431.

[15] Dennis T, He H, Todd K. Study of stability of time-domain features for electromyographic pattern recognition. J Neuroeng Rehabil. 2010;7:21.

[16] Bishop CM. Pattern Recognition and Machine Learning. New York: Springer; 2006.

[17] Saranya S, Poonguzhali S, Karunakaran S. Gaussian mixture model based clustering of Manual muscle testing grades using surface electromyogram signals. Phys Eng Sci Med. 2020;43(3):837–847.

[18] Dolatabadi E, Mansfield A, Patterson KK, Taati B, Mihailidis A. Mixture-model clustering of pathological gait patterns. IEEE J Biomed Health Inform. 2017;21:1297–1305. doi: 10.1109/JBHI.2016.2633000.

[19] Liao CF, Liaw LJ, Wang RY, Su FC, Hsu AT. Electromyography of symmetrical trunk movements and trunk position sense in chronic stroke patients. J Phys Ther Sci. 2015;27:2675–2681.

[20] Paternostro-Sluga, T, Grim-Stieger M, Posch M. Reliability and validity of the Medical Research Council (MRC) scale and a modified scale for testing muscle strength in patients with radial palsy. J Rehabil Med. 2008;40:665–671.

[21] Darby SA, Cramer GD. Muscles that influence the spine. In Clinical Anatomy of the Spine, Spinal Cord and ANS. 3rd ed. Missouri: Elsevier Inc., Mosby; 2017.

[22] Fan E, Ciesla ND, Truong AD, Bhoopathi V, Zeger SL, Needham DM. Inter-rater reliability of manual muscle strength testing in ICU survivors and simulated patients. Intensive Care Med. 2010;36:1038–1043.

[23] Benfica PDA, Aguiar LT, Brito SAF, Bernardino LHN, Teixeira-Salmela LF, Faria CDCM. Reference values for muscle strength: a systematic review with a descriptive meta-analysis. Braz J Phys Ther. 2018;22:355–369.

[24] Van HW, Blalock L, Merritt JL. Upper limb strength: study providing normative data for a clinical handheld dynamometer. PM&R. 2015;7:135–140.

[25] Andrews AW, Thomas MW, Bohannon RW. Normative values for isometric muscle force measurements obtained with hand-held dynamometers. Phys Ther. 1996;76:248–259.

[26] Garcés GL, Medina D, Milutinovic L, Garavote P, Guerado E. Normative database of isometric cervical strength in a healthy population. Med Sci Sports Exerc. 2002;34:464–470.

[27] Kuthe CD, Uddanwadiker RV, Ramteke AA. Surface electromyography based method for computing muscle strength and fatigue of biceps brachii muscle and its clinical implementation. Informatics Med Unlocked. 2018;12:34–43.

[28] Lippold CJ. The relation between integrated action potentials in a human muscle and its isometric tension. J Physiol.1952;117:492–499.

[29] Inman VT, Ralston HJ, Saunders JB, Feinstein B, Wright EW jr. Relation of human Electromyogram to muscular tension. Electroenceph Clin Neurophysiol. 1952;4:187–194.

[30] Li H, Zhao G, Zhou Y, Chen X, Ji Z, Wang L. Relationship of EMG/SMG features and muscle strength level: An exploratory study on tibialis anterior muscles during plantar-flexion among hemiplegia patients. Biomed Eng Online. 2014;13:1–15.

[31] Peter Fricker. Exercise increases muscle mass in those with low-back pain. Phys Sportsmed. 2002;30:15–16.

[32] Hettinger T. Physiology of Strength. Springfield, IL: Charles C Thomas Publisher; 1961.

13 IoT-Based Data Management and Systems for Public Healthcare

Ajay Sharma, Shashi Kala, Vandana Guleria and Varun Jaiswal

CONTENTS

DOI: 10.1201/9781003207856-13

13.1 INTRODUCTION TO THE HEALTHCARE SYSTEM

Healthcare systems, hospitals, clinics, and population wellness offices can be extremely dissimilar from other workplaces. Healthcare systems are troublesome, and there are numerous things you need to think about: Kinds of emergency clinic frameworks, patient considerations, protection, medical care suppliers, and other legitimate issues (Figure 13.1). A typical healthcare system consists of doctors, nursing staff, the hospital building, hardware utilized for therapy such as imaging machines (X-ray, UV, CT, MRI), and non-specialized supporting staff. In this section, the healthcare system, clinic framework, and patient framework are briefly described. The Internet of Things (IoT) plays a significant part in many of these services providing a medical services framework. Thus, it is important to find out how the medical services framework functions and where the IoT is now finding extension among current and conventional procedures.

13.1.1 Healthcare Systems

Figure 13.1 shows the relationship between the public healthcare team's hospital and community resource provider. There are several aspects of the healthcare system, including:

- Hospital systems
- Types of patient care
- Public health programs

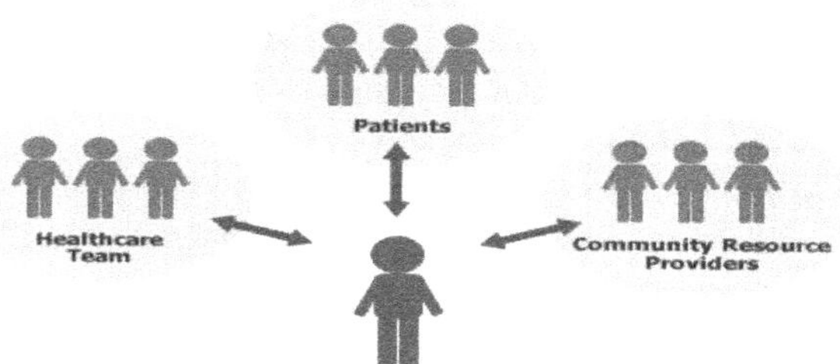

FIGURE 13.1 Healthcare relationships system.

13.1.2 Hospital Systems

A hospital system is a group of hospitals or services that work mutually to provide services to their communities. Different types of hospital systems have dissimilar types of ownership and financial goals. There are different types of hospital systems:

- **Public hospitals**
  Public clinics are supported and claimed by neighborhood, state, or central governments and receive cash from public authorities. Some open clinics are associated with clinical schools.
- **Non-profit hospitals**
  Non-profit hospitals are frequently community hospitals and may be associated with a religious denomination. The major goal of a non-profit hospital is to provide service to the community.
- **Private hospitals**
  Private clinics are owned by financial investors. They will probably acquire a benefit. Private clinics recommend more productive services, that is, restoration, elective or plastic medical procedures, or cardiology. They attempt to avoid nonbeneficial services, for example, crisis medication, which can lose cash because of uninsured patients.

13.1.3 Kinds of Patient Care

There are dissimilar types of care for patients, depending on their needs. Different types of patient care are:

- Primary care
- Specialty care
- Emergency care
- Urgent care
- Long-term care
- Mental health care

13.1.4 Healthcare Teams

Medical care is collaboration. Every medical care supplier is a group with a unique role. Some colleagues are specialists or professionals who help analyze illness. Others are specialists who treat illness or care for patients' physical and wellness needs. Healthcare colleagues include:

- Doctors
- Physician assistants
- Nurses

- Pharmacists
- Dentists
- Technologists and technicians
- Therapists and rehabilitation specialists
- Emotional, social, and spiritual support providers
- Administrative and support staff
- Community health workers and patient navigators

13.1.5 Internet of Things

The Internet of Things (IoT) describes the organization of actual "things" or items that have sensors, software, and different advancements. The motivation is associating and trading information with different procedures and frameworks over the web. The IoT can likewise be utilized in healthcare systems [1]. There are a numeral of genuine worries about danger in the development of IoT, particularly in the areas of protection and security; therefore, industry and administrative moves to address these concerns have started, including improvement of global standards [1, 2].

13.1.6 Applications of the Internet of Things

The wide variety of uses for IoT devices are regularly partitioned into buyer, business, mechanical, and foundation technologies. A growing sector of IoT devices are designed for shopper use, including vehicles, home computerization, wearable innovations, those associated with wellbeing, and machines with remote monitoring abilities. IoT devices are a piece of the bigger model which includes lighting, heating, air control, media, security frameworks, and camera systems [3, 4].

13.1.7 Organizational Applications

- The Internet of Medical Things (IoMT) is a use of the IoT for clinical- and wellbeing-related purposes, information assessment, examinations, and observations. The IoMT has been referred to as "Smart Healthcare," as it includes the innovation for creating a digitized medical healthcare system, interfacing available clinical resources and healthcare services [5, 6].
- IoT devices can be utilized to enable remote wellbeing checks and emergency notifications. These wellbeing-observing devices can change from pulse and heart rate monitors to advanced devices capable of checking specific devices, for example, pacemakers, FitBit electronic wristbands, and progressive listening devices [7].
- IoT devices can be utilized to screen and control the mechanical, electrical, and electronic frameworks utilized in different sorts of structures, for example, public, private, modern, organizational, and residential [7].

13.1.8 Industrial Applications

The Internet of Things is generally utilized in almost every field, including farming, fabricating, vehicles, heavy industry, delivery, and so on. In this section, we look at medical services. The IoT is broadly utilized in different types of automation in healthcare [8, 9].

- The IoT can connect different devices, for example, detecting individual proof, preparing communication, and organizing abilities. IoT-wise frameworks permit fast industrialization, enhancement of new products, and quick response to item requests.
- There are various IoT applications in farming, such as information on temperature, precipitation, humidity, wind speed, pest prevalence, and soil content. This information can be utilized to mechanize cultivating strategies, improve quality, and decrease the effort needed to manage crops.

13.1.9 How IoT Is Used in Different Fields of Healthcare

The IoT's versatility and network availability supply the best service because of its lower expense and ease of use. The primary focus of the Internet of Things in medical care services is to easily provide a rich client experience and improve patient satisfaction. A significant capacity of the IoT is to offer a network with clinical assets and dependable, successful, quality medical care services to mature patients who experience the ill effects of persistent illness. The IoT brings a smart medical care system into the clinical field that frequently includes smart sensors, a remote server, and the organization. This system can provide multi-dimensional highlights for observation and essential treatment ideas. A few applications used in healthcare systems are shown in Figure 13.2. IoT-based medical healthcare

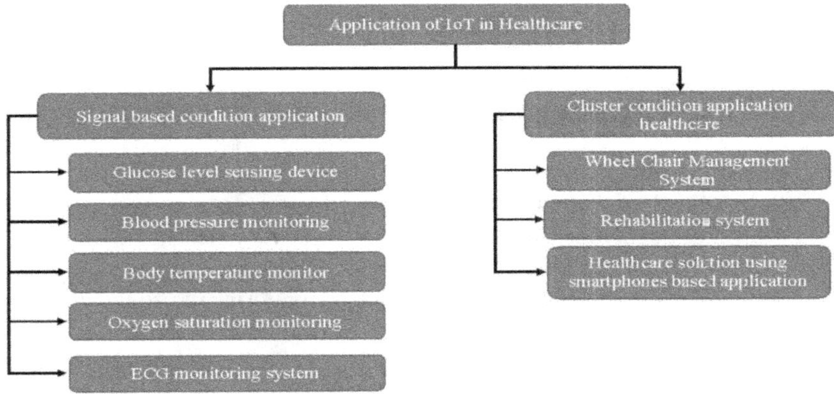

FIGURE 13.2 Classification of applications in IoT-based healthcare.

services are partitioned into two general classifications: Single-condition applications and clustered-condition applications [10–12].

13.1.9.1 Single-Condition Applications

Single-condition applications are divided into:

- **Glucose level sensing:** Diabetes is a metabolic disorder wherein the glucose level is higher than normal for a significant time. A blood glucose monitoring system checks individual blood glucose and assists with instructing the patient on the best preparation of meals, required exercises, and prescription times [11].
- **Blood pressure monitoring system:** Blood pressure determines the force with which the heart propels blood around the body. An IoT-based tool can check and control health requirements, for example, blood pressure (BP), hemoglobin (HB), sugar level in the blood, and cell improvement. IoT-based medical care systems are intended to screen pulse, diabetes, and obesity [13].
- **Body temperature monitoring:** Monitoring and estimating temperature is a fundamental part of healthcare. A body temperature monitoring system depends on the home being connected to the IoT system. It also assists in infrared identification and can have an radio-frequency identification module for checking and estimating internal body temperature
- **Oxygen saturation monitoring system:** A heartbeat oximeter is utilized for constant checking of oxygen saturation in the blood, and the use of the IoT with pulse oximetry is advantageous for innovation-based clinical care applications.
- **ECG (electrocardiogram) monitoring system:** ECG-observing devices can show ECG waves to the client/patient. These devices produce a clinical report for a patient by gathering ECG bio-flags and transferring the information to the cloud. This provides reasonable information to the user based on the composed data.

13.1.9.2 Clustered-Condition Applications

- **Wheelchair management system:** For seniors and disabled individuals, specialists have developed many different types of smart mechanized wheelchairs.
- **Rehabilitation system:** The IoT can develop rehabilitation systems regarding population development-related issues. Wheelchairs are furnished with different sensors which screen the assembling, position of seat with respect to patient and helps in the monitoring of patient/client's situation.
- **Lack of health expertise:** IoT sensors can recover the capacity of severely impaired individuals. A body sensor network is proposed to improve recovery. The philosophy of automated design holds that the

IoT can be an important medium for data connections. IoT-based recovery frameworks are designed software systems for adolescence, smart city clinical restoration, and incorporated application system for prisons in order to overcome from the lack of health expertise and to make them aware about the health issues.

- **Healthcare solutions using smartphones:** At present, cell phones can be used to control electronic devices with sensors. In the field of medical care systems, diverse applications for cell phones exist to help patients, outfit clinical instruction, and provide initial training. A few programming and hardware items have been created that communicate with the cell phone as a helpful device in medical care services.

13.1.9.3 Services of IoT in Healthcare

There are many services are provided by the IoT in healthcare, like living assistance and community healthcare such as children's healthcare. The following is a brief discussion on the services provided by the IoT in healthcare.

Ambient assisted living (AAL): In medical care systems, IoT innovations can help seniors as well as severely disabled individuals in daily life. The IoT in medical services can develop intelligent systems which can screen and record everyday activities of seniors or handicapped individuals residing in a smart environment. An AAL system depends on different sensors for estimating temperature, circulatory strain, glucose, oxygen, and weight. This system is generally adequate for patients with diabetes and cardiovascular arrhythmia. Ambient assisted living systems allow doctors and relatives to screen patients remotely.

Medical Internet of Things: Current advancements in information and communication technology (ICT) and IoT allow remote patient screening instead of diagnosing them in clinics. A patient can use specific sensors to gather wellbeing information and communicate it to data centers through the web so it is accessible for additional choices.

Community healthcare (CH): A community healthcare system is an organization that covers a local area. Local medical care can use a virtual health center, which is an IoT-based organization that screens the local area or housing area.

Children's health information (CHI): A children's health information system is a stage for kids to improve their health by changing their food habits when they are away from guardians and eating outside their homes. Kids can use cell phones to track food intake and receive notifications from their doctors or guardians. Clients can acknowledge food information through an augmented application.

IoT in healthcare: There are numerous fields in healthcare in which the Internet of Things can offer assistance, such as for patients, physicians, hospital staff, insurance agencies for the settlement of cases, and so forth. Smart devices have been created in various segments for the improvement of medical care, and they provide a superior and effective answer for the client instead of utilizing the traditional system.

- **IoT for patients:** Devices can be in the form of wearables like wellness apps and other remotely associated devices like circulatory strain monitors, pulse checkers, and glucometers. These devices can be tuned to help to remember carbohydrate levels, practice a check, monitor pulse changes, and much more. The IoT has changed people, particularly older patients, by allowing tracking of health conditions. This significantly affects individuals living alone and their families. On any incident or changes in the normal routine of an individual, the instrument conveys messages to relatives and concerned wellbeing providers such as health providers [14, 15].
- **IoT for physicians:** By utilizing wearables and other home checking gear installed with the IoT, doctors can monitor patients' wellbeing more successfully. They can follow patients' adherence to therapy plans or any requirements for clinical consideration. The IoT empowers medical service experts to be more careful and interact with patients proactively. Information gathered from IoT devices can assist doctors with determining the best treatment measures for patients to arrive at normal outcomes [14, 15].
- **IoT for hospitals:** Apart from checking patients' wellbeing, there are numerous different areas where IoT devices are extremely valuable in medical clinics. IoT devices labeled with sensors can be utilized to track the location of clinical hardware like wheelchairs, defibrillators, nebulizers, oxygen tanks, and other diagnostic gear. The position of clinical staff in various areas can likewise be examined in real time. The spread of diseases is a significant worry for patients in clinics. IoT-empowered cleanliness-observing devices help prevent patients from becoming infected [27]. IoT devices additionally help in resources like pharmacy stock control and ecological observation, for example, checking cooler temperature and humidity and temperature control. The IoT-based smart clinic is gaining more interest in the literature. Various investigations on IoT innovation and smart clinics are proposing new arrangements and mechanical innovations [14–16].
- **IoT for health insurance companies:** There are various advantages for health safety net providers with IoT-associated smart devices. Insurance agencies can use information captured by wellbeing-checking devices for their endorsing and claims activities. This information will empower them to discover fraud and recognize possibilities for endorsing. IoT devices provide guarantors and clients with accurate information for endorsing, valuing, dealing with cases, and hazard appraisal measures. Backup plans may offer motivation to their clients for using and sharing wellbeing information created by IoT devices. They can compensate clients for utilizing IoT devices to monitor their standard routines, adherence to treatment plans, and preventive health measures. This will assist insurers with decreasing cases overall. IoT devices can also enable insurance agencies to approve claims through the information captured by these devices [17, 18].

13.2 ROLE OF BIG DATA IN HEALTHCARE AND THE CHALLENGES ASSOCIATED WITH BIG DATA IN HEALTHCARE

Across industries, big data has changed the way we manage, analyze, and use data. Healthcare is one of the main fields where data analytics is having a significant impact. Indeed, healthcare analytics can lower medical rates, predict infectious outbreaks, prevent preventable illnesses, and increase the overall quality of life. The average lifespan for humans is rising around the world, posing new challenges to current care delivery methods. Researchers and health practitioners are capable of gathering large volumes of data and are looking for the best ways to use it [19].

Why and how can the IoT help? What are the barriers to its implementation? We'll look at some existing big data examples of healthcare that medical-based institutions can benefit from. But first, let's look at the fundamentals of big data analytics in healthcare. Big data in healthcare refers to vast amounts of data generated by the introduction of digital technology that captures patient records and aids in the management of hospital results that would be too broad and complex for traditional, conventional technologies [19, 20].

The use of big data analytics in healthcare has a number of lifesaving and positive implications. Big data, in essence, refers to the large amounts of digital data consolidated and analyzed using unique technology [21]. Healthcare data can help prevent outbreaks, cure disease, decrease costs, and so on. Treatment models have evolved as we have lived longer, and many of these changes are primarily informed by data [22]. Doctors try to learn as much as they can about their patients as early as possible in their lives. Prevention is better than cure when it comes to healthcare data analytics, and key success metrics, and being able to draw a comprehensive image of a patient, would enable insurers to have a customized plan. Patient data are everywhere and must be captured in bits and bytes and archived in hospitals, clinics, and procedures, among other places; see Figure 13.3. Indeed, collecting massive volumes of data for medical purposes has

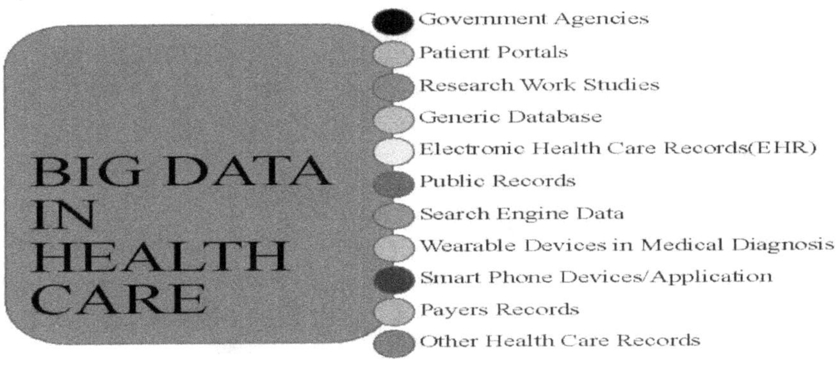
BIG DATA
IN
HEALTH
CARE
Government Agencies
Patient Portals
Research Work Studies
Generic Database
Electronic Health Care Records(EHR)
Public Records
Search Engine Data
Wearable Devices in Medical Diagnosis
Smart Phone Devices/Application
Payers Records
Other Health Care Records

FIGURE 13.3 Big data in healthcare.

been expensive and time consuming for years [23]. With today's ever-improving technology, it's easier to not only gather such data but also to generate detailed healthcare reports and transform them into critical insights to improve treatment. This is the goal of healthcare data analytics: To use data-driven results to not only anticipate and fix a problem before it's too late but also to evaluate methods and therapies more quickly, keep better track of accounts, and maintain patients' comfort by providing them with the resources they need to do so.

13.2.1 Five Vs of Big Data

In recent years, big data was defined by the "3Vs," but now there are "5Vs"; see Figure 13.4, which shows the 5 Vs of big data, also known as big data characteristics [24]:

1. **Volume:** The term "big data" refers to a massive amount of information. The term "volume" refers to a large amount of data. The size of data plays a critical role in determining its worth. When data are very large, they are called "big data." The volume of data therefore determines if a data collection can be considered a big data collection. Therefore, it is important to assume a certain volume when dealing with big data. For instance: The estimated worldwide mobile traffic in 2016 was 6.2 exabytes per month (6.2 billion GB). We will have nearly 40,000 exabytes of data by 2020.
2. **Velocity:** The term "velocity" denotes the rapid accumulation of data. Data comes in at a high rate from machines, networks, social media, cell phones, and other outlets for big data. A vast and incessant flow of data exists. This determines the data's potential, or how quickly data are produced and processed to meet demands. Data sampling can assist in dealing with issues such as velocity. For example, more than 3.5 billion searches per day are carried out on Google. In addition, Facebook users grow by approximately 22% annually.

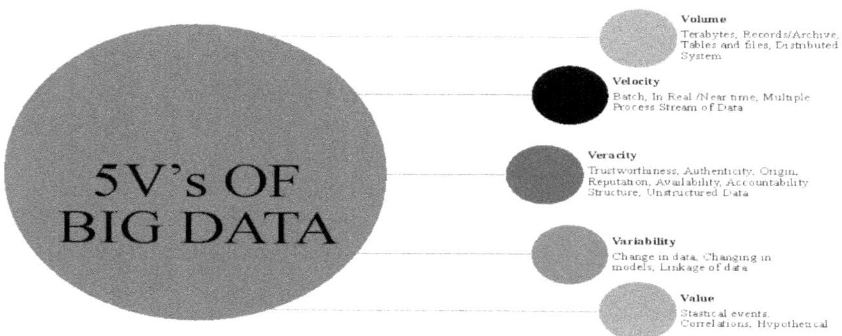
5V's OF
BIG DATA
Volume
Terabytes, Records/Archive, Tables and files, Distributed System
Velocity
Batch, In Real /Near time, Multiple Process Stream of Data
Veracity
Trustworthiness, Authenticity, Origin, Reputation, Availability, Accountability Structure, Unstructured Data
Variability
Change in data, Changing in models, Linkage of data
Value
Stastical events, Correlations, Hypothetical

FIGURE 13.4 Five Vs of big data.

3. **Variety:** Variety denotes structured, semi-structured, and unstructured data types. It may also apply to a variety of sources. Variety refers to the influx of data from new sources within and outside an organization. They can be organized, semi-organized, or unorganized:
   Structured data: These are data that have been organized. It refers generally to data that have been defined in terms of length and format.
   Semi-structured data: This type of data is semi-organized. It is a type of data that do not adhere to the formal structure of data. Log files are an example of this data type.
   Unstructured data: These data are essentially unorganized. It refers generally to data which do not properly fit a relational database's traditional row and column structure. Texts, images, and videos are examples of unstructured data that cannot be stored in the form of rows and columns.
4. **Veracity:** This denotes irregularities and uncertainty in data. Data that are available can sometimes become cluttered, and quality and accuracy are challenging to control. Big data is also variable due to the plethora of data dimensions resulting from a diverse set of data types and foundations. For example, bulk data may lead to confusion if less than half or incomplete data are transmitted.
5. **Value:** The majority of data with no value is useless to the company unless it is converted into something useful. Data alone are of no use or importance, but they need to be turned into something useful for information extraction. Value is thus the most significant of the 5 Vs.

13.3 CHALLENGES IN HEALTHCARE IoT

Several challenges, however, must be overcome. Stable, flexible, and interoperable systems can be developed for digital healthcare. We'll go over some of the present roadblocks to the extensive acceptance of digital healthcare. Big data storage technology has become critical in recent years for storing massive amounts of clinical data. Cloud storage becomes massive, and it is managed by big data. According to recent research, the combination of big data and the cloud is influencing remote healthcare. Amazon Elastic MapReduce (EMR) [25] offers a dissimilar way to manage large amounts of data and load them onto a cluster. The Amazon EMR has a separate function for loading data into the HBase cluster [26]. Loading sensor data from Amazon S3 to HBase can be done with the Apache Pig tool [27]. Apache Pig is used for analysis of the data in distributed databases that dramatically extend the scalable functionality to healthcare applications. Google Cloud Platform consoles are also developed as a lightweight model to simulate large data in IoT heterogeneous data [28].

The IoT has been used in a variety of ways to deliver different types of support for the healthcare system, such as patient monitoring and a smart home scheme for diabetic patients. The following are the major issues that occur in the healthcare system. IoT enables high flexibility; for example, if a patient needs continuous care, they can live at home rather than in a hospital and be observed regularly using IoT technology. Some wearable devices, such as sensors, are painful to the patient's body. Data from the sensors are transferred to the control unit and then to the monitoring center, which will affect data quality due to noise. An improved architecture aids in the transmission of data while preserving its integrity. A noise removal method can also be used to improve the data signal. The majority of existing ECG monitoring methods involve supervised signal analysis. This raises the cost and may result in detection errors [29–31]. Machine learning can be applied to signal analysis, thereby enhancing performance and reducing the costs, as we will see later. The processing of a higher number of sensors and devices necessitates more energy, which increases power leakage and energy consumption. To reduce energy consumption, an optimization algorithm can be used. The monitoring of a large number of IoT users requires more storage and mainframe resources, which can be prevented by storing cloud data. IoT cloud integration, however, increases the complexity. Another major problem in IoT is data protection, as devices are more susceptible to attack. These devices are resource poor and make it difficult to use encryption techniques.

- **Security and privacy:** IoT devices may pose a security and privacy threat to users. Unauthorized IoT device access could be a significant risk for the health and private information of patients. The connected devices collect, combined, process, and transfer medical data to the cloud, including medical and mobile devices. Cloning, spoofing, RF jamming, and cloud polling are vulnerabilities of the device layer. Traffic in the cloud polls can be redirected to permit man-in-the-middle command injections directly to a device. Distributed denial of service attack (DDoS) attacks may have a negative influence on health systems and impact the safety of patients. Although there is a common defense against a DDoS attack (the use of multiple devices on the network), duplication of resources may not always be possible in a healthcare environment, because certain devices are life critical. Due to the number and complexity of emerging vulnerabilities, software and hardware are still a challenge [32].

  We also saw a rise in the number of wearable electronic devices in recent years (including various embedded sensors and medical devices). The absence of security ethics and the availability of powerful search engines to locate devices connected to wearable devices make them vulnerable to all kinds of attacks. Recently, numerous wireless networking technologies have also been used in healthcare environments, including Wi-Fi, which is used to connect various types of medical devices and sensors. The protection against eavesdropping and attacks and security of these wireless and sensor technologies is a challenge. Centralized personal datasets, family history, electronic medical records, and genomic data should also be sheltered against hackers and malicious software, and their security and privacy should be ensured [32, 33].

Privacy and confidentiality are significant concerns for doctors, too. The sensitive nature of healthcare data means that patients may not wish to share or record their medical records (for example, cancer or HIV test results). There is concern about the possible confidentiality of health information with integration into the current medical information systems of connected technology. The anxiety that digital and associated technologies might attract hackers is responsible for these concerns about data security [33].

Recent research claimed that 25% of cyberattacks would target IoT devices by 2020:

- Infiltration with malware: 24%
- Phishing attacks: 24%
- Social engineering attacks: 18%
- Device misconfiguration issues: 11%
- Increasing privilege: 9%
- Credential robbery: 6%

- **Internal authentication and interoperability issues:** The creation of internal authentication for the performance of digital health transactions is critical for enterprises operating in different areas. Shibboleth is a federated identity solution that facilitates the authentication of entities within and between systems. Shibboleth has been deployed and successfully tested at the national level and is a system that provides inter-realm verification. A typical system allows a user of a digital healthcare system to authenticate to an identity provider and then sends a service application for a service provider (SP). However, due to the lack of facilities for hosting separate identity and service providers at the country level, not all of our digital health systems have these implementations and have all similar digital health infrastructure in the organization. Lack of IT expertise and the required Third World funding especially prevent system-ready implementation [33, 34].

The absence of interoperability between countries intending to cooperate with digital ICT infrastructures is another aspect which needs to be taken into account in the question of digital health. This weakness is due to the limited information technology infrastructures or lack of IT skills, as well as a failure of international cooperation policies to exchange sensitive medical information between nations that would make telemedicine easier and provide high-quality medical care remotely [34].

The lack of interoperability between heterogeneous inter-realm authentication platforms and standards is recognized as an impending vulnerability that can cause data privacy loss and compliance problems and interfere with retrospective compatibility with legacy systems. A lack of generalized digital health adoption, especially in countries with insufficient bandwidth, was reduced by sufficient standards for seamless, digital health transactions across several continents. The presence of a centralized X.509 digital certification authority (CA) enables both encryption and digital signing of patient prescriptions via public key data encryption to enable data integrity and verification. The presence of backend systems makes it easier for federated digital health systems to share authentication information. The architecture allows user attributes and authenticated entities to be declared. The confidentiality of claims on digital health status depends entirely on the strength of the computer board chip [33, 34].

- **Health information exchange (HIE) barriers:** The exchange of health information enhances the provision of healthcare by providing reliable and secure electronic communication of health information between various healthcare organizations. Currently, the following methods are used for HIE: Exchange, direct exchange, and question-based exchange mediated by the consumer [35].

  Consumer-mediated discussion provides patients access to their electronic data, enabling them to track their health conditions, detect incorrect billing or medical data, and modernize their reports. Vital information, such as laboratory test results and drug dosage, is transferred by healthcare organizations to other experts in the care of the same patient. Consultative exchanges typically take place in emergency medical care when a healthcare organization needs a new patient's previous health records. The HIE system is used to request access to these records [35].

  An important concern and an emerging threat to health information management system is the development of health cybercrime. Infringements of security in hospitals could cost them up to $7 million in damaged reputation, penalties, litigation, and so on. In organizations like Anthem, CareFirst, Premera, and UCLA Health Systems, major infringements have occurred. This resulted in 143 million records of patients being exposed through cyber-attacks, which represented 45% of the US population. In a cyber-safety analysis carried out by the Society for Healthcare Information and Management Systems in 2015, 64% of health organizations have been exposed to external cyber-attacks over the previous 12 months.

- **Device communication:** Communication is one of the biggest concerns for implementing intelligent or connected health. Now there are many devices with data collection sensors that frequently communicate with a server. There is a proprietary protocol for each manufacturer, meaning that instruments made by dissimilar producers cannot necessarily communicate with each other. In combination with privacy concerns, this fragmented software environment isolates valuable data islands, often undermining the key IoT idea.

  The presence of several devices also raises concerns related to the use of wireless network technologies to connect medical devices. For example, people who use a wireless personal area network (WPAN) device are expected to move freely, but the movement could cause collisions in similar frequency channels. WPAN collisions have several disruptive effects because of performance reduction and can lead to disasters, especially in the case of healthcare. There are therefore different types of wireless communication technologies which are essential to ensure that medical devices work properly if connected. The use of intelligent health systems by physicians is not always easy. A wide variety of features might sometimes complicate a system, which demotivates health workers in turn to learn how to use it. Both users and service providers need interoperability within and among IoT domains. This creates complex challenges because a diverse group of regulatory agencies regulates the different disciplines covered by IoT. In associated health situations, medical standards demand especially stringent rules, so this complexity is exacerbated further.

- **Collection and management of data:** IoT sensor devices face several challenges in the digital healthcare system. The data come from sensors used with or implanted into the human body. Due to the continuously changing state of the human body, a constant inflow of data occurs. Also, the data collected are varied (consisting of various data formats). Electrocardiograph data, for example, are frequently encoded in XML, while camera-based data are usually recorded in various image formats. A health-related scenario comprises interdependent, heterogeneous connected components and concerns, including devices, networks, systems (with large volumes of data), variety and speed (recovered from different sources), and truthfulness (uncertain data). To manage their continually varying cyber-physical components, digital health systems should be designed using appropriate data-driven training techniques. Proper data analyses can provide valuable information on the health conditions of patients. Over the past decade, researchers, pharmaceutical companies, and healthcare providers have been developing various tools for data analysis to enable usable knowledge to be quickly extracted from patient data. Due to the absence of standardized formats for data collection and the volume and speed of data generated in healthcare environments, several challenges exist. In terms of big data, integrity is also crucial. Incorrect information may give rise to wrong decisions and long-term strategic planning. Due to the frequent provenance of data form different sources in healthcare, robust authentication systems are necessary to ensure the provision of healthcare data from actual registrars and hospitals. It is difficult enough to collect information in a healthcare system that is clean, formatted, thorough, and accurate. Moreover, the definitions of healthcare and metrics are complex, and the healthcare industry continues to change.
- **Design and implementation based on multi-disciplinary knowledge:** A digital health system is developed with many fields of expertise, including embedded systems, network design, database analysis,

and bioengineering. Digital health is also being developed. Knowledge about disease in many fields is essential to the creation and employment of such a heterogeneous system. The system must also constantly evolve to meet changing needs. For example, smart health systems with certain healthcare systems such as ultrasound and CAT scans are currently being limitedly integrated.

- **Compatibility and interoperability of different IoT systems [36]:** According to market analysts at McKinsey, we accomplish interoperability between different IoT systems by between 40% and 60% of total values. It is problematic to maintain interoperability with numerous vendors, OEMs, and service providers between various IoT systems. The IoT's integral components are sensors and networking. Not every machine has the ability to communicate and share data effectively using advanced sensors and networking capabilities. In addition, sensors with different capacity and safety standards incorporated in legacy machines cannot achieve the same results.
- **Identification, authentication and integration of technologies with IoT platforms:** According to a Gartner report (2020) there are currently around 20 billion connected devices, and connecting these devices does not just involve complexity but significant security risks. A large number of connected devices must be formalized and system architecture implemented on one platform to identify and authenticate such devices. Companies need to integrate different IoT-connected products with the right IoT platforms to successfully implement IoT applications. Failure to integrate properly could lead to function and efficiency abnormalities in giving clients value. The major challenge here is not to use too many IoT endpoints and statements to add sensor data and pass them on to IoT platforms. Only with deep integration can companies use big data to gain insight and predict the results.
- **Handling unstructured data [37]:** The challenges of managing unstructured data in terms of volume parameters, speed, and variety are increasing with increasingly connected devices. The real challenge for companies, however, is to determine the value of the data, as only data of high quality can be used. A survey found that 80% of current data are unstructured data, and therefore the data can't be stored in SQL format. Stored in NoSQL format, unstructured data make data recovery somewhat complicated. The problems and difficulty of handling unstructured data have decreased somewhat with the launch of big data frameworks such as Hadoop and Cassandra, but big data itself is so large that, combined with the IoT, managing it is a huge task. Also, there are no standard data and metadata retention and use guidelines.
- **Intelligent analytics:** We are currently translating data into meaningful information, that is, to the IoT itself. A data or data model defect could lead to false-positive and false-negative results. We must understand that

the information is not an insight itself; rather, the correct questions must be asked from the exact data to gain insight.

- **Delivering value:** According to the Forbes Insights Survey, the quality of IoT technology is the major challenge for 29% of management in building IoT capabilities. These data reveal the struggle of IoT development firms to provide their consumers value. So, a business must clearly define what value through what capacity before IoT applications are developed and how their solution improves efficiency, productivity, and customer satisfaction. Since the IoT is concerned with "connected things," IoT projects require a high degree of support throughout the process. Approximately 50% of IoT-initiated companies are strong suppliers of IT services and consulting companies that rely on them to provide solutions and advice on business.

13.3.1 Applications of Big Data in Healthcare

Now that you understand the importance of big data, let's explore the real-world applications showing how an analysis can improve processes, improve patient care, and eventually save lives [38, 39].

- **Patient predictions for improved staffing:** We will look to the traditional issue of shift managers, our first big-data example in healthcare: How many people do I employ in a certain period? You risk superfluous labor costs if you employ too many workers. Too few employees can achieve poor customer service results or even be fatal to patients in this industry. At least in a few Paris hospitals, big data helps to solve this problem. An Intel White Paper details how four hospitals in Paris use data from a range of sources to predict the number of patients expected to be admitted every day and hour. One of the key tools data scientists use is time series analysis. These analyses enable scientists to see relevant admission rate patterns. Then, you can find the most precise algorithms that forecast future admission trends using machine learning. The data science team has developed a web-based user interface that forecasts the burden of patients and helps to plan the assignment of resources using online data visualization to improve overall patient care [20, 39].
- **Real-time alerting:** Additional instances of healthcare data analytics segment one key feature, real-time alertness. Clinical decision support (CDS) software analyzes on-site medical data to provide advice to health professionals on prescription choices. Doctors, however, wish to keep patients away from hospitals so that costly treatments are avoided. Analytics has the potential to form part of the new strategy and was already one of the keywords for business intelligence in 2019. Wearables continuously collect health information from patients and transmit it to the cloud. Further, this information is accessible within the general public health database, which allows physicians to compare and modify delivery strategies in

a socio-economic context. Organizations and advanced healthcare management tools are used to track this massive stream of data and to react when there are troubling results. If, for instance, the patient's blood pressure increases alarmingly, the doctor is sent a real-time alarm and can take action to reach the patient and reduce the pressure [39].

- **Enhancing patient engagement:** Many consumers are already interested in intelligent devices that record their steps, heart rate, sleep habits, and so on. Many consumers are also potential patients. All this essential information can be combined with other trackable information to identify potential health risks. Chronic insomnia and high heart rate can indicate, for example, the risk for future cardiac disease. Patients are directly involved in health monitoring, and health insurance incentives can lead them to a healthy lifestyle. Another way to do this is to develop new wearables, track specific trends in health, and transfer them to the cloud, where doctors can monitor them. Patients with asthma or blood pressure can benefit from this, be more independent, and reduce unnecessary visits to doctors [20, 39].
- **Prevent opioid abuse/provide tracking and monitoring of illegal drugs:** Another instance of big data healthcare addresses a problem in the United States. This is a sobering fact: This year, overdoses of misused opioids in the United States have caused more accidental deaths than road accidents, which had been the most common cause of accidental death. It became such a problem for Canada that opioid abuse was declared a "national health crisis," and in the United States, President Obama allocated $1.1 billion to develop solutions to this problem during his time in office. Again, applying big data analysis in healthcare may be the answer for everyone: Blue Cross Blue Shield data scientists have started to work with fuzzy logic analysis experts to address the problem [39].
- **Using health data for informed strategic planning:** Based on better insight into people's motives, the use of big data can aid strategic planning in the field of care. Care managers can analyze the results of monitoring among people in dissimilar population groups and identify which factors prevent people from receiving treatment. Google Maps and free public health data were utilized by the University of Florida to prepare heat maps that address a range of problems, including chronic diseases and population growth. Researchers then compared the available health services to the most heated areas with this information [39].
- **Big data might cure cancer [40]:** An interesting example of the use of large-scale data in healthcare is the Cancer Moonshot Program. Before his second term, President Obama had a program that aimed to find a successful cure for cancer. Medical scientists can use large numbers of cancer patient treatment plans and recovery rates to look for trends and treatments in the highest real-world success rates. For instance, in biobanks connected to patient therapy records, researchers could examine tumor samples. Using these data, researchers can look at things such as

how certain mutations and cancer proteins interact with various treatments. These data may also have unforeseeable advantages, such as the finding that the antidepressant desipramine has the ability to treat certain lung cancer types. Patient databases from different institutions, such as hospitals, universities, and non-profit organizations, should, however, be linked in order to make these insights available. For instance, researchers could then access other institutions' patient biopsy reports. Genetically sequencing cancer tissue samples from patients from clinical trials and providing these data for the broader cancer database were among the potential large cases of data use in healthcare.

- **Predictive analytics in healthcare [29, 40]:** Two years in succession, we have already recognized that predictive analysis is one of the largest trends in business intelligence, but potential applications go much further than business. Optum Labs, a collaborative US research firm, collected EHRs of more than 30 million patients for predictor analysis instruments that improve care provision. Online corporate intelligent healthcare aims to enhance patient treatment by helping doctors make data-based decisions in seconds. This is especially useful in patients suffering from multiple conditions with complex medical histories.
- **Telemedicine:** Telemedicine has been available on the market for 40 years now, but it has only been able to flourish today with the arrival of online video lectures, smartphones, wireless appliances, and wearables [41]. The term refers to the provision of technologically remote clinical services. It is first and foremost used in consultations, remote patient monitoring, and healthcare professionals' medical education. Telesurgery is more specific; doctors are able to perform robotic operations and have access to a fast real-time data supply if they cannot actually be at a patient's location. Clinicians use telemedicine to provide individualized treatment plans and prevent re-admission or hospitalization. This use of data analysis in healthcare can be linked to the previously seen use of extrapolative analysis. Clinicians are able to prevent deterioration in inpatient conditions and predict acute medical events in advance. Telemedicine helps reduce costs and enhance the quality of service by keeping patients out of hospitals. Patients can avoid waiting in lines, and doctors will not waste their time on inconvenient consultations and red tape. Telemedicine also enhances the availability of care, since patient condition can be monitored, and patients can consult a doctor anywhere [42].
- **Integrating big data with medical imaging:** Medical imagery is dynamic, and some 600 million imaging procedures are conducted every year in the United States. The manual analysis and storage of these images is time and money consuming, as radiologists are essential to individually check each image, while hospitals require several years of storage. Provider of medical imagery Carestream explains how large-scale health analytics can change the way images are read: An algorithm has developed analysis such that specific images could be identified by

hundreds of thousands pixel patterns and converted to numbers that help doctors diagnose them. It may be that radiologists do not have to look at the images anymore but rather analyze algorithms that study and remember more images. That would undoubtedly affect the role, education, and skills of radiologists.

- **Suicide, self-harm prevention, advanced risk, and disease management:** Almost 800,000 people worldwide die each year as a result of suicide. Furthermore, 17% of the people of the world will self-harm at some point in their lives. Although this issue is very difficult to address, the use of big data in healthcare helps to affect suicides and self-harm positively. Health institutions can use data analysis to view large numbers of patients daily to identify people who may harm themselves. To deal with a hospitalization risk in certain patients with chronic diseases, big data and healthcare are essential. By studying types of drugs and symptoms, medical institutions can provide accurate prevention and ultimately reduce hospital admissions.
- **Improved supply chain management:** If the supply chain of a medical institution is weakened or fragmented, the rest of the system will likely suffer in terms of long-term care, treatment, and finances. For big data in health instances, however, analytics focus on the value of maintaining the supply chain efficiently every day. By using analytical tools to track the metrics of the supply chain and making accurate, data-based decisions regarding operations and expenditure, hospitals can save up to $10 million per annum. Descriptive and predictive analytical models can improve price negotiations, reduce supply variation, and optimize the whole ordering process. This allows medical institutions to prosper in the long term while providing patients with vital treatment without potentially catastrophic delays, snags, or encounters.
- **Developing new therapies and innovations:** The last example of our health analysis is working in the medical industry for a brighter and bolder future. Big data is powerful in healthcare to help in the development of new therapies and innovative drug findings. Health professionals' use of historical, detailed, and predictable metrics as well as a cohesive combination of data visualization techniques can detect potential strengths and weaknesses in trials or processes. Big data analysis can play a key role in developing ground-breaking new medicines and future-oriented therapies in healthcare by analyzing genetic information and predicting reactions in patients. Healthcare data analytics can streamline, innovate, secure, and save lives. It provides trust and clarity and is the way to progress.

13.3.2 How to Use Big Data in Healthcare

Overall, trends have been identified in the field of healthcare analytics: A dramatic increase in patient experience, including quality of therapy and satisfaction levels, sustainable overall population health improvements, and a significant reduction in operational costs [43–45]. Let us now look at a particular example of how data analytics can be used in medical care:

- **Big data in healthcare applied on a hospital dashboard:** This health dashboard gives you an impression as a director of the hospital or institutional manager. In a core point, you have a large picture of your hospital that will be of great assistance for its smooth operations, gathering all the data on each division and its nature, costs, and so on. The most important indicators of various aspects are shown here: The number of hospitalized patients, how long they stayed and where, the cost of treatment, and the average wait time in emergencies. This holistic perspective helps top management recognize eventual bottlenecks, tendencies, and patterns over time. [45].
- **Big data healthcare applications in patient care:** Our dynamic patient dashboard is another realistic application of large data analysis in healthcare, designed for enhancing service standards and treatment accuracy throughout departments. It is visually balanced. Medical institutes can achieve synchronization between departments by offering a combination of patient-centered information in a central place and streamline care developments in a wealth of critical areas. For example, bed occupancy rate metrics provide a window on where resources may be required, and senior management provides information about how they need to reduce expensive patient display system while tracking cancelled or missed appointments. In this section, you can find all you need to improve patient attention in real time and on a long-term basis [45].

13.3.3 Healthcare Systems for Public Health

IoT technology helps hospitals track staff and patients through remote monitoring and virtual access; IoT medical devices make chronic disease care easier; IoT automates the workflow of patient care and quickly processes the collection and analysis of data so everyone is on the same page, thereby reducing inefficiencies and errors. Figure 13.5

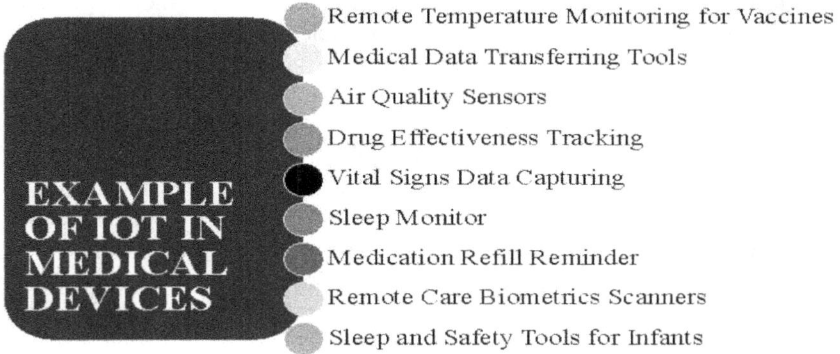

EXAMPLE OF IOT IN MEDICAL DEVICES
Remote Temperature Monitoring for Vaccines
Medical Data Transferring Tools
Air Quality Sensors
Drug Effectiveness Tracking
Vital Signs Data Capturing
Sleep Monitor
Medication Refill Reminder
Remote Care Biometrics Scanners
Sleep and Safety Tools for Infants

FIGURE 13.5 Examples of IoT medical devices.

shows an example of IoT devices in different healthcare areas. They can enhance pharmaceutical manufacturing processes, which can result in reduced prices for drugs. Health costs can even be reduced by streamlining the overall process.

13.3.4 Healthcare Monitoring Devices

IoT devices provide health professionals a number of new possibilities for monitoring patients, as well as for supervising patients. In addition, the range of wearable IoT devices offers healthcare workers and their patients a wide range of benefits and challenges [46].

- **Remote patient monitoring:** The most popular use of IoT healthcare equipment is remote patient monitoring. In IoT systems, the need to travel to providers or for patients to collect them themselves can be eliminated automatically by taking health metrics such as cardiac rate, blood pressure, temperature, and much more from patients who do not have to physically be in health facilities. When a patient's data are collected by an IoT device, it transfers information to a software application where health workers and/or patients can view it. To recommend treatments or to generate an alert, data analysis may done be using algorithms. An IoT sensor, for example, that detects an unusually low cardiac rate in a patient may create an alert for healthcare professionals. One major challenge for remote patient monitoring devices is to ensure safe and private data collection by these IoT devices.
- **Glucose monitoring:** Glucose monitoring has traditionally been difficult for the over 30 million Americans with diabetes. It is not only uncomfortable to check the glucose level and record results manually, but that also reports the level of glucose in a patient just at the exact time of the test. Periodic tests may not be adequate to detect problems if the levels fluctuate widely. IoT instruments can help tackle these difficulties by continuing automatic glucose monitoring in patients. Glucose monitors eliminate manual recording requirements and can alert patients to problems with glucose levels. These experiments include the design of a glucose monitoring IoT device that is sufficiently small to continuously monitor the patient without causing disruption and uses less power so that it doesn't need to be recharged frequently. However, these are no insurmountable challenges, and these devices promise to revolutionize the way patients handle the monitoring of glucose.
- **Heart rate monitoring:** Even for patients who are in health facilities, heart rate monitoring, like glucose, may be challenging. Periodic controls on the heart rate do not protect against rapid heart rate fluctuations, and the conventional cardiac monitoring devices used in hospitals require that patients be permanently attached to wired machines that impair their mobility. A variety of small IoT device systems for cardiac monitoring are now available, allowing patients to move freely while

continuously monitoring their hearts. It is a challenge to ensure ultra-accurate results, but most modern devices can provide accuracy rates of approximately 90% or better.

- **Hand hygiene monitoring:** Historically, there hasn't been a reliable way to guarantee that physicians and patients within a healthcare institution cleaned their hands correctly to reduce the danger of transmitting disease. Many hospitals and other healthcare facilities now employ IoT devices to remind individuals to clean their hands before entering hospital rooms. The gadgets can also offer recommendations on how to sterilize in order to reduce a specific danger for a certain patient. One significant limitation is that these gadgets can only remind individuals to wash out their hands; they cannot do it for them. Using these devices can lower infection rates in hospitals.
- **Depression and mood monitoring:** Additional data, which are usually problematic to collect continuously, include information on depression symptoms and the general mood of patients. Healthcare providers could ask patients regularly how they feel but cannot predict sudden mood changes, and patients often don't report their sensations accurately. "Mood-aware" IoT devices can tackle these challenges. Information such as cardiac rate and blood pressure can be collected and analyzed to provide information about a person's mental state. Advanced mood-monitoring IoT devices can even monitor data, for example, eye movement.
- **Parkinson's disease monitoring:** IT healthcare providers should be able to evaluate how serious symptoms fluctuate throughout the day to treat patients with Parkinson's most effectively. IoT sensors promise to facilitate this task by continuously gathering data about the symptoms of Parkinson's disease. The devices simultaneously allow patients to spend longer periods in hospitals to observe them and live in their own homes.
- **Connected inhalers:** Disorders like asthma and COPD often involve sudden, unpredictable attacks. Patients can benefit from IoT-connected inhalers that monitor attack frequency and collect environmental data to assist healthcare providers in understanding what led to a heart attack. Connected inhalers can also warn when you leave your inhaler, risk an attack without your inhaler, or misuse the inhaler.
- **Ingestible sensors:** Data collection within the human body is usually difficult and very disruptive. You wouldn't like a camera or a test, for example, stuck in your digestive tract, but the data from digestive and other systems can be collected much less intrusively with ingestible sensors. For example, they provide insight into the Ph levels of the stomach or help identify the source of internal bleeding. These instruments must be small enough to be easily swallowed. They must also be able to smoothly dissolve or go through the human body. Some companies are working hard on ingestible sensors that meet these standards.
- **Connected contact lenses:** Intelligent contact lenses provide an additional chance for the passive, non-intrusive collection of medical data.

Incidentally, they could also have micro-cameras which enable wearers to take photos with their eyes effectively, which is perhaps why companies such as Google have patented connected contact lenses. Intelligent lenses promise to transform the human eyes into a powerful digital interaction tool, whether used for health or other purposes.

- **Robotic surgery:** Surgeons can perform complex processes in human bodies that are difficult to manage using human hands by using small robots with the Internet. At the same time, small IoT surgeries may reduce the incisions required for surgery, resulting in less invasive processes and a quicker recovery for patients. These devices have to be sufficiently small and reliable to conduct minimally disruptive surgery. They also need to be able to interpret complex conditions within the correct decision-making process in human bodies on how to operate. However, IoT robots are already used in operation and surgery and show the ability to meet these challenges.

13.4 CLOUD COMPUTING VS. FOG COMPUTING IN HEALTHCARE

By 2020, it is predicted that the number of IoT devices will be around 30 trillion worldwide, and by 2025, according to Statista, the figure will exceed 75 billion connected items. All these devices generate enormous amounts of data that need quick and sustainable processing. Fog computing is being implemented to meet the growing demand for IoT solutions. At certain things, fog is even better than cloud computing [47].

13.4.1 Cloud Computing

We've already become familiar with the technical term "cloud," which is an Internet network of multiple devices, computers, and servers [48–50]. Such a computing system can be figuratively divided into two parts:

The frontend—consists of client devices (computers, tablets, mobile phones).

The backend—consists of data storage and processing systems (servers) that can be located far from the client devices and make up the cloud itself.

These two layers communicate directly with each other via wireless links. Cloud computing technology offers different types of services divided into three groups, as shown in Figure 13.6:

You can reach these services from anywhere from different devices by connecting your device to the cloud-based system. Therefore, the greatest benefit is availability. In addition, local servers need not be maintained, and the provider takes care of downtime, saving you money. The cloud integration of the Internet

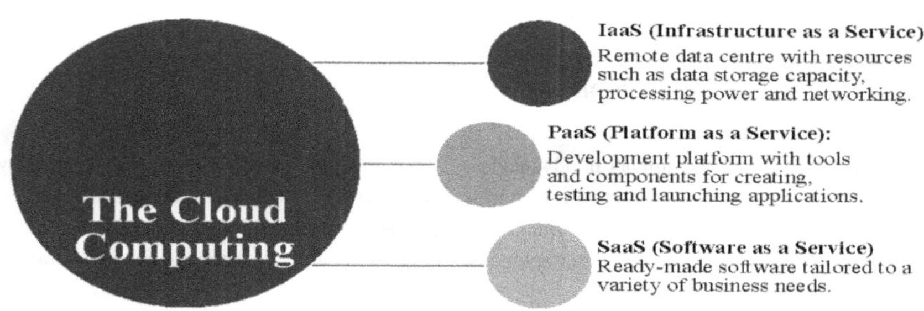

The Cloud Computing
IaaS (Infrastructure as a Service):
Remote data centre with resources such as data storage capacity, processing power and networking.
PaaS (Platform as a Service):
Development platform with tools and components for creating, testing and launching applications.
SaaS (Software as a Service)
Ready-made software tailored to a variety of business needs.

FIGURE 13.6 Cloud computing services.

TABLE 13.1
Pros and Cons of Cloud Computing in the Internet of Things

Pros	Cons
With the limited storage and processing capacity of connected devices, cloud computing is helpful in the integration of:	Nothing is perfect, and cloud technology, in particular for Internet services, has its disadvantages.
Improved performance: Communication between IoT sensors and systems of data processing is at a fast rate.	**High latency:** More and better IoT applications require very little latency, but because of the distance between customer devices and data processing centers, the cloud cannot guarantee it.
Storage capacities: Very scalable and endless storage space can integrate and aggregate a huge amount of data and share it to different platforms in the cloud.	**Downtime:** Technical problems and network interruptions may occur for whatever reason and cause customers to fail; many companies are using several connection channels with automated failure recovery to prevent problems.
Processing capabilities: Remote data centers for professing provide an on-demand virtual capability.	**Security and privacy:** Your private data are transmitted along with thousands of gigabytes of information from other users via global connected channels.
Reduced costs: The license fees are lower than the on-site cost and maintenance of the equipment.	

of Things is an economical way to do business. Off-site services offer scalability of data collected on connected devices and the flexibility to accomplish and analyze data on special platforms (e.g. Google Cloud IoT services, IBM Watson, AWS, Azure IoT Suite), allowing designers and developers to build IoT apps without any major hardware and software investments.

13.4.2 Fog Computing

In 2014, Cisco coined the term "fog computing" or "fogging," so it's new to the public. Fog and cloud computing are interrelated with each other. In nature, the fog is closer to the earth than clouds; in technology, fog is closer to the

TABLE 13.2
Pros and Cons of Fog Computing

Pros	Cons
The fogging approach has a number of advantages for the Internet of Things, big data, and in real time. Here are the main advantages of cloud computing: **Low latency:** Fog is closer to users geographically and can provide immediate answers. **No problems with bandwidth:** Instead of sending them together via one channel, pieces of information are collected at different points. **High security:** Data are processed in a complex distributed system through a large number of nodes. **Power efficiency:** Edge nodes run power-efficient Bluetooth, Zigbee, or Z-Wave protocols.	No apparent disadvantages to the technology, but certain deficiencies can be identified: **A more complicated system:** Fog is a supplementary data processing and storage system layer. **Additional expenses:** Enterprises should purchase edge equipment, including routers, hubs, and gateways. **Limited scalability:** Fog is not as scalable as a cloud system.

user, which leads to cloud capacity. The fog consists of several edge computing nodes connected to physical devices. These nodes are much closer physically to devices than centralized data centers, so they can provide immediate connections. The significant processing power of edge nodes enables them to compute large amounts of data themselves without sending them to remote servers. They aim to support high-resource IoT apps requiring low latency. The main difference is that cloud is a centralized system, and fog is a distributed decentralized infrastructure. Fog computing is an intermediary between remote servers and hardware. It controls the information to be transmitted to the server and handled, processing it locally. In this way, the fog is a smart gateway that unloads clouds, which can store, process, and analyze data more effectively. It is important to note that fog networking is not a separate architecture that replaces cloud computing but instead supplements it and gets as close as possible to the source of information. Another approach similar to fog computing is data processing edge computing. It is essential to process data on devices directly without sending it to other nodes or data centers. Edge computing offers bandwidth savings and improves data security, which is especially useful for IoT projects. The new technology will probably have the biggest impact on IoT, embedded AI, and 5G solutions, as they need agility and smooth connections more than ever before [51–53].

13.4.3 Fog Computing vs. Cloud Computing: Key Differences

The concepts of cloud versus fog are very much parallel. But there is still a difference in certain parameters between cloud and fog computing. A fog and cloud computing comparison is available here point by point [54, 55].

13.5 MACHINE LEARNING-BASED PROSPECTIVE IN HEALTHCARE

Machine learning, in short, is a kind of artificial intelligence that is programmed for computers to learn information without any human intervention. In machine learning, computational statistics are the basis for the development of the underlying algorithms. Computers provide data, followed by computers that learn from the input data. The computer reveals its complex patterns and the algorithms underlying them. The bigger the dataset, the more accurate the output will be. Machine learning is being increasingly used in healthcare and helps patients and clinicians in many ways. There are many examples of machine learning and health concepts being used in medicine. Researchers at MD Anderson developed the first algorithm to predict acute toxicity in radiation therapies for head and neck cancers. In radiology, the use of deep learning (DL) in medicine automatically identifies complex patterns from images and assists radiologists in making smart decisions in images such as conventional X-rays, CT, MRI, PET images, and reports. Google's health apps for machine learning have been trained in breast cancer detection and have achieved a precision of 89% or more than radiologists [56, 57].

Nearly 80% of the information held or "locked" in electronic health record systems is unstructured health data for machine learning. These are not data elements but documents or text files, which could not be analyzed in the past without human reading. Human language is a very complex language, lacking uniformity, and it has enormous ambiguity. Machine learning (ML) in healthcare usually relies on natural language processing (NLP) programs to convert these medical image data into more useful and analyzable data. Most deep learning with NLP requires some form of medical machine learning in healthcare applications. There are many cases of healthcare uses for machine learning [58].

Machine learning: Machine learning is a subset of an artificial intelligence (AI) application that offers the system the ability to learn and improve its experience without being programmed at this level. Machine learning uses the information to train and obtain precise results. Machine learning focuses on developing software that accesses and uses the data to learn from itself. ML is a type of AI in which a computer is trained to automate tasks that are exhausting or impossible for human beings. It is the best tool for analysis, comprehension, and identification of data patterns based on computer algorithm studies [58]. In comparison with machine learning, artificial intelligence uses information in order to provide an algorithm to understand the relation between input and output.

Deep learning: Deep learning is a subset of machine learning in which an artificial neural network (ANN) is connected. The algorithms are just like machine learning, but they are composed of more algorithms. All these algorithm networks are commonly known as an artificial neural network. More simply, it just replicates the concept of learning exactly like the human brain, in the way all the neuron networks are connected in the brain. With the help of algorithms and their processes, it solves complex problems. It is a subset of machine learning and is known as deep learning because it uses deep neural networks. To learn from data, the machine uses different levels. The model depth is shown by the number of layers in the model. The new state of the art in the realm of AI is profound learning. The learning phase is performed via a neural network in deep learning. A neural network is an architecture in which each layer is stacked [59, 60].

13.5.1 Machine-Learning Process

A program that recognizes objects is supposed to build them. A classifier is used to train the model. A classifier uses the characteristics of an object to attempt to determine its class, such as car, boat, airplane, cat, dog, elephant, bus, deer.

These things are the class that must be recognized by the classifier. You need some data as input to construct a classifier and give it an input as a label. The algorithm takes these data, finds a pattern, and categorizes the data into the appropriate class. This task is referred to as supervised learning. Training an algorithm requires following a few standard steps; see Figure 13.7.

In the first step, the algorithm will succeed or fail to choose the correct data. You choose to train the model as a function. The features are the pixels of the images in the object: Every image is a row of the data, and every pixel is a column. The dataset contains a column of 784 if your image is 28 × 28. Each image is transformed into a functional feature vector in the picture. This label tells the computer what the object in the picture is.

This training data are intended to be used to classify the object type. The next step is to create columns for the features. The third step consists of choosing a model training algorithm. When the training is completed, the model predicts which picture matches which object. It is easy to predict new images using the model afterward. The machine predicts the class it belongs to for each new image fed into the model. For example, the model passes through an entirely new image without a label. For a human being, it is trivial to classify the image as a car. To predict whether the image is a car, bus, or train, the system will uses the knowledge it acquired during training of the ML model [60].

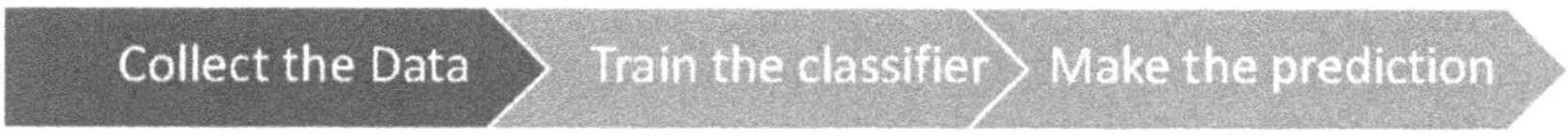

FIGURE 13.7 Overview of ML application architecture.

TABLE 13.3
Difference between Machine Learning and Deep Learning

Sr. No	Machine Learning	Deep Learning
1	Machine learning is a superset of deep learning.	Deep learning is a subset of machine learning.
2	The data in machine learning are completely different from deep learning because it uses structured data.	In deep learning, the data representation is very different because it uses neural networks.
3	Machine learning is an evolution of AI.	Deep learning is a development of machine learning. That's how profound the deep learning process is.
4	Machine learning consists of thousands of data points.	Big data: Millions of data points.
5	Outputs: Numerical value, like classification of score.	Anything from numerical values to free-form elements, such as free text and sound.
6	Uses several types of automated algorithms, using models and predicting future data action.	Uses the neural network, which transmits information through layers to interpret data characteristics, relations, and features.
7	In order to investigate specific variables in datasets, data analyzers detect algorithms.	When used in production, algorithms are largely self represented for data analysis.
8	Machine learning is used for teaching a machine that how to make accurate prediction and learn new things.	Deep learning solves complex problems in machine learning.

13.5.2 Deep Learning Process

The learning phase is performed via a neural network in deep learning. A neural network is an architecture that stacks layers on top of each other. Take the previous example of the same image. The image training set would be supplied and fed to a neural network. Each input is placed in a neuron and is weighed. The multiplication result flows to the next layer and becomes the input for that layer. For each layer of the network, this procedure is repeated. A mathematical algorithm is used by the neural network to improve the weight of all neurons. When the value of the weight gives a realistic output, the neural network is fully trained. For example, a neural network which is well trained can recognize the object in a picture with greater precision than the traditional neural network used in other DL/ML models [60, 61].

13.5.3 Applications of Machine Learning in Healthcare

The increasing number of machine learning applications in healthcare allows us to look at a future in which data, analytics, and invention work to help many patients without their even realizing it. Soon, ML-based applications will be

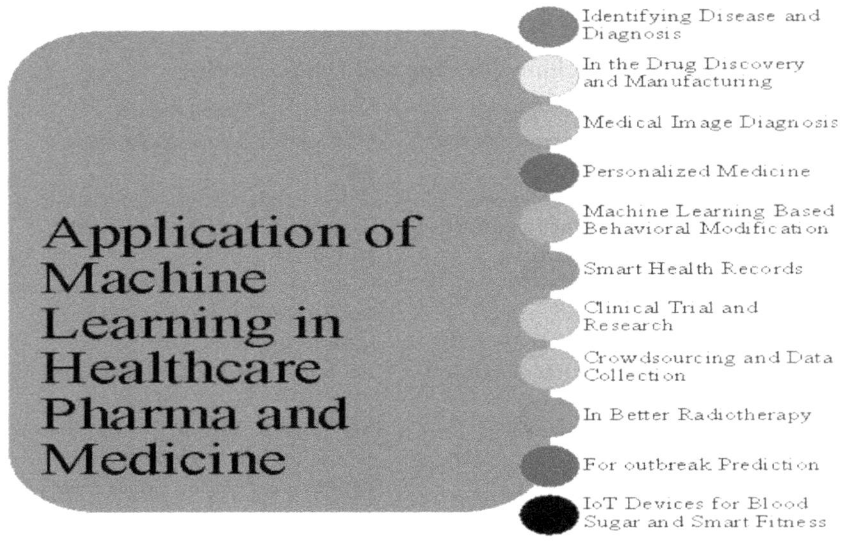

FIGURE 13.8 Application of ML in healthcare, pharma and medicine.

found in several countries with patient information in real time, thus enhancing the effectiveness of new, previously unavailable treatment options [57, 62].

Here are the top ten applications of machine learning in healthcare (see Figure 13.8):

1. **Identifying diseases and diagnosis**: Disease identification and diagnosis of diseases that are normally considered difficult to diagnose is a major ML application in healthcare. Cancer can include anything that is difficult to catch in the early stage to other genetic diseases. IBM Watson Genomics is a prime example of how the integration of cognitive computing with tumor sequencing for genomes can contribute to a rapid diagnosis. Berg, the biopharmaceutical giant, leverages AI in areas such as oncology to develop treatment.
2. **Drug discovery and manufacturing**: An early stage of major clinical applications in the drug discovery process is machine learning. This includes R&D technology such as next-generation sequencing and precision medicine that can help find alternative approaches to multifactor disease therapy. Machine-learning techniques currently involve unsupervised learning that allows patterns to be identified in data without predictions. Microsoft's Hanover project utilizes ML-based technologies to undertake several initiatives, including AI-based treatment technology and acute myeloid leukemia (AML) custom combinations.
3. **Medical imaging diagnosis**: Computer vision is an advanced technology that is responsible for machine and deep learning. It is used by

the Microsoft InnerEye initiative, which works with imaging analysis tools. As machine learning becomes easier and grows in its descriptive capability, it will become part of this artificial intelligence diagnostic process as more databases are created from different medical images.

4. **Personalized medicine**: Individual healthcare and predictive analysis can not only be more effective but will also be ready for further research and better disease assessment. Doctors are currently limited to selecting or evaluating patients' risk based on their history of symptoms and on the information available from a specific series of diagnoses. However, machine learning in healthcare is making great strides and, through the use of patient history to create several treatment options, IBM Watson Oncology is at the forefront of this movement.
5. **Machine learning-based behavioral modification**: Constant change is a significant part of preventive medication, which has resulted in countless start-ups in the area of cancer detection, identification, prevention, patient care, and so on, with the proliferation of machine learning in healthcare. Somatix is a data analytics company with an ML-based application to recognize our daily actions to enable us to understand our unconscious behavior and make necessary changes.
6. **Smart health records**: Keeping health records updated is a complex procedure, and while technology has helped make it much easier to enter data, the truth is that even now, most procedures take a lot of time. Streamlining processes to reduce time, effort, and money is the key role of machine learning in medical care. MIT is today at the cutting edge of developing a new generation of intelligent health archives that include ground-based ML rates to support diagnoses, clinical therapy, and so on.
7. **Clinical trials and research**: In clinical trials and research, machine learning has several potential applications. Clinical testing, as anyone in the pharmaceutical industry would tell you, costs a lot of time and money and may take many years to complete. Using predictive analytics based on ML to detect applicants for a possible clinical trial may draw a pool from a range of data points, including previous visits to a doctor, social networks, and so on. Machine study also has used the best sample size to be tested to ensure real-time monitoring, data access, and the power to reduce data-based errors in electronic records.
8. **Crowdsourced data collection**: Crowdsourcing is all the rage in the medical field today to allow scientists and practitioners access to a wide range of personal information. Live health data have great consequences for how medicine is perceived throughout the whole process. Apple's Research Kit enables users with interactive apps to try to treat Asperger's and Parkinson's disease using ML-based facial recognition. IBM has recently partnered with Medtronic to decrypt, collect, and disclose crowd information in real time, based on diabetes and insulin data.
9. **Better radiotherapy**: One of the most popular applications in the field of radiology is machine learning in healthcare. The analyses of

medical images have many discrete variables which can develop at any given time. There are many lesions, cancer focuses, and so for which complex equations cannot be modeled. Since ML-based algorithms are learned from a multitude of available samples, diagnosis and variables are easier. The classification of objects such as lesions into categories like normal or abnormal is one of the most popular uses for machine training in analyzing medical images. Google's DeepMind Health supports researchers at UCLH to actively develop algorithms that detect the difference between benign and malignant tissues and improve their treatment with radiation.

10. **Outbreak prediction**: In the monitoring and predicting of epidemics around the world, AI technology and machine learning are also used today. Scientists now have access to a large amount of satellite data, updates to social media in real time, information on websites and so on. Artificial neural networks contribute to the collection of this information and predict everything from malaria outbreaks to serious chronic diseases. In third world countries, predicting such outbreaks is particularly helpful, as they lack essential medical and educational infrastructure.

13.6 CONCLUSION/FUTURE RECOMMENDATIONS

- This chapter describes the importance of technology in healthcare, including the concept of the IoT in various domains of the healthcare industry, patient care, doctor assistance, and hospital maintenance or regulation.
- Data are everywhere, so we can develop new solutions with the help of information technology and the IoT regarding how to smartly and efficiently handle the data generated in the healthcare industry.
- Machine learning and deep learning are now emerging technologies and have the capability to change the future of the healthcare industry, and many advancements are going on this field.
- Due to space and relevance limitations, the authors can't include algorithms. Those who want to enhance their knowledge about these technologies can study the core mathematics and behavior of ML/DL algorithms like support vector machine, random forest, neural networks, convolutional neural networks, reinforcement neural networks, and so on.

ACKNOWLEDGMENTS

As Steve Jobs said, "Great things in business are never done by one person. They're done by a team of people." The same applies in the field of research and education, so with this in mind, this chapter is dedicated to all the reviewers who gave their time to review it. The authors would like to acknowledge coursera's (www.coursera.org) course "Machine Learning" by Stanford University, "Deep Learning Specialization: by Andrew NG. The authors would like to thank Shoolini University, where the idea came to start the writing this chapter.

AUTHOR CONTRIBUTIONS

All authors contributed equally. Writing and framing the basic concept of the chapter took place at Shoolini University, Department of CSE. Dr. Vanda Guleria prepared the introductory section of the book chapter. Ms. Shashi Kala prepared the IoT section and contributed to the big data section. Ajay prepared the sections on deep learning and machine learning and big data, and Dr. Varun, along with Ajay, did major revisions and checks for the chapter.

REFERENCES

[1] Rouse, M., *Internet of Things (IoT).* IOT Agenda, 2020.

[2] Brown, E., *21 Open source projects for IoT.* Linux.com., 2016.

[3] Vongsingthong, S. and S. Smanchat, *Internet of Things: a review of applications and technologies.* Suranaree Journal of Science and Technology, 2014. **21**(4): p. 359–374.

[4] Prajapati, C.D., et al., *An elementary research scope and constraints with IoT.* International Journal of Multidisciplinary and Current Research, 2020. **8**.

[5] da Costa, C.A., et al., *Internet of Health Things: toward intelligent vital signs monitoring in hospital wards.* Artificial Intelligence in Medicine, 2018. **89**: p. 61–69.

[6] Kang, W.M., S.Y. Moon, and J.H. Park, *An enhanced security framework for home appliances in smart home.* Human-centric Computing and Information Sciences, 2017. **7**(1): p. 1–12.

[7] Dey, N., et al., *Internet of Things and big data analytics toward next-generation intelligence (Vol. 35).* 2018, Berlin: Springer (Studies in Big Data).

[8] Yang, C., W. Shen, and X. Wang, *The Internet of Things in manufacturing: key issues and potential applications.* IEEE Systems, Man, and Cybernetics Magazine, 2018. **4**(1): p. 6–15.

[9] Younan, M., et al., *Challenges and recommended technologies for the industrial Internet of Things: a comprehensive review.* Measurement, 2020. **151**: p. 107198.

[10] Gupta, P., et al., *IoT and cloud-based healthcare solution for diabetic foot ulcer.* In *2020 sixth international conference on Parallel, Distributed and Grid Computing (PDGC).* 2020, IEEE.

[11] Prabha, R., et al., *IoT based smart healthcare monitoring systems: a literature review.* European Journal of Molecular & Clinical Medicine, 2021. **7**(11): p. 2761–2769.

[12] Aceto, G., V. Persico, and A. Pescapé, *Industry 4.0 and health: Internet of Things, big data, and cloud computing for healthcare 4.0.* Journal of Industrial Information Integration, 2020. **18**: p. 100129.

[13] Qadri, Y.A., et al., *The future of healthcare Internet of Things: a survey of emerging technologies.* IEEE Communications Surveys & Tutorials, 2020. **22**(2): p. 1121–1167.

[14] Kadhim, K.T., et al., *An overview of patient's health status monitoring system based on Internet of Things (IoT).* Wireless Personal Communications, 2020. **114**: p. 2235–2262.

[15] Uslu, B.Ç., E. Okay, and E. Dursun, *Analysis of factors affecting IoT-based smart hospital design.* Journal of Cloud Computing, 2020. **9**(1): p. 1–23.

[16] Bangui, H., M. Ge, and B. Buhnova, *Improving big data clustering for jamming detection in smart mobility.* In *IFIP international conference on ICT systems security and privacy protection.* 2020, Springer (Advances in Intelligent Systems and Computing [AISC]).

[17] Ahmad, M.A., et al., *Fairness in machine learning for healthcare.* In *Proceedings of the 26th ACM SIGKDD international conference on knowledge discovery & data mining.* 2020.

[18] Kavitha, M. and P.V. Krishna, *IoT-cloud-based health care system framework to detect breast abnormality.* In *Emerging research in data engineering systems and computer communications.* 2020, Springer (Advances in Intelligent Systems and Computing book series (AISC, volume 1054)). p. 615–625.

[19] Agrawal, R. and S. Prabakaran, *Big data in digital healthcare: lessons learnt and recommendations for general practice.* Heredity, 2020. **124**(4): p. 525–534.

[20] Dhungel, B., *Big data in healthcare: The role of big data in cardiology.* 2020.

[21] Nazir, S., et al., *A comprehensive analysis of healthcare big data management, analytics and scientific programming.* IEEE Access, 2020. **8**: p. 95714–95733.

[22] Khanra, S., et al., *Big data analytics in healthcare: a systematic literature review.* Enterprise Information Systems, 2020. **14**(7): p. 878–912.

[23] Rghioui, A., J. Lloret, and A. Oumnad, *Big data classification and Internet of Things in healthcare.* International Journal of E-Health and Medical Communications (IJEHMC), 2020. **11**(2): p. 20–37.

[24] Sagiroglu, S. and D. Sinanc, *Big data: A review.* In *2013 international conference on collaboration technologies and systems (CTS).* 2013, IEEE.

[25] Deyhim, P., *Best practices for Amazon EMR.* 2013, Technical report, Amazon Web Services Inc.

[26] Vora, M.N., *Hadoop-HBase for large-scale data.* In *Proceedings of 2011 international conference on computer science and network technology.* 2011, IEEE.

[27] Fuad, A., A. Erwin, and H.P. Ipung, *Processing performance on Apache Pig, Apache Hive and MySQL Cluster.* In *Proceedings of International Conference on Information, Communication Technology and System (ICTS) 2014.* 2014, IEEE.

[28] Sabharwal, N. and P. Pandey, *Introduction to GCP automation.* In *Pro Google cloud automation.* 2021, Springer. p. 1–21.

[29] Anand, S. and S.K. Routray, *Issues and challenges in healthcare narrowband IoT.* In *2017 International Conference on Inventive Communication and Computational Technologies (ICICCT).* 2017, IEEE.

[30] Farahani, B., F. Firouzi, and K. Chakrabarty, *Healthcare IoT.* In *Intelligent Internet of Things.* 2020, Springer. p. 515–545.

[31] Selvaraj, S. and S. Sundaravaradhan, *Challenges and opportunities in IoT healthcare systems: a systematic review.* SN Applied Sciences, 2020. **2**(1): p. 1–8.

[32] Hwang, Y.H., *Iot security & privacy: threats and challenges.* In *Proceedings of the 1st ACM workshop on IoT privacy, trust, and security.* 2015.

[33] Zhou, J., et al., *Security and privacy for cloud-based IoT: Challenges.* IEEE Communications Magazine, 2017. **55**(1): p. 26–33.

[34] Bertino, E., *Data security and privacy in the IoT.* In *EDBT.* 2016.
[35] Hamdan, R., *Human factors for IoT services utilization for health information exchange.* Journal of Theoretical and Applied Information Technology, 2018. **96**: p. 2095–2105.
[36] Hatzivasilis, G., et al., *The Interoperability of Things: Interoperable solutions as an enabler for IoT and Web 3.0.* In *2018 IEEE 23rd International Workshop on Computer Aided Modeling and Design of Communication Links and Networks (CAMAD).* 2018, IEEE.
[37] Blumberg, R. and S. Atre, *The problem with unstructured data.* Dm Review, 2003. **13**(42–49): p. 62.
[38] Raghupathi, W. and V. Raghupathi, *Big data analytics in healthcare: promise and potential.* Health Information Science and Systems, 2014. **2**(1): p. 1–10.
[39] Murdoch, T.B. and A.S. Detsky, *The inevitable application of big data to health care.* JAMA, 2013. **309**(13): p. 1351–1352.
[40] Savage, N., *Bioinformatics: big data versus the big C.* Nature, 2014. **509**(7502): p. S66-S67.
[41] Yellowlees, P.M., *Successfully developing a telemedicine system.* Journal of Telemedicine and Telecare, 2005. **11**(7): p. 331.
[42] Galletta, A., et al., *An innovative methodology for big data visualization for telemedicine.* IEEE Transactions on Industrial Informatics, 2018. **15**(1): p. 490–497.
[43] Baro, E., et al., *Toward a literature-driven definition of big data in healthcare.* BioMed Research International, 2015. **2015**.
[44] Feldman, B., E.M. Martin, and T. Skotnes, *Big data in healthcare hype and hope.* Dr. Bonnie, 2012. **360**: p. 122–125.
[45] Dimitrov, D.V., *Medical Internet of Things and big data in healthcare.* Healthcare Informatics Research, 2016. **22**(3): p. 156.
[46] Kim, J., et al., *Wearable biosensors for healthcare monitoring.* Nature Biotechnology, 2019. **37**(4): p. 389–406.
[47] Kumari, A., et al., *Fog computing for Healthcare 4.0 environment: opportunities and challenges.* Computers & Electrical Engineering, 2018. **72**: p. 1–13.
[48] Hayes, B., *Cloud computing.* 2008, ACM, New York.
[49] Antonopoulos, N. and L. Gillam, *Cloud computing.* 2010, Springer.
[50] Armbrust, M., et al., *A view of cloud computing.* Communications of the ACM, 2010. **53**(4): p. 50–58.
[51] Yi, S., C. Li, and Q. Li, *A survey of fog computing: concepts, applications and issues.* In *Proceedings of the 2015 workshop on mobile big data.* 2015.
[52] Yi, S., et al., *Fog computing: Platform and applications.* In *2015 Third IEEE workshop on hot topics in web systems and technologies (HotWeb).* 2015, IEEE.
[53] Iorga, M., et al., *Fog computing conceptual model.* 2018.
[54] More, P., *Review of implementing fog computing.* International Journal of Research in Engineering and Technology, 2015. **4**(6): p. 335–338.
[55] Saharan, K. and A. Kumar, *Fog in comparison to cloud: a survey.* International Journal of Computer Applications, 2015. **122**(3).
[56] Ngiam, K.Y. and W. Khor, *Big data and machine learning algorithms for healthcare delivery.* The Lancet Oncology, 2019. **20**(5): p. e262–e273.
[57] Erickson, B.J., et al., *Machine learning for medical imaging.* Radiographics, 2017. **37**(2): p. 505–515.
[58] Giger, M.L., *Machine learning in medical imaging.* Journal of the American College of Radiology, 2018. **15**(3): p. 512–520.

[59] Goodfellow, I., Y. Bengio, and A. Courville, *Deep learning*. Vol. 1. 2016, MIT Press, Cambridge, MA.

[60] Géron, A., *Hands-on machine learning with scikit-learn and tensorflow: Concepts*. In *Tools, and techniques to build intelligent systems*, 2017.

[61] LeCun, Y., Y. Bengio, and G. Hinton, *Deep learning*. Nature, 2015. **521**(7553): p. 436–444.

[62] Rajkumar, A., J. Dean, and I. Kohane, *Machine learning in medicine*. New England Journal of Medicine, 2019. **380**(14): p. 1347–1358.

14 Biosensors in Healthcare

C. Chandralekha

CONTENTS

DOI: 10.1201/9781003207856-14

14.1 INTRODUCTION

Leland C. Clark originated biosensors in his first experiment and found oxygen by using platinum electrodes. The enzyme glucose oxidase was kept close to the platinum surface by catching it against the electrodes using a piece of dialysis membrane. Based on the concentration of oxygen present in the environment, the activity of the enzyme was altered. Gluconic acid was produced by reacting glucose with glucose oxidase and reducing glucose oxidase by manufacturing two electrons and two protons. This produces oxidized glucose oxidase and hydrogen peroxide by making the highly available glucose oxidase react with more glucose. When the glucose content is higher, the consumption of oxygen is higher, and when glucose content is lower, the production of hydrogen peroxide is greater. Hence, the concentration of glucose can be measured either by increasing hydrogen peroxide or by decreasing oxygen.

In recent days, the medical industry has placed more stress on finding primary risks, preventing various diseases, finding new techniques for healthcare and emphasizing people's need to take care of their health. This is due to the evolution of emerging factors like the rise in population, several chronic diseases and the nature of treatment. Many people dislike visiting a doctor for consultation, which means more time spent for waiting in rooms and high fees, and physicians have to spend their entire day listening to and diagnosing patients. Also, continuous care of older people with chronic diseases is required. Major advancements in science and technology like wireless communication, biomedical sciences and information technology in recent years and the development of several wearable biosensors are improving quality in the medical care industry through the application of these new technologies [1]. These biosensors are utilized in keeping track of athletes, psychiatric patients, premature infants, people who need very close attention and people located away from medical and health services. Biosensors are used in control and the timely treatment and prevention of diseases.

14.2 PRINCIPLES OF BIOSENSORS

The word "biosensor" means "biological sensor," which is a device consisting of a transducer and biological elements like nucleic acid, an antibody or an enzyme. The transducer produces an electric signal by interacting with a biological element or a bioelement with an analyte. A biological component acting as the sensor and an electronic component for detection and transmission of signal are present in every biosensor. Several names exist for biosensors based on their applications, like chemical canaries, optrodes, biochips, glucometers, immunosensors, biocomputers and resonant mirrors. Microprocessors can analyze the message format of the result obtained by the reaction of the biosensor with a particular substance [2].

When we compare biosensors with any other presently existing diagnostic device, biosensors are advanced in selectivity as well as sensitivity. Applications of biosensors mainly include checking ecological pollution control in the agricultural field as well as uses in food industries. The main features of biosensors are stability, cost, sensitivity and reproducibility.

Each biosensor consists of a biological component acting as sensor and an electronic component for detecting and transmitting signals. Several substances, like nucleic acids, enzymes and antibodies in proteins; lectins; and complex materials such as microorganisms and tissue slices can be utilized as the bioelement in biosensors. Electrical, optimal or thermal signals are generated when there is interaction between analyte and the sensor. These signals are then converted into electrical parameters like voltage or current using an appropriate transducer.

14.2.1 Elements of Biorecognition

Analyses are not carried out in chemistry labs exclusively, but calculation of analytes in biological fluids can be done in the hospital or at home by patients. Hence, bioanalytical sensors are appropriate for several new applications, which makes biosensors more attractive than techniques used for spectroscopy and chromatography.

Biosensors provide platforms that are advanced in nature for biomarker analysis and have the advantages of easy, fast and robust utility, besides providing the testing capability of multianalytes. Biomarkers are considered molecules that are assessed as a sign of disease processes and pharmacologic reaction to therapeutic interruption.

In 1962, Clark and Lyons created the first biosensor for measuring glucose in blood. Enzyme-based biosensors were developed as the first generation of biosensors, and in the succeeding years, several biosensors for clinically significant materials were created. Hence, biosensors may be classified in accordance with their detection of biological elements like enzymes: Those for DNA are known as whole-cell biosensors, and signal transduction methods, including optical, thermal and electrochemical, are known as mass-based biosensors [4] (Figure 14.1).

Factors like ease of isolation of an enzyme, utilizing enzymes in combination for identification of a target analyte [5], availability for commercial purposes and applications in medicines have prompted an increase in the number of published works on enzyme-based biosensors in the literature.

In various studies of biosensors [6], several enzymes like alkaline phosphatase, glucose oxidase and horseradish peroxidase were used. A benefit of enzyme-based biosensors is their capability to alter the properties of catalysts, and a disadvantage is the absence of precision in classifying compounds belonging to the same classes [7]. In last few years, focus has been given to affinity biosensors, which provide details of bonding between antigens and antibodies, ligands and cell receptors. The particular interaction of immunosensors is understood by a

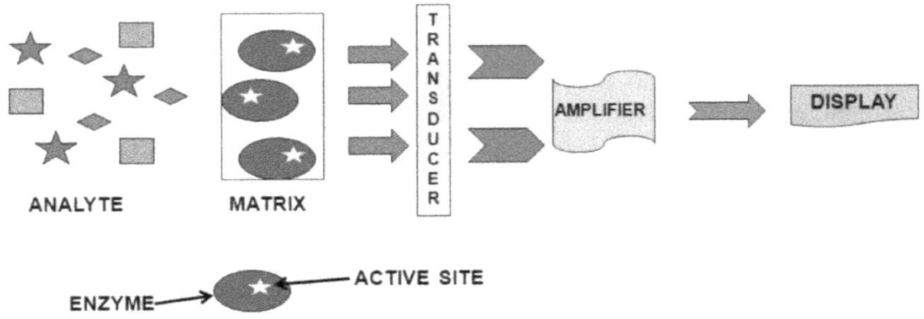

FIGURE 14.1 Schematic of a biosensor.

transducer, and calculations may be done directly within a few minutes, compared to obtaining visual results of the ELISA test, which may require many hours. Sensors operating directly are called homogeneous immunosensors, and sensors operating indirectly are called heterogeneous immunosensors. The specificity and sensitivity provided by antibodies is a critical part of immunosensors, which are more adaptable than enzyme-based biosensors since antibodies are more discerning and distinct. Today, immunosensors are frequently utilized in diagnosis of infectious diseases.

A significant application of biosensors in clinical chemistry is DNA analysis. In the sample, DNA biosensors combine oligodeoxynucleotides with complementary target DNA [8]. Infiltration or hybridization may be done either in solution or on solid support. The system may be utilized for repeated analysis, since the nucleic acid ligands can be transformed to reverse binding and then restored [9]. More research is required to develop techniques for finding highly sensitive DNA in organisms and human blood [8]. DNA biosensors are used in the diagnosis of infectious diseases, cancer testing, diagnosis of genetic diseases, calculation of resistance to drugs and identifying the circulation of cancer cells. Whole-cell biosensors act as recognition elements based on the metabolic nature of yeasts, fungi, bacteria, plants or animal cells. Whole cells can be altered to absorb and degenerate new substrates. The capability of cells to absorb and detect many chemicals depends on lot of enzymes and co-factors that exist in the cells [10].

14.2.2 Technology of Transduction

The interaction between bioreceptor and analyte converts the information into a signal that is measurable. Several feasible transducer methods are available in the development of biosensor technology. Some common methods are piezoelectric, optical and electrochemical [11]. In the case of interaction between analytes and the sensing surface of the detecting electrode, the electrochemical changes that occur are measured by electrochemical sensors. Since the electrochemical reactions take place at the interface of electrode and solution, the electrochemical method is considered reliable and simple. For these reasons and cost determination, according to reports in the literature, many biosensors are based on electrochemical transducers. The electrical changes may be potentiometric, which means an alteration in the voltage calculated between reference electrodes and the indicator; amperometric, which means an alteration in the current calculated at a particular applied voltage; or conductometric, which means an alteration in the capability of the sensing material for transporting charge. This electrochemical platform is appropriate for DNA/RNA and enzyme-based sensors, hand-held field monitoring applications and in implantable biosensors.

Optical transducers may be used to detect affinity reactions like applying quantitative antigenic species in clinical chemistry to learn the interactions between DNA and the affinity of antigen–antibody. Light going through an optical device is passed through optical fibers and directed to a sensing surface, which is reflected back from it. This reflected light is observed by utilizing a detector like a photodiode, which gives details about the physical events happening at the sensing surface. Such optical signals may consists of surface plasmon resonance, fluorescence, absorbance and chemiluminescence. Many optical methods need a spectrophotometer to monitor the changes in the signal.

Mass sensors can generate signals depending on the mass of chemicals that communicate with the sensing film, which is a vibrating piezoelectric quartz crystal. Acoustic wave devices consisting of piezoelectric substances are commonly used sensors that bend on applying voltage to the crystal. The operation of acoustic wave sensors works by the application of oscillating voltage at the resonant frequency of the crystal and calculating the alterations in resonant frequency during the interaction of the target analyte with the sensing surface.

14.3 TYPES OF BIOSENSORS

Several varieties of biosensors are used depending on the sensor device and the biological material, explained in the following.

14.3.1 Electrochemical Biosensors

Electrochemical biosensors depend on an enzymatic catalysis reaction which absorbs electrons. These types of enzymes are called redox enzymes. Three electrodes, reference, working type and counter, are present in the substrate of this biosensor.

There are four types of electrochemical biosensors:

- Amperometric biosensors
- Potentiometric biosensors
- Impedimetric biosensors
- Voltammetric biosensors

14.3.1.1 Amperometric Biosensors

Depending on the current resulting from oxidation, an amperometric biosensor is considered a self-contained incorporated device. These types of biosensors have higher sensitivities, ranges for energy and reaction times when compared to potentiometric-biosensors. A "Clark oxygen" electrode is a frequently utilized amperometric biosensor. The quantity of current flowing to the counter electrode and functioning motivated by a redox response at the operational electrode drive the operation of this type of biosensor.

14.3.1.2 Potentiometric Biosensors

A logarithmic reply is provided by this biosensor through a high energetic range. Electrode prototypes present on a synthetic substrate-covering polymer with connected enzymes are produced by these types of biosensors. These biosensors consist of two electrodes, which are more reactive and powerful.

14.3.1.3 Impedimetric Biosensors

Currently, impedimetric biosensors are rising in popularity. The methods used in impedimetric sensors are used to differentiate biosensor invention and to examine the responses of enzymes like receptors, antibodies, lectins and nucleic acids. Electrochemical impedance spectroscopy (EIS) is considered an indicator for response in a variety of chemical and physical properties.

14.3.1.4 Voltammetric Biosensors

This biosensor consists of four groups of iron (Fe) along with Hb (hemoglobin) and has a carbon glue electrode which gives oxidation in reverse and has a procedure for reducing Hb (Fe).

14.3.2 Physical Biosensors

These biosensors are widely used and are considered the most basic biosensors. Whenever there is a response to outside physical stimuli due to touch, hearing or sight, any device that responds to the physical presence of a medium is called a physical biosensor, and they are differentiated into two types: Piezoelectric and thermometric biosensors.

14.3.2.1 Piezoelectric Biosensors

These sensors consist of analytical devices based on the functioning of the law of "affinity interaction recording." The law of oscillation transformation is applied to the platform of a piezoelectric sensor. After analysis, the modified surface of this biosensor has an antibody or antigen and a polymer, which are molecularly stamped. The detection parts are combined normally by the usage of nanoparticles.

14.3.2.2 Thermometric Biosensors

The foundation of these types of biosensors is various types of biological reactions, which are coupled with the origination of heat. These biosensors are also called thermal biosensors, and in general, they are utilized to calculate the cholesterol in serum. As cholesterol obtains oxidized through the enzyme cholesterol oxidize, then the heat will be generated that can be measured. These biosensors can also be used for the evaluation of penicillin G, urea, glucose and uric acid.

14.3.3 Optical Biosensors

Optical measurement principles are applied in optical biosensors. Optoelectronic transducers and fiber optics are utilized in this type of biosensors. The terms optical and electrode are combined to form the term optrode. Enzymes like transducing elements and antibodies are involved in these sensors. There are two types of optical biosensors: Labeled optical detection biosensors and direct optical detection biosensors.

14.3.4 Wearable Biosensors

Recently, a digital device called a wearable biosensor has been developed. These are able to be worn on the human body as different wearable systems such as tattoos, smart watches and smart shirts, which permit regulation of levels of glucose in blood, blood pressure, heart rate and so on. These wearable sensors indicate a signal for the improvement of human health. They provide a better experience for patients in finding the status of their real-time fitness. These types of sensors help to identify the health issues of humans in advance so that hospitalization can be prevented. Such sensors also reduce admissions and readmissions to the hospital, which will create a positive awareness among the public in the future. Besides, information reveals that these sensors will become the most cost-effective equipment in the health world. One of the major challenges the world is facing is the increase in the population of aged people, particularly in developed countries. In the next 20 years, this aged population may increase by 20%, so the requirement to provide high-quality healthcare services will become significant.

Research on elderly people suggests they are not interested in the usage of wireless systems, and even if they learn, they forget them very soon, and they are frightened of working with such technology. Hence, systems whose operation is simple and that are adaptable from a social perspective must be given to such groups [12]. One of the new technologies that meets these conditions is the medical smart shirt. These shirts help the elderly to be independent, but they cannot replace nurses.

One study [13] discussed belts containing respiratory sensors, temperature sensors, two skin electrodes, an accelerometer sensor and an electrocardiogram, with the capability to provide valuable information on people's activities like resting, running, walking and falling. Physiological factors can be calculated for telediagnostics, particularly in elderly people's houses. Two decades ago, researchers designed digital clothing for military purposes which consisted of sensors and optical fibers in the fabric and had the ability to calculate heart rate and breathing rate. The position of a bullet inside the body of a wounded soldier can be shown by this smart clothing. In order to find out whether the soldier was wounded, an optical signal was passed from one side to the other, and if the signal did not reach the other side, then it meant the soldier was wounded. If the light returned, then it showed the bullet [14]. Research by Reinzo (2005) explained smart vests consisting of conductive fabric. These vests are able to calculate the heart and breathing rates during resting and working time and can pass the information to the processing center. In such a way, health checkups can be given even after discharge from the hospital [15].

Researchers [16] have recommended various applications of biosensors for continuously monitoring the health of athletes. The Mehr News Agency stated that remote monitoring of patients using smart biosensors can reduce the patient's referral to care centers by up to 30% [17]. Researchers from eight European countries designed smart shirts for chronic obstructive pulmonary disease (COPD) patients. In these shirts, sensors are connected to smartphones to transfer the health information of patients to the doctor, who may quickly diagnose the patient's data by utilizing smart software [17].

Researchers have referred to the good performance of such wearable biosensors in physical medicine and in the action of restoring someone to health or normal life through training and therapy after an illness. Significant vital signs may be received by metallic nanoparticles present in smart clothing designed by Iranian researchers. In such clothing, the processors and sensors implanted within it produce important signs of blood temperature and heart rate, and this critical information can be passed to the doctor in case of an emergency or when any critical conditions are met [18]. In their article, the researchers [19] noted these shirts can be washed and are very lightweight, which allows very easy movement, making them fitting for miners, astronauts, soldiers and firefighters.

Research has shown that biosensors are able to send data to an ambulance in emergency warning situations. Suppose a person living alone suffers a stroke or heart failure. The data will be transmitted to the ambulance, which reduces the time needed to check the patient. In a research article, researchers [20] suggested that smart shirts can be utilized for assessment and monitoring of data processing devices. The applications of smart shirts include sports and fitness, battlefield situations, health monitoring and public security. Accelerometers are present in smart shirts, which enables them to record electrocardiograph signals when the patient uses a treadmill at various speeds. The smartest shirts in the world are called Om-signal T-shirts, as described by Jam News Scientific Services. In these shirts, several sensors are sewn inside the fabric and are used to check the health status of the user regularly. Such shirts are utilized in finding various operations like movement, movement intensity, breathing, breathing capacity, heart rate variability and calories burned. The user can monitor their body operation by keeping track of the data stored in a small black box. These shirts, in addition to the use for bodybuilding exercises, can be worn during the day in offices. Such shirts can give a report about the extent of stress a person undergoes. These Om-signal T-shirts can either be worn alone or in combination with other clothes [21]. Various studies in recent years have shown that smart clothing technology may be used for monitoring patients in operation theatres. Research has shown that smart wearable sensors applied in clothes must be very thin, flexible and adaptable with the textile or should be fabricated utilizing textile technology or new fibers containing particular properties like electrical, mechanical and optical features.

14.3.5 Telemedicine Sensors

Telemedicine sensors are made up of 2 × 2-mm silicon chips. A thermal sensor and a slim strip of lithium battery are present in these chips, and they need much less power to initiate the circuit, process and pass electronic signals. On receiving a command from the monitor to send data, the antenna present inside the chip passes the data by radio signals [22]. Computation of heart rate, blood pressure and oxygen level in blood are a few applications of these types of sensors. In order to develop a collection of chips for displaying and monitoring the activities of the body and pass on the results to the appropriate medical centers, these sensors were developed. These telemedicine sensors can be attached to various parts of the human body, like the fingertip; several important parameters can be recorded; and the results can be reported [23].

The vital signs of soldiers present in war zones can be sent to a remote control register center by attaching these telemedicine sensors as a sticky substance to various parts of the soldier's body. These sensors have the ability to transmit physiological data to a mini-monitor fixed on another soldier's hat connected through wireless transmission. In such cases, if the data reveal any physical injury, then the monitor will produce an alarm so that the injury may be attended to in a short span of time. Moreover, the monitor has the ability to transmit and receive signals from a global positioning system (GPS) so that the location of the incident can be accessed quickly [24].

14.4 APPLICATIONS OF BIOSENSORS

Today, biosensors are becoming very popular and are being applied in various fields, as shown subsequently.

Agriculture, veterinary, military, measurements of metabolics, offense detection, clinical psychotherapy, common healthcare checking, ecological pollution control and diagnosis of disease are some of the applications of biosensors.

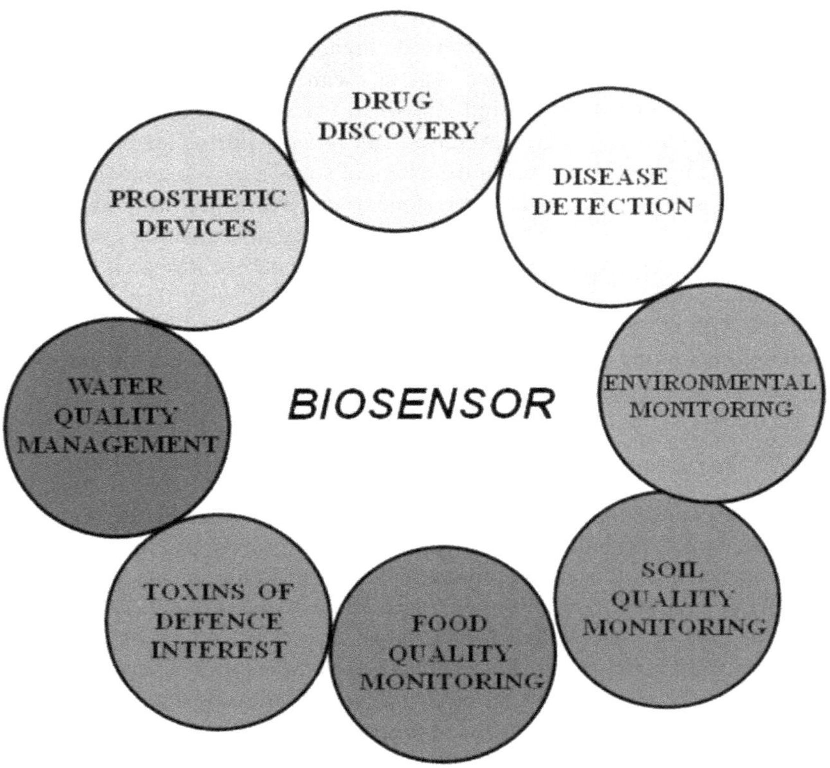

FIGURE 14.2 Applications of biosensors.

14.5 BIOSENSOR APPLICATIONS FOR HUMAN DISEASES

14.5.1 Nanoelectronic Biosensor Applications

In recent years, one of the major area of research is the application of nanoelectronic biosensors in medicine. This happens due to the capability of nanoparticles to spread throughout specific tissues inside the body. Several techniques for nanoelectronic biosensors capable of diagnosing, addressing and monitoring the progress of human diseases have been devised by biomedical engineers and nanomedical scientists. Nanoelectronic biosensors are able to pass electric signals between the remote device and the sensor. They are utilized by physicians as a helping tool for monitoring and diagnosing the health condition of the patients.

Nanoelectronic biosensors heavily rely on conduction to send electric signals between the sensor and the remote device. They are usually administered by physicians prior to the onset of any disease, as a helpful tool in diagnosing and monitoring the patient's condition. They are used for identification of growth of infectious cells, location of disease and predictions about the disease.

14.5.2 Cancer Applications

The standard methods used for identification of cancer include magnetic resonance imaging, digital rectal examination, biopsy, antigen tests and transrectal ultrasound, which are sometimes more risky and ineffective because they produce side effects to the human body. Due to the fast spread of cancer all over the human body, quick medical treatment that incorporates identification and therapy of the cancer is required. Advancements in nanotechnology like the optical and electrical features found in nanoelectronic biosensors can be utilized to identify and treat cancer like prostate cancer. Nanoparticles act as imaging agents that provide good access in finding cancerous tissues.

There are five types of nanoelectronic biosensors which can be utilized for the early detection and treatment of cancer. They are as follows:

- *Gold nanoparticles (GNPs)*—These sensors absorb and scatter well when compared to standard treatment techniques.
- *Quantum dots (QDs)*—These sensors are called luminescent nanosensors and are capable of tracking the motion of molecules in the cellular environment.
- *Magnetic nanoparticles*—These are mainly utilized in the imaging of cancer cells.
- *Carbon nanotubes (CNTs)*—In recent research, these sensors have been used in cancer diagnosis, specifically in the destruction of cancer cells.
- *Nanowires (NWs)*—These possess good electrical conduction and better functionalization of their surface; hence, they provide good results for images.

The effective improvements in signal, standard output identification and lower cost of application in these nanoelectronic biosensors make them a leading technology in the future of cancer detection and treatment.

Various invasive techniques that depend on cell morphology utilizing microscopy and staining are used in detecting cancer. The removal of tissues can mean missing the beginning stage of cancer cells. Cancer diagnosis based on biosensors is more practical and has more advantages, such as being user-friendly, faster and less expensive, and it demands fewer techniques when compared to proteomic analyses. Cancer is one of the dreadful diseases that gives rise to death in several developing and economically developed countries. The global increase of such a disease is due to several factors, like aging and the increase in smokers around the globe. Breast cancer is the most frequently detected cancer among females, and lung cancer is common among males because of smoking. Death due to cervical cancer [25] has increased today, comparable with breast cancer, which is a common cause of death of females in economically developing countries. Carelessly ignoring the earlier detection and treatment of solid cancers leads to death. There are several genetic and environmental factors that cause death due to cancer. Exposure to radiation, bacterial (e.g. stomach cancer) and viral infections (e.g.

cervical cancer), carcinogenic chemicals and toxins (aflatoxin; e.g. liver cancer) can lead the way to the development of cancer [26].

Cancer has become very common, and clinical testing is cumbersome. Various genetic and epigenetic changes can be the origin of the development of cancer cells. In this process, not even a single gene is changed, but a group of them brings trouble during detection and diagnosis. Modifications occurring either in tumors from various locations or inside tumors from the same location are difficult to detect and diagnose. Hence, several biomarkers can be examined to diagnose the disease. Such biomarkers can be manufactured either by the tumor or by the body reacting to the presence of cancer [27]. The presence of disease can be found by analyzing the presence of biomarkers in body fluids like urine and blood.

14.5.3 Cardiovascular Disease Applications

Cardiovascular diseases, even though they are highly avoidable, are a crucial reason for the increase in human deaths throughout the world. One of the major significant reasons for the rise of cardiovascular disease and cardiac arrest is the rise in aggregation of blood cholesterol [28]. Regular analysis of the levels of cholesterol in the blood is mandatory in clinical applications. Biomarkers have replaced electrocardiographic findings. Cardiac troponin is an unique marker utilized recently, since it is determined from myocardial tissue which can be found easily and is helpful for the healing process.

In recent years, 17 million deaths have occurred due to cardiovascular diseases (CVDs). Even though various technologies are used in the detection and treatment of cardiovascular diseases, many challenges exist, such as more information being needed for surgery, regeneration of tissues, imaging of single cells and particular therapeutic methods. During the assessment of cardiovascular disease using nanoelectronics, three chips are used in general. The first chip allows initial sensing and operation of the inspected molecular activity in the desired area. The second and third chips are called standard microcontrollers and have various functional features which provide quick results. These nanoelectronic biosensors are best at measuring the levels of C-reactive proteins (CRPs) in the blood.

14.5.4 Psychological Disorder Applications

The functionality of the brain is a significant field to be addressed in research. Assessment of neural functions at various molecular and cellular levels will provide a clear idea about diagnostic applications which can be applied for several psychological and neurological disorders. Recently available empirical proofs say that nanoelectronics can be utilized in the treatment of several mental illnesses and depression.

14.5.5 Diabetes Applications

Many people in the world are affected by diabetes, which is today a major cause of death, and the death rate is increasing faster recently. Diabetes is caused by metabolism problems, which increase the level of sugar in blood. Not monitoring glucose levels in the blood may result in kidney failure, disorders in the neurological system, a rise in blood pressure, heart disease, stroke, blindness and still more difficulties related to health. Such issues can be decreased by educating patients to undergo systematic checkups and constant monitoring of the glucose level in blood [29]. Efficient management of diabetes by patients includes calculating the glucose level in the blood. Estimation of glucose content is mandatory, since it is the major biomarker of diabetes. According to the American Diabetes Association, insulin-dependent type 1 diabetics should check their blood glucose at least three to four times every day, and insulin-dependent type 2 diabetics should check their glucose at least once every day [30].

However, keeping track of glucose levels by patients at the prescribed times is cumbersome and can cause trouble and pain when measuring with traditional methods. There are various techniques for analyzing glucose levels in blood, but most of these involve difficult processes and cost much more. Hence, it is essential to produce easy, exact, less expensive methods for analyzing glucose that are suitable for fast field examinations and can also be a substitute for the prevailing techniques. Many glucose biosensors, like implantable sensors used for calculating glucose levels in tissue or blood, were developed after the first biosensor [31].

Nowadays, glucose sensors are mostly used for calculating substitutional glucose levels in subcutaneous fat. In the glucose monitoring process, there are various requirements for a sensor, including compactness of the instrument, long-term stability, removal of dependency on oxygen, user comfort and compatibility with tissue without producing any toxic or immunological response when the body is exposed to it. Sensor activity is lost when spreading low-molecular-weight substances over a polyurethane sensor's outer membrane. A solution for this problem is microdialysis or ultrafiltration technology methods joined with glucose biosensors. Many sensors produce exact results, even though several sensor errors, like delay of the interstitial sensor value, drift and calibration errors exist in the blood value. Glucose biosensors are an example of an electrochemical biosensor that depends on a disposable amperometric electrode. Such a biosensor is commonly used around the world for testing of glucose at home so that the diagnosis is brought to door increasing the convenience of diabetes patients.

14.6 WEARABLE BIOSENSORS AND THEIR APPLICATIONS

14.6.1 Treatment of Depression Using Helmets

A new helmet was designed by Danish researchers which aids in regenerating segments associated with depression and provides fast relief for patients by transmitting weak electrical pulses to the brain. These electrical pulses operate on blood vessels copying the body's treatment mechanism so as to form new blood vessels. These electrical pulses are not felt by the patients when compared to electroconvulsive therapy (ECT), where electrical pulses are severe, which may result in memory loss in a few cases. Researchers in Copenhagen University found that these electrical pulses reduce the symptoms of depression in many patients after seven days, and they secure good scores on depression tests. Mild nausea is a major side effect of this helmet, which can be overcome when the treatment is completed. Using the results obtained in these studies aids in the evolution of new methods of treatments for various disorders, like posttraumatic stress disorder (PTSD) [32].

14.6.2 Smart Shirts

A smart shirt consists of special sensors to keep track of significant signs of the body. A smart shirt provides a skeleton for tracking sensing. The sensors can be placed in appropriate positions on the human body based on their shapes and sizes. Washing this smart shirt is quite easy and can be done without any harm. These smart shirts aid in keeping track of temperature, rates of respiration and heart rate. A fiber grid that is conductive in nature and integrated sensors are fixed in the shirt and contain shirt band connectors. On finding any unusual parameters, these connectors pass a signal to either a Bluetooth device, personal digital assistant or personal controller wireless system, which will execute the next process of medical care.

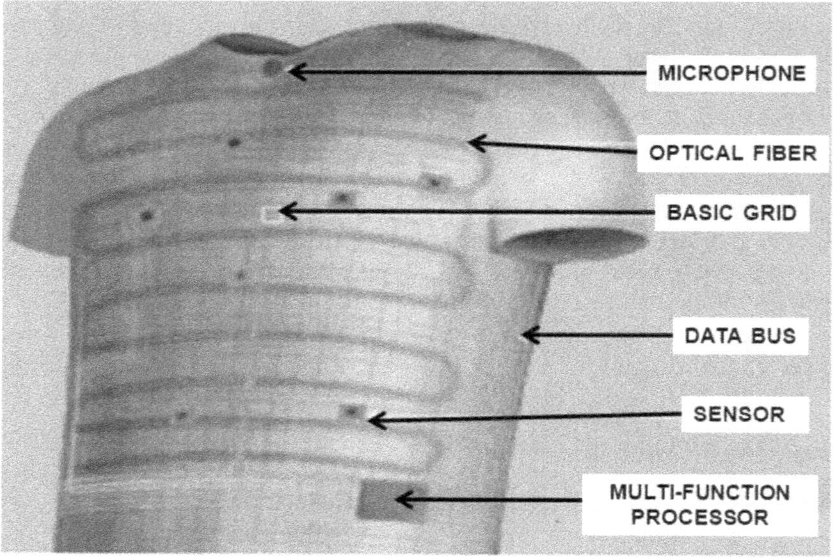

FIGURE 14.3 Smart shirt sensory architecture.

(From https://www.ijeat.org/wp-content/uploads/papers/v9i6/E9703069520.pdf.)

14.6.3 Smart Socks

Smart socks are utilized by parents to monitor the health of their infants by using a mobile application. These smart socks are also called *owlets* and can send information on the infant's quality of sleep, skin temperature oxygen level, heart rate and sleeping position to the parents' smartphones. The manufacturers of smart socks say that this technology has the capability to monitor the daily health of babies so as to detect sudden infant death syndrome. De-identified data are passed to the company, so a database can be created by the manufacturers to help in finding the problems and pass early warning signs to the parents [33].

Sensors within smart socks are able to control the way the feet are kept on the ground in various conditions and in walking. Wearing these smart socks plays a vital role in balancing while walking, and they are mainly utilized by elder patients who have trouble with walking. Children who are starting to learn to walk can utilize these socks as a training tool since they help avoid injuries that may be caused while walking. The recorded data in sensors can be passed to user's computer by wireless system so that it can be examined by a program and an alarm can be set if required for the person [34].

14.6.4 Smart Shoes

Researchers have designed smart insoles containing sensors that fit internally which aid in correcting deformities in movement for people with foot fractures (see Figure 14.5) or those with hip replacements or artificial legs and for correcting people's walking style. Walking patterns are changed with the help of a special gel insole containing sensors for monitoring pressure. Reports on walking style can be seen by using an accelerometer or internal gyroscope. Users are able to see the data given by the smart insole using a wireless software program in their smartphones. These data are used by physiotherapists for correcting discrepancies in motion using concurrent instructions either by audio or video. This technology is utilized as one of the major techniques for improvement of bone fractures and any temporary paralysis of the legs [35].

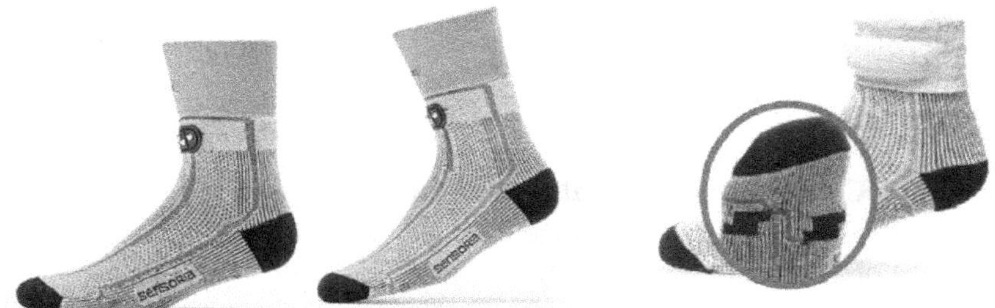

FIGURE 14.4 Smart socks for monitoring balance in walking.

(From https://www.odtmag.com/contents/view_online-exclusives/2016-01-28/smart-socks-monitor-gait-improve-balance-and-track-rehab/.)

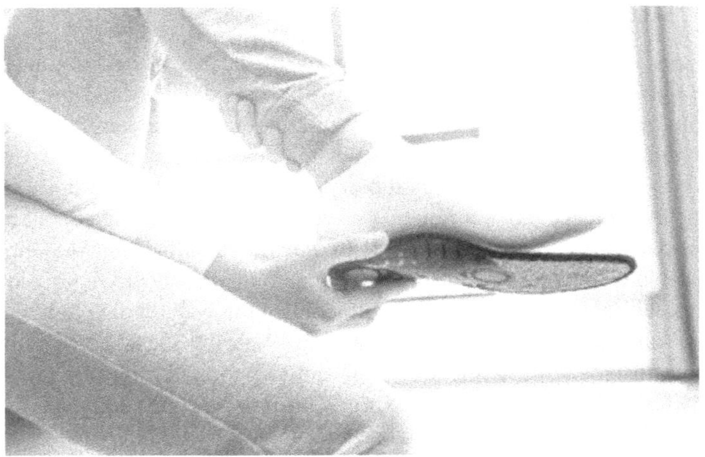

FIGURE 14.5 Smart shoes—biosensor insole for balancing foot fracture.

(From https://www.flawlessfeet.net/blog/10-conditions-that-may-mean-you-need-orthotics.)

14.6.5 Smart Clothing

14.6.5.1 Monitoring Premature Babies

Annually more than 10 million premature babies are born around the globe. Among them, about 1 million undergo psychological and physical difficulties because of dehydration. Smart clothing was successfully designed by Polish researchers that premature babies can wear. This type of clothing consists of two layers: An ordinary fabric and one with a skin that stops excessive sweating.

14.6.5.2 Prevention of Bedsores

A new type of clothing has been designed by scientists to evaluate the circulation of nutrients, oxygen and blood needed for various parts of the body. This clothing consists of a set of electrodes which give light shocks to certain parts of body whenever required for raising the flow of blood to that part; hence, the possibility of bedsores will be drastically lowered [36].

14.6.5.3 Children's Health Status Monitoring

Parents of newborn babies can utilize smart clothing to keep track of the physical status of their baby. Smart clothing consists of various sensors, transmitters and receivers using Wi-Fi or Bluetooth to constantly keep track of the state of the body; temperature; breathing rate; and activity levels like sleeping, playing or awake. A memo application must be installed on the smartphone to access all these activities. This clothing keeps parents informed about their children's health and notifies them immediately when anything unnatural occurs [37].

14.6.5.4 Stress-Measuring T-Shirt

A new T-shirt containing sensors has been designed by Canadian researchers that is able to monitor the levels of stress in daytime depending on breathing, motion, sleep and heart activity. Data from this T-shirt are passed to a smartphone in a wireless manner. This device calculates the activity levels and stress throughout the day, and it also guides in planning schedules for athletes' training programs [38].

14.6.5.5 Examination of Mental Conditions with Digital Clothing

Small sensors embedded in this clothing can determine people's mental state, temperature and heart rate. These data are passed to a database using a mobile phone, where suitable data are sent based on the prevailing situation. A screen containing light-emitting diode (LED) lamps is embedded in the clothing and is able to display confident statements during depression or when people panic in certain situations. Some speakers are present in the helmet, which can play suitable music and send hopeful messages or even jokes from the patient's family [39].

14.7 CONCLUSION

A rapid diagnosis is necessary for a treatment to be successful and to ensure speedy recovery of patients. Methods used for diagnosis should be sensitive and easy and must have the ability to find various biomarkers that are present in lower concentrations in biological fluids. All these requirements can be satisfied with biosensors. This chapter explained the principles of biosensors and their various categories. Several applications of biosensors in medical fields like treatment of psychological disorders, cancer, diabetes and cardiovascular diseases have become common recently. The study of many kinds of wearable biosensors, like smart shirts, socks, shoes and helmets, was also dealt with in this chapter. It is expected that usage of smart clothing will become common, like smartphones, and this future is not too distant. Very soon, these wearable biosensors will find their way into all clinical applications. Today, numerous companies have started developing and producing such wearable products, and we can say that the future of the medical world will significantly involve wearable tools.

REFERENCES

[1] Ajami, S., & Bagheri-Tadi, T. (2013). Health information technology and quality of care. Journal of Information Technology and Software Engineering, Vol. S7, p. e003.

[2] Flow Sensors in Medicine. Available from: www.medicblog.ir/post-1425.aspx.

[3] Hall, E.A.H. (1990). Biosensors. Open University Press, Cambridge, UK, ISBN-10: 0335151612.

[4] Wanekaya, A.K., Chen, W. & Mulchandani, A. (2008). Recent biosensing developments in environmental security. Journal of Environmental Monitoring, Vol. 10, No. 6, pp. 703–712.

[5] D'Orazio, P. (2003). Biosensors in clinical chemistry. Clinica Chimica Acta, Vol. 334, No. 1–2, pp. 41–69.

[6] Laschi, S., Franek, M. & Mascini, M. (2000). Screen-printed electrochemical immunosensors for PCB detection. Electroanalysis, Vol. 12, No. 16, pp. 1293–1298.

[7] Buerk, D.G. (1993). Biosensors: Theory and Applications. Technomic Publishing Company, Lancaster, UK, ISBN 0-87762-975-7.

[8] Palecek, E. (2002). Past, present and future of nucleic acids electrochemistry. Talanta, Vol. 56, No. 5, pp. 809–819.

[9] Ivnitski, D., Abdel-Hamid, I., Atanasov, P. & Wilkins, E. (1999). Biosensors for detection of pathogenic bacteria. Biosensors and Bioelectronics, Vol. 14, No. 7, pp. 599–624.

[10] Ding, L., Du, D., Zhang, X. & Ju, H. (2008). Trends in cell-based electrochemical biosensors. Current Medicinal Chemistry, Vol. 15, No. 30, pp. 3160–3170.

[11] Collings, A.F. & Caruso, F. (1997). Biosensors: recent advances. Reports on Progress in Physics, Vol. 60, No. 11, pp. 1397–1445.

[12] Flow Sensors. [Last accessed on 2015 Jun 14]. Available from: http://persian-expert.com/thread789.html.

[13] Sardini, E. & Serpelloni, M. (2010). Instrumented wearable belt for wireless health monitoring. Procedia Engineering, Vol. 5, pp. 580–583.

[14] Become Familiar with a Variety of Smart Clothes. [Last accessed on 2015 Jun 13]. Available from: www.yjc.ir/fa/news/4469479.

[15] Di Rienzo, M., Rizzo, F., Parati, G., Ferratini, M., Brambilla, G., & Castiglioni, P. (2005). A textile-based wearable system for vital sign monitoring: Applicability in cardiac patients. Conference Computers in Cardiology, Vol. 32, pp. 699–701.

[16] Perego, P., Moltani, A., & Andreoni, G. (2012). Sport monitoring with smart wearable system. Studies in Health Technology and Informatics, Vol. 177, pp. 224–228.

[17] Picture a Fancy Dress for the Patient/Physician Patient Transfer. [Last accessed on 2015 May 27]. Available from: www.mehrnews.com/detail/News/1636657.

[18] Design and Construction of Smart Clothes for Critical Signals. [Last accessed on 2014 Jun 13]. Available from: www.danakhabar.com http://danakhabar.com/fa/news/1160016.

[19] Pandian, P.S., Mohanavelu, K., Safeer, K.P., Kotresh, T.M., Shakunthala, D.T., Gopal, P., et al. (2008). Smart vest: Wearable multi-parameter remote physiological monitoring system. Medical Engineering & Physics, Vol. 30, pp. 466–477.

[20] Leea, Y.D. & Chung, W.Y. (2009). Wireless sensor network based wearable smart shirt for ubiquitous health and activity monitoring. Sensors & Actuators, B: Chemi cal, Vol. 140, pp. 390–395.

[21] Wear This Shirt to Stay Healthy. [Last accessed on 2014 Jun 13]. Available from: www.jamnews.ir/detail/News/349977.

[22] Flow Sensors. [Last accessed on 2015 Jun 14]. Available from: http://persian-expert.com/thread789.html.

[23] Flow Sensors. [Last accessed on 2014 Jun 14]. Available from: www.dezmed.com/old/news.php?extend.507.36.

[24] Flow Sensors and Wearable in Biomedical Engineering. [Last accessed on 2014 Jun 17]. Available from: http://vista.ir/article/258815.

[25] Jemal, A., Bray, F., Center, M.M., Ferlay, J., Ward, E. & Forman, D. (2011). Global cancer statistics. CA: A Cancer Journal for Clinicians, Vol. 61, doi:10.3322/caac.20107.

[26] Vineis, P., Schatzkin, A. & Potter, JD. (2010). Models of carcinogenesis: an overview. Carcinogenesis, Vol. 31, No. 10, pp. 1703–1709.
[27] Robert, J. (2010). Polymorphismes génétiques. Bulletin du Cancer, Vol. 97, No. 11, pp. 1253–1264.
[28] Franco, M., Cooper, R.S., Bilal, U. & Fuster, V. (2011). Challenges and opportunities for cardiovascular disease prevention. American Journal of Medicine, Vol. 24, No. 2, pp. 95–102.
[29] Turner, A.P.F. & Pickup, J.C. (1985). Diabetes-mellitus—biosensors for research and management. Biosensors, Vol. 1, No. 1, pp. 85–115.
[30] American Diabetes Association. (1997). Clinical practice recommendations 1997—introduction. Diabetes Care, Vol. 20, No. Suppl 1, pp. S1–S70.
[31] Clark Jr., L.C. & Lyons, C. (1962). Electrode systems for continuous monitoring in cardiovascular surgery. Annals of the New York Academy of Sciences, Vol. 102, No. 1, pp. 29–45.
[32] Hat for Depression Treatment. [Last accessed on 2015 Jun 13]. Available from: www.migna.ir/vdccspqi.2bq0s8laa2.html.
[33] Check Vital Signs. Smart Baby Socks. [Last accessed on 2015 Jun 15]. Available from: www.tebyan.net/newindex.aspx?pid=256221.
[34] Wearable Technology Is Smarter. [Last accessed on 2015 Jun 12]. Available from: www.tabnak.ir/fa/news/383033.
[35] Smart Shoes Momentary Reports of Abnormalities of Gait. [Last accessed on 2015 Jun 15]. Available from: http://isna.ir/fa/news/91082213611/.
[36] Special Intelligent Design of Premature Infants. [Last accessed on 2015 Jun 15]. Available from: www.irna.ir/fa/News/80868812.
[37] Wearable Gadget. [Last accessed on 2015 Jun 15]. Available from: http://dbportal.ir/portal/topic/tag/.
[38] Measure Stress Levels and Sleep with a T-Shirt. [Last accessed on 2015 Jun 15]. Available from: www.mehrnews.com/detail/news/2142634.
[39] Special Intelligent Design of Premature Infants. [Last accessed on 2015 Jun 15]. Available from: www.irna.ir/fa/News/80868812.

15 Early Detection of Autism Spectrum Disorder Using EEG, MRI and Behavioral Data

A Review

A.K. Jayanthy and Qaysar Mohi Ud Din

CONTENTS

15.1 INTRODUCTION

Autism spectrum disorder (ASD) is a neurodevelopmental disorder, which is characterized by impairments in social interaction and communication, restricted and repetitive behaviors or interests and alteration in sensory processing. Its prevalence has increased in the last two decades from 2 to 5 per 10,000 to 1 in 54 children, and the prevalence in males is four times greater than in females [1]. Co-occurring neurological or psychiatric disorders are commonly present in people with autism, including attention deficit hyperactivity disorder, anxiety, epilepsy and depression [2]. Individuals with ASD may have different signs and symptoms; however, the disorder is characterized by core features in two main areas, social communication and restricted, repetitive sensory-motor behaviors. The *Diagnostic and Statistical Manual of Mental Disorders* (DSM-5) criteria of the American Psychiatric Association was published in 2013 to make the diagnosis of ASD straightforward. Autism spectrum disorder can be diagnosed by pediatricians, psychiatrics and

DOI: 10.1201/9781003207856-15

psychologists. Ideally, inputs from various disciplines are taken. Some standardized diagnostic instruments include the Screening Tool for Autism in Toddlers and Young Children (STAT) and Autism Diagnostic Observation Schedule (ADOS) [3].

ASD is influenced by both genetic and environmental factors which affect brain development. Neuropathologic studies have revealed differences in cerebellar connectivity and architecture; frontal, temporal and cortical lobe alterations; and limbic system abnormalities. An increase in cortical size and extra-axial fluid have been found in subjects with autism spectrum disorder [4]. The onset symptoms of ASD are observed before three years of age, whereas changes in social behavior and other autistic features can be noticed as early as in the first few months of life. Brain development is rapid during the initial years of life, and a combination of genetics and biological and environmental conditions leads to typical neurodevelopment. Brain development that may lead to ASD can give rise to symptoms months after the occurrence of the brain development. A lot of time will be wasted between the appearance of symptoms and the occurrence of the brain development which leads to ASD if the diagnosis of ASD is only based on behavior. Therefore, identification of biomarkers for early detection of ASD is important for early intervention for the disease.

In this chapter, detection of ASD based on MRI, behavioral data and EEG is discussed.

15.2 MRI-BASED DETECTION TECHNIQUES

Almost all the studies based on MRI data examined in this chapter collected data from the Autism Brain Imaging Data Exchange (ABIDE) database, which is an international collaborative project for collecting and sharing neuroimaging data. Brain images can be used to find functional connectivity and blood flow fluctuations in different brain regions. Wang et al. used the MRI images of 54 ASD subjects and 57 control subjects from the ABIDE database and proposed a canonical correlation analysis-based graph-matching space group lasso (GMSGL) feature selection technique for classifying ASD. The results indicated that the proposed method outperformed the previously used methods for classifying ASD [5]. A study conducted by Yao et al. on data obtained from the NYU Langone Medical Center, which is a collection site of ABIDE, consisted of 79 ASD and 105 typical development children [6]. Pearson's correlation coefficient was calculated, and based on that, covariance matrices of each subject were calculated. The functional connectivity of subjects with ASD showed weak connectivity for a longer time in comparison to typically developed children according to the T values, and ASD showed more divergent connectivity strength of the brain state than the typically developed children [6]. Data have also been collected from the ABIDE database to develop a novel framework that uses short-term activation patterns of brain connectivity for detecting disease-induced disruptions of brain connectivity [7]. A clustering algorithm was used for decomposing resting-state fMRI time series data into different clusters with similar spatial distributions of neural activity, and it outperformed conventional networks by at least 7% [7]. Data were collected from the ABIDE database, which included data from 240 adolescent subjects, 112 with ASD and 128 neurotypical controls. In the slow-5 (0.01–0.02 Hz) and slow-4 (0.027–0.073 Hz), the whole brain functional connectivity networks were constructed. An accuracy of 79.17% was achieved by using a support vector machine (SVM). A significant correlation was found between social and communication deficits based on the connectivity between the default mode network and cingulo-opercular network [8].

Data consisting of a primary sample of 48 subjects with ASD and 48 typically developing control subjects was selected from the ABIDE dataset. The white matter hypointensity (WMH) was calculated from high-resolution T1-weighted scans. The WMH volume was compared with an independent, multi-site sample consisting of 80 ASD cases and 80 typically developed children (TDC) cases. The results showed that periventricular WMH was associated with restricted repetitive behaviors and was elevated in ASD [9]. The MRI and fMRI data of 54 ASD subjects and 57 typical controls under the age of 15 years was obtained from the ABIDE database. The brain space was then parceled into 116 ROIs by applying the automatic anatomical labeling (AAL) atlas to each image. A feature weighting and fusion method called hierarchical supervised local canonical correlation analysis (HSL-CCA) was proposed to effectively identify ASD patients from typical controls. Experiments on the multimodal ABIDE database showed that the proposed method achieved superior performance [10]. A deep neural network was developed for high-dimensional resting-state functional patterns of the whole brain for classifying ASD. The dataset obtained from the ABIDE I database contained samples of 55 ASD subjects and 55 typically developing control subjects. Features with high discriminating power were selected by the model and then used by sparse autoencoders. A classification accuracy of 86.36% was achieved by this approach [11].

Another study was conducted to compare the abnormalities detected in ASD subjects in comparison with subjects with other developmental disorders. Thirty-two subjects with ASD and 16 with other developmental disorders, including intellectual disability and language disorder, were recruited for this study. Whole brain T1-weighted spoiled gradient echo volumes were acquired for each subject. The results showed an over-connectivity pattern in ASD in networks, mostly in fronto-temporal nodes and basal ganglia. The results indicated different connectivity patterns in ASD and other developmental disorders [12]. The MRI images of 59 subjects in which 18 subjects were female and 41 were male were acquired during natural sleep. The data were then preprocessed. Two hundred eighty regions of interest were calculated, and then pair-wise Pearson correlation coefficients were generated. For classification, data of one infant was removed for testing the model, and the remaining 58 were used as a training set. All the classification analysis was performed in MATLAB's Statistics and Machine Learning Toolbox [13]. fMRI data and the blood oxygen level-dependent (BOLD) signals generated from fMRI images have also been used for detection of ASD. The fMRI data (consisting of 1,035 subjects) collection and BOLD preprocessing was performed by the ABIDE consortium. A classification accuracy of 78.6% was achieved for adolescent males and 85.4% for adult males. Ninety-five percent classification was achieved for adult females and 86.7% for adolescents. The classification accuracies for females were higher than those for males [14]. A computer-aided diagnosis (CAD) system used magnetic resonance brain images and segmented the cerebral cortex and cerebral white matter using a 3D joint model. Spherical harmonics (SPHARM) was applied to the reconstructed meshes of the cerebral cortex to derive four matrices for each mesh point. All extracted shape features were fed to a deep network for feature fusion. The performance of the CAD system was evaluated using subjects from ABIDE databases (8–12.8 years), achieving an accuracy of 93%, and from a National Institute of Mental Health data archive (NDA) database (16–51 years), an accuracy of 97% was achieved [15].

Several methodologies were presented for using phenotypic data with resting-state fMRI data in a single deep learning network for classifying ASD. The long short-term memory-based architecture was used, and the fMRI data were used as input. The neural network models were executed using Keras, and tenfold cross-validation was used for evaluation. A classification accuracy of 70.01% was achieved on the ABIDE dataset [16]. A deep transfer learning neural network framework was developed to classify whole-brain functional connectivity patterns. Resting-state fMRI data were obtained from ABIDE repository. A stacked sparse autoencoder was trained and used for classification. The results suggested that this approach achieved improved performance compared to traditional models [17]. A deep belief network was executed to perform binary classification using fMRI data obtained from the ABIDE I and ABIDE II datasets. A subsample of 185 participants, which included data from 116 individuals with ASD and 69 control subjects, was selected. The fMRI images were segmented into 116 regions of interest (ROIs) based on the automated anatomical labeling template. With fMRI data, an accuracy of 60.56% was achieved, and with fusion of fMRI, grey matter and white matter, a maximum accuracy of 65.56% was achieved [18]. The ABIDE dataset, consisting of 1,111 scans, including 573 typical controls and 538 ASD subjects, was considered for the study. The maximum accuracy achieved by fivefold cross-validation for ABIDE data was 0.614 [19]. The ABIDE datasets included resting-state fMRI images, t1 structural brain images and phenotypic information of 505 ASD subjects and 530 matched controls (typical controls; TC). The data were slice-time corrected and motion corrected, and the voxel intensity was also normalized. The deep neural network achieved a mean classification accuracy of 70% (sensitivity 74%, specificity 63%) from cross-validation folds and a range accuracy of 66% to 71% in individual folds. The support vector machine algorithm (SVM) classifier achieved a mean accuracy of 65% (from 62% to 72%), sensitivity of 68% and specificity of 62%; the random forest classifier achieved a mean accuracy of 63% (sensitivity 69%, specificity 58%) [20].

A subset of T1w MRI images provided by the Autism Brain Imaging Data Exchange 1 (ABIDE 1) site, which included 182 subjects with T1w images consisting of 78 subjects with ASD and 104 typically developing subjects, was used. The tenfold cross-validation method was used to evaluate the proposed system. The proposed method achieved the highest classification accuracy when the top 3,000 features were selected. The accuracy, sensitivity and specificity were 90.39%, 84.37% and 95.88%, respectively [21]. A model has also been designed using an autoencoder and single-layer perceptron to improve the quality of extracted features. To produce synthetic datasets, a data augmentation strategy based on linear interpolation was designed. This method achieved an accuracy of 82% and outperformed other state-of-the-art methods for ASD classification. The dataset used in this study was collected from the ABIDE database [22]. Multi-institutional fMRI data of 198 school-aged subjects were obtained from the ABIDE II database, and stacked autoencoders were used to classify those with ASD from typically developing children. The results obtained showed an accuracy of 96.62%, and the classification results were higher than previous studies [23]. A convolutional neural network model was proposed for classifying ASD by using resting-state functional magnetic resonance imaging data obtained from the ABIDE I and ABIDE II databases. Transfer learning was used in combination with a mixture of expert and simple Bayes approaches for analysis of the data. The accuracy obtained by using the Adamaz optimization technique was 0.72, and the accuracy achieved by using the Adam optimization technique was 0.70. It was concluded that this approach can also be used for analyzing resting-state fMRI data related to brain dysfunctions [24].

A method called ASD-DiagNet was proposed for the classification of subjects with ASD from healthy control subjects using a preprocessed ABIDE-I dataset that was provided by the ABIDE initiative. The resting-state fMRI data from 505 subjects with ASD and 530 typical controls was used, and the data were parceled into 200 functionally homogenous regions which were generated using a spatially constrained spectral clustering algorithm. An autoencoder was used to extract a lower-dimensional feature representation. The synthetic minority over-sampling technique (SMOTE) was used as the data augmentation technique which uses the nearest neighbor of a sample for generating synthetic data. An ASD-DiagNet model was evaluated using *k*-fold cross-validation. ASD DiagNet achieved 70.3% accuracy when tenfold cross-validation was performed on whole ABIDE-I dataset [25]. Classification algorithms such as logistic regression, linear discriminant analysis, K-nearest neighbour (KNN), classification and regression trees, naive Bayes and support vector machine (SVM) were implemented on the data obtained from ABIDE. Linear discriminant analysis (LDA) achieved the peak accuracy, ranging from 74.86% to 85.16%. KNN achieved an accuracy range of 68.42% to 76.12% [26]. An auto-ASD network model was proposed to classify subjects with autism from typical subjects using fMRI and MRI data generated from 1,112 typical control and ASD subjects provided by ABIDE. The SMOTE algorithm was used for data augmentation for generating artificial data and to avoid overfitting to increase the classification accuracy. The discriminative power of features extracted using multi-layer perceptron was investigated by feeding the features to an SVM classifier. The highest accuracy of 80% was achieved using the model [27].

Resting-state functional connectivity MRI and behavioral data were collected from 167 subjects, of which 15 had ASD. At 12 and 24 months, higher scores of ritualistic behavior were found to be associated with less positive functional connectivity among visual and control networks [28]. A multi-site adaption framework via low-rank representation decomposition (MALRR) for the detection of

ASD based on functional MRI was proposed. A dataset consisting of 1,112 subjects, including 539 ASD subjects and 573 typical controls was collected from the ABIDE database. When the proposed MALRR method which aims to reduce the differences in data distributions was used with SVM and KNN classifiers, it outperformed the compared methods in terms of accuracy, positive predictive value and negative predictive value [29]. A study was conducted to develop a model for the automated classification of ASD using a convolutional neural network (CNN) with rs-fMRI data, The data were obtained from the ABIDE database. The results indicated that the proposed model achieved an accuracy of 70.22%. The proposed CNN model's fewer parameters and results indicated that it could be used to prescreen ASD subjects [30].

Functional and structural information have been merged to improve the detection of autism spectrum disorder. The data were collected from the ABIDE database, and the dataset included data from 368 ASD subjects and 449 control subjects. Stacked autoencoders were trained in an unsupervised manner, and a classification accuracy of 85.06% was achieved [31]. A multichannel deep-attention neural network has also been designed for the automated diagnosis of ASD. The resting-state fMRI data were collected from the ABIDE database. The dataset contained data of 408 ASD subjects and 401 typically developing subjects. The proposed model achieved an accuracy of 0.732 in classifying ASD by combining brain functional connectomes and personal characteristic data. K-fold and leave-one-out cross-validation were done to evaluate the model [32].

15.3 DETECTION METHODS BASED ON BEHAVIORAL DATA AND OTHER DETECTION TECHNIQUES

Behavioral data is yet another biomarker considered for the detection of ASD. A study was conducted on 226 subjects who had been diagnosed with ASD and 163 subjects with attention-deficit/hyperactivity disorder, language disorders, intellectual disability and emotional disorders to examine the effectiveness of the Child Behavior Checklist (CBCL) for screening ASD. The results indicated misclassifications when CBCL profiles were used for the screening of ASD [33]. Classification and regression trees (CART), which is a data mining procedure, was used on the data collected from 660 participants (1.5–1.3 years of age) to distinguish subjects with ASD and subjects without ASD. The classification accuracy achieved by this model was more than 80% and was in agreement with ADOS classification [34]. The possibility of saliva-based miRNA serving as a potential diagnostic screening tool for autism spectrum disorder was investigated. Purified salivary miRNA was collected from 24 ASD subjects and 21 age-matched control subjects. By using RNA-seq, a total of 246 miRNA were detected. The results indicated that the 14 miRNA were differentially expressed in autism spectrum disorder subjects, and 95% accuracy was achieved in classifying ASD subjects based on these 14 miRNA by using a best-fit logistic regression model [35]. Fifteen subjects without any developmental concerns and 11 suspected subjects with ASD were examined, and a video recording was also made. More red flags were shown by suspected ASD subjects during structural evaluations [36]. A screening observation scale was developed for screening ASD which can be used in primary care, and a study was developed. The subjects were divided into three groups, an ASD group with 37 subjects, intellectual disability with 23 subjects and typically developing with 26 subjects. Fisher's exact tests were used for performing pair-wise group comparisons. The results indicated that the subjects with ASD had an overall higher score in observations than the typically developing subjects [37].

Data were collected from a previous study and from six subjects with autism. The subjects were wearing three-axis wireless accelerometers. The results showed that this method can provide accurate stereotypical motor movement detection using CNN [38]. For 56 high-risk children and 26 age-matched low-risk children at 24 months, CBCL/I1/2–5 scores were analyzed. The CBCL scores at 24 months were compared for high risk and low risk children. The results indicated that 13 of the 56 children in the HR group were diagnosed with ASD and 43 were not diagnosed at 24 months of age. The HR group also obtained higher CBCL scores than the LR group [39]. At four and nine months of age, 12,179 infants were followed and screened with the Program for Research and Studies on Autism (PREAUT) grid to predict ASD. The checklist for autism in toddlers was completed for a sample of 1,835 infants. The results indicated that the PREAUT grid can help in the detection of ASD and, when combined with the Checklist for Autism in Toddlers (CHAT), can improve the early detection of autism spectrum disorder [40]. The 512 participants, including 223 ASD subjects and 289 non-ASD subjects, used for this study were from three separate projects and were recruited through the early intervention programs, ASD-related networks and pediatric practices. The ROC plots which described the relationship between Brief Infant Toddler Social Emotional Assessment (BITSEA) ASD scores and the ASD diagnosis were plotted, and the results indicate the BITSEA is an effective screening tool for ASD [41].

The screening accuracy of the BITSEA was evaluated and compared with the Pervasive Developmental Disorders Screening Test-II and Developmental Clinic Screener (PDDST-II-DCS) in diagnosis of ASD in toddlers born at less than 30 weeks gestation. The caregivers of 555 children, including 94% mothers, completed the questionnaires. Four percent of children had an ASD diagnosis. The results indicated that the accuracy of the BITSEA was better than that of the PDD-II-DCS [42]. Two-tiered screening was examined by combining the modified checklist for autism in toddlers, and a screening tool for autism in toddlers and young children improved the detection of autism early in life. One hundred nine subjects who had received level 1 screening were screened using level 2 screening. The results indicated that the combination of level 1 and level 2 for screening reduced the false positive rate [43]. Two machine-learning algorithms were trained on parent-reported questionnaire and behavioral data. The results were then combined using a combination algorithm to increase the accuracy of diagnosis. A validation set consisting of data from 162 subjects was then used to check the performance, and the findings suggested that the machine-learning method is a reliable method for the detection of ASD [44]. The specificity and sensitivity of the Modified Checklist for Autism in Toddlers (MCHAT) and the Parent's Observations of Social Interactions (POSI) were compared. Both MCHAT and POSI displayed sensitivities above 70% for the subjects of the age group between 16–30 months. The results indicated that both methods had acceptable sensitivity for the evaluation of autism in subjects at the age of 48 months [45]. At 14 months, around 200 subjects were observed, of which 119 subjects had ASD. For 59% of the subjects, clarity in diagnosis of ASD was found, while the other subjects had to do a follow-up [46]. Forty subjects with ASD and 40 typically developing subjects participated in a study in which the mean scores of the autism group were higher than normal group [47]. The ASD classification was done based on social relationship, emotional response, communication, behavioral patterns, sensory aspects and cognitive component. Discriminant analysis was used to classify children with autism from typical children. The results indicated that fast and accurate diagnosis of autism (FADA) is a reliable tool for the assessment of subjects with autism [47]. A computational method, variable analysis, was proposed that considered feature-to-class correlations and also reduced feature-to-feature correlations. The data were collected through a mobile app for this study. The results showed that variable analysis derived fewer features from different screening methods and showed good accuracy [48].

The psychometric properties of the systematic observation of red flags were examined in a sample of 228 infants, including 84 subjects with ASD, 82 subjects with developmental delay and 62 typically developing subjects [49]. A total score summing all the items, domain score and number of red flag items were calculated. The results indicated that Systematic Observation Of Red Flags (SORF) can be used as an alternative to other screening methods [49]. Fifty caregivers participated in a study and received a questionnaire. It was found that significant agreement existed between the age and stages questionnaires: social emotional and child behavior checklist, and significant agreement was also found between the BITSEA and child behavior checklist. When their agreement with the modified checklist for autism in toddlers was examined, it was found that the BITSEA had significant agreement with it and could be used as a screener for ASD [50]. Motor skills were examined by using Peabody developmental motor scales in 140 subjects 6 months of age who were at high and low risk of developing ASD. The results indicated that motor skills at 6 months predicted ASD at 24–26 months and predicted expressive language at the age of 30 to 36 months [51]. A study was also conducted to develop an automated system using acoustic and text features to decrease the time required for classifying ASD. Data were taken form 70 subjects with ASD and 35 typically developing subjects. A classification accuracy of 75.71% was achieved, but the results also showed that the subject ratings were higher than this model [52].

The EMR records of 1,397 ASD subjects and 94,741 non-ASD subjects were collected from the Israeli Health Maintenance organization, and a tenfold cross-validation technique was used to evaluate the prediction accuracy. The average accuracy achieved was 98.18%, and it showed that such methods can enhance the ability to detect ASD at an early stage and in a large population [53]. Using near-infrared spectroscopy, spontaneous hemodynamic fluctuations were obtained from the temporal cortex and bilateral inferior frontal gyrus of 25 subjects with ASD and 22 typically developing children. A multilayer neural network, complex gated recurrent neural networks (CGRNN), which is a combination of convolution neural network and a gate recurrent unit, was used for feature extraction and classification. This technique achieved an accuracy of 92.2%, which indicated that the multilayer neural network CGRNN can be used for the classification of ASD subjects and typically developing subjects [54]. Diffusion tensor images were acquired from 118 typically developing subjects aged 0–8 years and from 31 subjects with autism spectrum disorder, recruited at Beijing Children's Hospital. The diffusion tensor image metrics were used to measure the microstructure of every major white matter tract and tract group. When they kept typically developing white matter curves as reference, it was observed that there was a higher residual variance of white matter microstructural maturation in all the major tracts in the 0–8-year age group [55].

In yet another trial, cry voices were recorded from 31 ASD subjects and 31 TD subjects, and the features were extracted using a subset instance classifier. The sensitivity and precision for male subjects were 85.71% and 92.85%, respectively. The sensitivity and precision for female subjects were 71.42% and 85.71%, respectively [56]. A simulated interaction task, which is a digital tool for the automatic quantification of biomarkers of social interaction deficits, was presented to 37 subjects with ASD and 43 control subjects. With the help of machine-learning tools, an accuracy of 73% was achieved based on facial expressions and vocal characteristics [57]. A clustering-based autistic trait classification (CATC), which is a semi-supervised machine-learning framework, was proposed. The proposed method identifies autism subjects based on similarity traits. The results indicated that the CATC has higher predictive accuracy compared to other classification approaches [58]. A continuous-wave functional near-infrared spectroscopy (FNIRS) system was used to scan 25 subjects with ASD and from 22 age-matched subjects, and the parameters measured were the concentration changes in HbO_2, Hb and total hemoglobin. An integrated deep learning model, consisting of long-short term memory and a convolutional neural network, was constructed. The proposed model performed well even with FNIRS data of only one variable. This study mainly emphasized the combination of long short-term memory (LSTM) and CNN and the integration strategy. Though accurate classification was achieved, the size of the dataset was lower [59].

15.4 DETECTION TECHNIQUES BASED ON EEG DATA

EEG is also one of the biomarkers used to detect ASD. Several features of EEG signals have been used for the detection of ASD. EEG was recorded in a resting state while the eyes were closed using the Deymed Truscan 32 EEG system. The results revealed that autistic subjects had less absolute delta power than control subjects. The relative delta power was reduced in autistic children as compared to control subjects [60]. Another study was conducted to confirm the occurrence of epileptic seizures and EEG abnormalities in ASD subjects. Data from 1,014 autistic subjects were obtained. A 32-channel digital EEG was recorded every six months during sleep. A source derivation method, topography and dipole analysis were used for EEG analysis. Epilepsy was found in 37% of subjects, and epileptic discharges were found in 85.8% of subjects [61]. Resting-state EEG data with eyes-closed data recorded from nine ASD children and eight non-ASD subjects were obtained from Atieh Comprehensive Center for Psych and Nerve Disorders, Tehran. A radial basis function neural network (RBFNN) classifier was used for classification. An accuracy of 90% was obtained by using the RBFNN classifier [62]. To classify TD and HR groups, a multiclass support vector machine algorithm was used. Multi-scale entropy differences appeared to be greatest at ages 9 to 12 months. At the age of 9 months, infants were classified into control and high risk for autism groups with over 80% accuracy, and for boys, the classification accuracy was 100% [63]. A study was conducted to investigate the linear and fractal EEG features in autistic children and children with intellectual disabilities. Three EEG recordings were taken from 19 autistic children and 19 children with intellectual disability. An increase in delta activity was observed in the right posterior delta region in autistic subjects as compared to subjects with intellectual disability, and higher delta and gamma activity was observed during sleep [64]. Regularized Fisher's linear discriminant (RFLD) analysis was conducted for the detection of autism in subjects using EEG signals. The EEG recordings were taken from eight ASD subjects and four non-ASD subjects. Fast Fourier transform was used for the extraction of features. The classification accuracy obtained using RFLD analysis was 92% [65]. Fuzzy synchronization likelihood was obtained between different EEG signals, which were obtained from nine ASD subjects and nine non-ASD subjects in a resting state recorded at Atieh Comprehensive Center, Tehran, Iran. An enhanced probabilistic neural network was used as a classifier, and the classification accuracy achieved was 95.5% [66].

Data from 19 patients with ASD and 19 age- and gender-matched control subjects were obtained. Spectral and relative power were computed. The results showed that the relative gamma power was higher in ASD subjects when compared with control subjects [67]. Neural responses to speech and non-speech sounds in 14 ASD children who were intellectually able and 11 TD children were investigated. A semi-synthesis speech generation method was utilized for stimuli, six different kinds of stimuli were used and EEG was recorded. The results suggested that children with ASD failed to activate right hemisphere mechanisms [68]. A dataset was obtained from King Abdul Aziz University. A discrete wavelet transform (DWT) was used for the decomposition the signals, and EEG subbands were obtained. Shannon entropy was used to construct the feature vector. An artificial neural network was used to classify the EEG signals. The highest classification accuracy of 99.71% was achieved with the combination of discrete wavelet transform and Shannon entropy [69]. The EEG was recorded in a resting condition with eyes open and eyes closed from 15 children with ASD and 10 control subjects. The implicit function as squashing TIME (I-FAST) algorithm was applied to the EEGs of 15 subjects with autism and 10 control subjects. The I-FAST algorithm, which consists of a squashing phase, noise elimination phase and classification phase, is shown in Figure 15.1. By using a training testing protocol, the predictive capability of the model was 100%, and by using the leave-one-out protocol, the best results were obtained by using a random forest machine-learning system with an overall accuracy of 92.8% [70].

Oscillatory activity of the alpha band associated with attentional capture in ASD subjects and typically developing children was examined. Continuous resting-state EEG from 21 subjects with ASD and 21 typically developing age- and nonverbal IQ-matched subjects was recorded. The subjects with ASD didn't show electrophysiological evidence of attentional capture by distracters or behaviorally relevant targets regardless of whether they shared a task-relevant feature. ASD subjects showed reduced resting alpha power [71]. In another study, EEG signals recorded from 188 children were decomposed using wavelet transform into multiple frequency bands. Nine nonlinear functions were calculated for each frequency band. Leave-one-out cross-validation was used for the prediction of ASD and non-ASD. The results showed that the ASD subjects were distinguished from low-risk control subjects with a sensitivity of 100% [72]. Continuous EEG data were recorded from 59 subjects with ASD and 39 TD subjects for two minutes in a dark room and while bubbles were being displayed on a computer screen. Some electrode pairs were found to be different in autism spectrum disorder subjects. The correlation was not found for long-range connectivity [73]. Power spectrum analysis was performed on EEG data recorded from 52 subjects with ASD and 52 control subjects using artifact-free EEG data in MATLAB. Entropy and bicoherence were also evaluated. An accuracy of 91.38% was obtained using an SVM classifier, and this method can be used to help in the detection of autism spectrum disorder [74].

A dataset which contained EEG data from 16 ASD subjects and 46 typically developing subjects was obtained from Boston Children's Hospital, Harvard

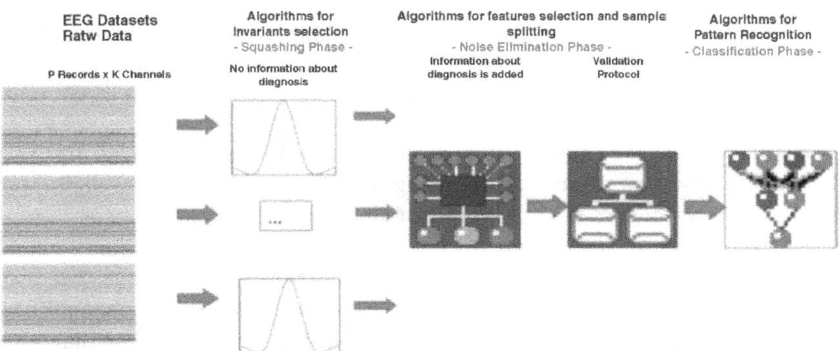

FIGURE 15.1 Implicit function as squashing TIME algorithm used for ASD detection.

(From Enzo Grossi et al. 2017.)

Medical School and Semel Institute, University of California. Recurrence quantification analysis was performed on continuous resting-state EEG segments. The results indicated that an accuracy of 92.9% was achieved using leave-one-out classification with a non-linear support vector machine classifier [75]. Empirical mode decomposition was used to obtain intrinsic mode functions nonlinearly from 64-channel EEG data collected from 60 ASD subjects and 60 typically developing subjects with ages between 4 and 13 years. The results indicated that an accuracy of 94.4% was obtained with the neural network classification based on second-order difference plot features [76]. A study was conducted to evaluate the EEG and eye movement data for the diagnosis of ASD. The data were recorded from 52 subjects, of which 24 subjects had ASD and 28 were control subjects. The preprocessed signals were divided into windows of size 40, and discrete fast Fourier transform was computed for each window. An accuracy of 100% was achieved by using an SVM with Shannon entropy. An accuracy of 71% was achieved with logistic regression [77].

Different feature extraction and EEG classification techniques for assisting in epilepsy and ASD detection were investigated. An EEG dataset which included data from ten typically developing subjects and nine autistic subjects was collected from King Abdul Aziz University, Saudi Arabia. DWT and cross-correlation approaches were used to extract features from the EEG signals. The results indicated that an overall classification result of 94.6% was obtained by the combination of DWT, Shannon entropy and *k*-nearest neighbor techniques [78]. The Biosemi Activetwo 128-channel 24-bit resolution system was employed to obtain the five-minute EEG recordings from 19 patients with ASD and 19 control subjects with eyes closed. The spectral power of independent components was used for the evaluation of the degree of synchronization of neural activity. In this study, gamma-band abnormalities in ASD were successfully characterized from resting-state EEG data [79]. Motor-related gamma oscillations in ASD subjects were investigated by using magneto-encephalography. From 14 ASD children and 15 typically developing children, magneto-encephalography signals were recorded during a motor task. The ASD children showed slightly longer button response time and also reduced amplitude of motor evoked magnetic fields. In the bilateral primary motor cortex, the subjects with autism showed reduced power of motor-related gamma oscillations. The linear discriminant analysis showed a high classification accuracy of 86.2% [80].

Data were gathered from 88 subjects composed of 44 subjects with ASD and 44 typically developing subjects. By using a Nihon-Kohden system, digital ten-channel EEG was recorded. No significant alpha peak frequency, power between the groups or effect of age in typically developing controls on the alpha frequency were observed. An increase of alpha frequency and power with the age of the participant was found by the linear method approach [81]. Sixty-four-channel EEG data was also obtained from 99 subjects whose older siblings had been diagnosed with ASD and 89 control subjects aged 3 to 36 months. Non-linear features computed from EEG were given as an input to the statistical learning methods. The classification of ASD subjects from low-risk controls was performed with nearly

100% sensitivity, and the predicted severity scores also highly correlated with the actual scores [82]. From 16 subjects with ASD, 42 high-risk subjects without ASD and 43 low-risk subjects, EEG data and cognitive and behavioral assessments were acquired. The high-risk subjects without ASD showed reduced baseline frontal gamma power compared to the low-risk subjects. Increased frontal baseline gamma power was observed with ASD subjects [83]. Thirty-six children were recruited and divided into groups with mild and severe ASD containing 18 subjects each. Multicsale entropy features and patterns were identified in 64-channel EEG data collected from the subjects. The averaged multiscale entropy values of subjects with autism spectrum disorder were higher in subjects with mild ASD than subjects with severe ASD in right frontal, right parietal and central cortical areas. The results indicated that subjects with mild ASD had increased sample entropy values compared to subjects with severe ASD [84].

EEG data were recorded from 39 ASD subjects and 16 age-matched subjects while watching videos of bubbles, and the perceived rating scale was used to rate the state of subjects. The results indicated that ASD subjects had higher perceived state ratings (PSRs) than the typically developing subjects, and the typical subjects had more alpha power than ASD subjects [85]. A study was conducted to evaluate the phenotypic characteristics, potential correlations between EEG abnormalities and cognitive variables and prevalence of EEG abnormalities. For this study, 69 subjects with ASD underwent language assessment, development testing and behavioral skills evaluation, and EEG recordings were taken. EEG abnormalities were found in 39.13% of the subjects and were correlated with several phenotypic features [86]. One hundred twenty-nine-channel EEG data and eye tracking data were obtained from 14 ASD subjects and 14 TD subjects to examine the differences in neural processing of dynamic cartoons that contained human-like social interactions. The results indicated that impairments in brain regions were present from an early age in ASD [87]. EEG data and eye tracking data were taken from 32 children with ASD and 32 TD children. The results indicated that theta power was low in subjects with ASD, indicating that ASD can be associated with dopaminergic activity, which may contribute to theta-band power [88].

EEG data in a resting state were recorded from 36 children who were grouped into a mild ASD group and severe ASD group. The 35 feature sets obtained were given to an artificial neural network with Levenberg-Marquardt back-propagation. An overall accuracy of 97.2% was obtained [89]. One hundred forty-three subjects at a high and low familial risk of ASD watched videos of toys spinning and women singing rhymes while EEG was being recorded. At 14 months, association between higher functional connectivity was replicated, and at 36 months, there was a greater severity of repetitive and restricted behaviors for subjects who met the criteria for ASD [90]. From 58 ASD subjects and 39 TD subjects, EEG data were collected. The covariate-adjusted region-referenced generalized functional linear model (CARR-GFLM) was used for the analysis of data. The T8 electrode showed the highest contribution for the log-odds for diagnosis of ASD [91]. Frontal EEG asymmetry was examined in response to direct gaze in 21 ASD, 19 typically developing and 17 children with intellectual disability in a study that was part of an autism and gaze research project. Four-way ANOVA was used for the analysis. The asymmetry scores were higher in ASD subjects and for the static stimuli; three-way ANOVA did not show any significant main effects [92]. The EEG data of normal subjects were obtained from BCI competition IV, and the autistic dataset was obtained from BNCI Horizon and University of Pompeu, Fabra. The dataset contained data of 20 typical subjects and 10 autistic subjects. Daubechies-eight with eight-level discrete wavelet transform was used to extract features, and the EEG signals were divided into different frequency bands. The best accuracy of 92.8% was achieved by the time domain using subspace KNN, while an accuracy of 87.3% was achieved by the frequency domain [93].

EEG recordings were obtained from eight subjects with ASD and nine risk control subjects. Power spectra were generated for data from each electrode by using frequency band decomposition and wavelet transforms. The results indicated that a classification accuracy of 92% was achieved using non-linear models, and an accuracy of 56% was achieved using linear models [94]. The data were recorded from 15 subjects who included 10 subjects with ASD and 5 control subjects. Statistical features were obtained from the EEG signals. Discrete wavelet transform was executed and relevant features were selected using correlation-based feature selection. Using random forest and correlation-based features, an accuracy of 93% was obtained [95]. EEG was recorded from 86 subjects, including 43 children with ASD and 43 typically developing children. Using the Renyi permutation entropy method, it was found that at 4 years of age, there was a significant difference in the central part and in the frontal and central cortex by using sample entropy for the 5-year-old group. The results showed that the entropy values of the ASD subjects were lower than those for typically developing subjects in frontal, left temporal, central and right temporal, which showed the reduced complexity in ASD children [96]. Sixty children (30 control subjects and 30 ASD subjects) varying in ages from 4 to 8 years were tested. An animation was shown for five minutes after a two-minute registration of baseline. Visibility graphs were drawn and topological features were extracted using a complex network called the average degree (AD). The KNN algorithm was used for classification. The results showed that the average degree of nodes in almost 75% of the control group sample exceeded that of the ASD group sample [97]. Microstate analysis was used to investigate the differences in four temporal parameters (mean duration, frequency of occurrence, time coverage and global explained variance). The dataset used was obtained from a previous study (Hames et al., 2016). Segmentation of the data was done by carrying out a two-step spatial cluster analysis. The results showed that six template maps best described the complete dataset with 83% of the global variance [98]. The general input formulations of EEG signals for deep learning and machine learning algorithms is shown in Figure 15.2.

EEG recordings were taken from 9 subjects with ASD and 17 subjects without ASD. The absolute and relative powers were calculated. The results showed the differences centrally and parieto-occipitally on both the left and right sides in the alpha band. The primary finding of this study was that tuberous sclerosis

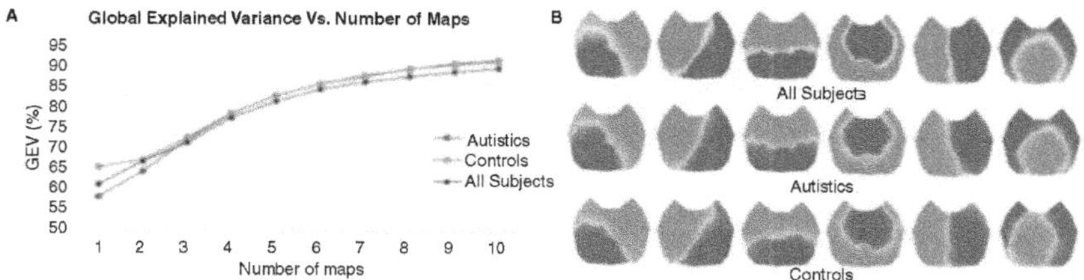

FIGURE 15.2 General input formulations employed for neurological disease detection using EEG.

complex subjects with ASD significantly showed higher levels of alpha relative power during stage 2 sleep [99]. Longitudinal EEG measurements were taken from 3- to 36-month-old children at low and high risk of ASD to analyze how and when EEG power distinguishes ASD and the risk by the age of 3 years. The power trajectories consistently discriminated infants with ASD from others. The results indicated the importance of developmental timings in understanding the pathophysiology and classification of ASD [100]. Resting-state EEG and eye-tracking data from 97 children were used as input for an SVM to identify autism spectrum disorder. A power spectrum analysis was performed on EEG data and areas of interest. The classification was performed using the minimum redundancy maximum relevance feature selection method and support vector machine classifiers, and a classification accuracy of 85.44% was achieved [101].

Fast periodic visual stimulation and EEG were combined to assess the neural sensitivity to detect facial expressions. Twenty-three subjects with ASD and 23 typically developing subjects were involved in this study. The stimuli were given in the form of front images of 14 individuals. The EEG data were recorded by using a BIOSEMI active-two amplifier system. The results indicated that both groups showed equal neural synchronization and neural responses to happy and sad faces. The classification accuracy of this method was 87% [102]. Data from 34 subjects with ASD and 11 typically developing subjects were obtained in cooperation with Noor-e-Hedayat Center, Iran. Linear and non-linear features such as power spectrum and wavelet transform were extracted from the EEG signal. An accuracy of 99.91% was achieved using an SVM, and an accuracy of 72.77% was achieved using KNN [103]. A 64-channel EEG was recorded from the entire brain for 20 minutes in a resting state with a sampling frequency of 500 Hz. The higher-order spectra (HOS) bispectrum was obtained, and non-linear features were extracted from the HOS bispectrum. Run-length-matrix-based features like log energy, Kapoor entropy and max entropy were extracted. These extracted non-linear features were reduced using locality sensitivity discriminant analysis (LSDA). An accuracy of 98.70%was achieved by the probabilistic neural network classifier, and the tenfold cross-validation technique was used for evaluation of the performance of the classifier. The results indicated that this method can be used to assist in diagnosing autism [104].

15.5 CONCLUSION

Different approaches have been used for the detection of ASD. The studies included in this chapter indicate that autism spectrum disorder can be detected by extracting features from data. When features were extracted from MRI data, the studies showed good accuracy, suggesting this approach can assist in detection of ASD. The results from studies using EEG data look very promising. More research needs to conducted so that ASD can be detected as early as possible and to find a biomarker for ASD detection.

REFERENCES

[1] Shaw, K.A., et al., "Early Identification of Autism Spectrum Disorder among Children Aged 4 Years—Early Autism and Developmental Disabilities Monitoring Network, Six Sites, United States, 2016." MMWR Surveillance Summaries, vol. 69, March 2020.

[2] Lord, Catherine, et al. "Autism Spectrum Disorder." *Nature Reviews Disease Primers*, vol. 6, no. 1, 2020, doi:10.1038/s41572-019-0138-4.

[3] Lord, Catherine, et al. "Autism Spectrum Disorder." *The Lancet*, vol. 392, no. 10146, 2018, pp. 508–520.

[4] Hodges, Holly, et al. "Autism Spectrum Disorder: Definition, Epidemiology, Causes, and Clinical Evaluation." *Translational Pediatrics*, vol. 9, no. S1, 2020, doi:10.21037/tp.2019.09.09.

[5] Wang, Liye, et al. "Multi-Task Feature Selection via Supervised Canonical Graph Matching for Diagnosis of Autism Spectrum Disorder." *Brain Imaging and Behavior*, vol. 10, no. 1, 2015, pp. 33–40, doi:10.1007/s11682-015-9360-1.

[6] Yao, Zhijun, et al. "Resting-State Time-Varying Analysis Reveals Aberrant Variations of Functional Connectivity in Autism." *Frontiers in Human Neuroscience*, vol. 10, 2016, doi:10.3389/fnhum.2016.00463.

[7] Wee, Chong-Yaw, et al. "Diagnosis of Autism Spectrum Disorders Using Temporally Distinct Resting-State Functional Connectivity Networks." *CNS Neuroscience & Therapeutics*, vol. 22, no. 3, 2016, pp. 212–219, doi:10.1111/cns.12499.

[8] Chen, Heng, et al. "Multivariate Classification of Autism Spectrum Disorder Using Frequency-Specific Resting-State Functional Connectivity—A Multi-Center Study." *Progress in Neuro-Psychopharmacology and Biological Psychiatry*, vol. 64, 2016, pp. 1–9, doi:10.1016/j.pnpbp.2015.06.014.

[9] Blackmon, Karen, et al. "Periventricular White Matter Abnormalities and Restricted Repetitive Behavior in Autism Spectrum Disorder." *NeuroImage: Clinical*, vol. 10, 2016, pp. 36–45, doi:10.1016/j.nicl.2015.10.017.

[10] Zhao, Feng, et al. "Feature Fusion via Hierarchical Supervised Local CCA for Diagnosis of Autism Spectrum Disorder." *Brain Imaging and Behavior*, vol. 11, no. 4, 2016, pp. 1050–1060, doi:10.1007/s11682-016-9587-5.

[11] Guo, Xinyu, et al. "Diagnosing Autism Spectrum Disorder from Brain Resting-State Functional Connectivity Patterns Using a Deep Neural Network with a Novel Feature Selection Method." *Frontiers in Neuroscience*, vol. 11, 2017, doi:10.3389/fnins.2017.00460.

[12] Conti, E., et al. "Network Over-Connectivity Differentiates Autism Spectrum Disorder from Other Developmental Disorders in Toddlers: A Diffusion MRI

Study." *Human Brain Mapping*, vol. 38, no. 5, 2017, pp. 2333–2344, doi:10.1002/hbm.23520.

[13] Emerson, Robert W., et al. "Functional Neuroimaging of High-Risk 6-Month-Old Infants Predicts a Diagnosis of Autism at 24 Months of Age." *Science Translational Medicine*, vol. 9, no. 393, 2017, doi:10.1126/scitranslmed.aag2882.

[14] Subbaraju, Vigneshwaran, et al. "Identifying Differences in Brain Activities and an Accurate Detection of Autism Spectrum Disorder Using Resting State Functional-Magnetic Resonance Imaging: A Spatial Filtering Approach." *Medical Image Analysis*, vol. 35, 2017, pp. 375–389, doi:10.1016/j.media.2016.08.003.

[15] Ismail, Marwa, et al. "A New Deep-Learning Approach for Early Detection of Shape Variations in Autism Using Structural MRI." *2017 IEEE International Conference on Image Processing (ICIP)*, 2017, doi:10.1109/icip.2017.8296443.

[16] Dvornek, Nicha C., et al. "Combining Phenotypic and Resting-State FMRI Data for Autism Classification with Recurrent Neural Networks." *2018 IEEE 15th International Symposium on Biomedical Imaging (ISBI 2018)*, 2018, doi:10.1109/isbi.2018.8363676.

[17] Li, Hailong, et al. "A Novel Transfer Learning Approach to Enhance Deep Neural Network Classification of Brain Functional Connectomes." *Frontiers in Neuroscience*, vol. 12, 2018, doi:10.3389/fnins.2018.00491.

[18] Aghdam, Maryam Akhavan, et al. "Combination of Rs-FMRI and SMRI Data to Discriminate Autism Spectrum Disorders in Young Children Using Deep Belief Network." *Journal of Digital Imaging*, vol. 31, no. 6, 2018, pp. 895–903, doi:10.1007/s10278-018-0093-8.

[19] Sen, Bhaskar, et al. "A General Prediction Model for the Detection of ADHD and Autism Using Structural and Functional MRI." *PLoS ONE*, vol. 13, no. 4, 2018, doi:10.1371/journal.pone.0194856.

[20] Heinsfeld, Anibal Sólon, et al. "Identification of Autism Spectrum Disorder Using Deep Learning and the ABIDE Dataset." *NeuroImage: Clinical*, vol. 17, 2018, pp. 16–23, doi:10.1016/j.nicl.2017.08.017.

[21] Kong, Yazhou, et al. "Classification of Autism Spectrum Disorder by Combining Brain Connectivity and Deep Neural Network Classifier." *Neurocomputing*, vol. 324, 2019, pp. 63–68, doi:10.1016/j.neucom.2018.04.080.

[22] Eslami, Taban, et al. "ASD-DiagNet: A Hybrid Learning Approach for Detection of Autism Spectrum Disorder Using FMRI Data." *Frontiers in Neuroinformatics*, vol. 13, 2019, doi:10.3389/fninf.2019.00070.

[23] Wang, Mingliang, et al. "Identifying Autism Spectrum Disorder With Multi-Site FMRI via Low-Rank Domain Adaptation." *IEEE Transactions on Medical Imaging*, vol. 39, no. 3, 2020, pp. 644–655, doi:10.1109/tmi.2019.2933160.

[24] Xiao, Zhiyong, et al. "Computer-Aided Diagnosis of School-Aged Children with ASD Using Full Frequency Bands and Enhanced SAE: A Multi-Institution Study." *Experimental and Therapeutic Medicine*, 2019, doi:10.3892/etm.2019.7448.

[25] Aghdam, Maryam Akhavan, et al. "Diagnosis of Autism Spectrum Disorders in Young Children Based on Resting-State Functional Magnetic Resonance Imaging Data Using Convolutional Neural Networks." *Journal of Digital Imaging*, vol. 32, no. 6, 2019, pp. 899–918, doi:10.1007/s10278-019-00196-1.

[26] Eslami, Taban, et al. "ASD-DiagNet: A Hybrid Learning Approach for Detection of Autism Spectrum Disorder Using FMRI Data." *Frontiers in Neuroinformatics*, vol. 13, 2019, doi:10.3389/fninf.2019.00070.

[27] Song, Yuqing, et al. "Characterizing and Predicting Autism Spectrum Disorder by Performing Resting-State Functional Network Community Pattern Analysis." *Frontiers in Human Neuroscience*, vol. 13, 2019, doi:10.3389/fnhum.2019.00203.

[28] Eslami, Taban, and Fahad Saeed. "Auto-ASD-Network." *Proceedings of the 10th ACM International Conference on Bioinformatics, Computational Biology and Health Informatics—BCB '19*, 2019, doi:10.1145/3307339.3343482.

[29] Mckinnon, Claire J., et al. "Restricted and Repetitive Behavior and Brain Functional Connectivity in Infants at Risk for Developing Autism Spectrum Disorder." *Biological Psychiatry: Cognitive Neuroscience and Neuroimaging*, vol. 4, no. 1, 2019, pp. 50–61, doi:10.1016/j.bpsc.2018.09.008.

[30] Sherkatghanad, Zeinab, et al. "Automated Detection of Autism Spectrum Disorder Using a Convolutional Neural Network." *Frontiers in Neuroscience*, vol. 13, 2020, doi:10.3389/fnins.2019.01325.

[31] Rakić, Mladen, et al. "Improving the Detection of Autism Spectrum Disorder by Combining Structural and Functional MRI Information." *NeuroImage: Clinical*, vol. 25, p. 102181, 2020, doi:10.1016/j.nicl.2020.102181.

[32] Niu, Ke, et al. "Multichannel Deep Attention Neural Networks for the Classification of Autism Spectrum Disorder Using Neuroimaging and Personal Characteristic Data." *Complexity*, vol. 2020, 2020, pp. 1–9, doi:10.1155/2020/1357853.

[33] Havdahl, K. Alexandra, et al. "Utility of the Child Behavior Checklist as a Screener for Autism Spectrum Disorder." *Autism Research*, vol. 9, no. 1, 2015, pp. 33–42, doi:10.1002/aur.1515.

[34] Cohen, Ira L., et al. "Using the PDD Behavior Inventory as a Level 2 Screener: A Classification and Regression Trees Analysis." *Journal of Autism and Developmental Disorders*, vol. 46, no. 9, 2016, pp. 3006–3022, doi:10.1007/s10803-016-2843-0.

[35] Hicks, Steven D., et al. "Salivary MiRNA Profiles Identify Children with Autism Spectrum Disorder, Correlate with Adaptive Behavior, and Implicate ASD Candidate Genes Involved in Neurodevelopment." *BMC Pediatrics*, vol. 16, no. 1, 2016, doi:10.1186/s12887-016-0586-x.

[36] Chambers, Nola J, et al. "Early Detection of Autism Spectrum Disorder in Young IsiZulu-Speaking Children in South Africa." *Autism*, vol. 21, no. 5, 2016, pp. 518–526, doi:10.1177/1362361316651196.

[37] Haglund, Nils, et al. "The Observation Scale for Autism (OSA): A New Screening Method to Detect Autism Spectrum Disorder before Age Three Years." *Journal of Intellectual Disability—Diagnosis and Treatment*, vol. 3, no. 4, 2016, pp. 230–237, doi:10.6000/2292-2598.2015.03.04.9.

[38] Rad, Nastaran Mohammadian, and Cesare Furlanello. "Applying Deep Learning to Stereotypical Motor Movement Detection in Autism Spectrum Disorders." *2016 IEEE 16th International Conference on Data Mining Workshops (ICDMW)*, 2016, doi:10.1109/icdmw.2016.0178.

[39] Rescorla, Leslie A, et al. "Autism Spectrum Disorder Screening with the CBCL/1½-5: Findings for Young Children at High Risk for Autism Spectrum Disorder." *Autism*, vol. 23, no. 1, 2017, pp. 29–38, doi:10.1177/1362361317718482.

[40] Olliac, Bertrand, et al. "Infant and Dyadic Assessment in Early Community-Based Screening for Autism Spectrum Disorder with the PREAUT Grid." *PLoS ONE*, vol. 12, no. 12, 2017, doi:10.1371/journal.pone.0188831.

[41] Kiss, Ivy Giserman, et al. "Developing Autism Screening Criteria for the Brief Infant Toddler Social Emotional Assessment (BITSEA)." *Journal of Autism*

and Developmental Disorders, vol. 47, no. 5, 2017, pp. 1269–1277, doi:10.1007/s10803-017-3044-1.

[42] Boone, Kelly M., et al. "Screening Accuracy of the Brief Infant Toddler Social-Emotional Assessment to Identify Autism Spectrum Disorder in Toddlers Born at Less Than 30 Weeks' Gestation." *Child Psychiatry & Human Development*, vol. 49, no. 4, 2017, pp. 493–504, doi:10.1007/s10578-017-0768-2.

[43] Khowaja, Meena, et al. "Utilizing Two-Tiered Screening for Early Detection of Autism Spectrum Disorder." *Autism*, vol. 22, no. 7, 2017, pp. 881–890, doi:10.1177/1362361317712649.

[44] Abbas, Halim, et al. "Machine Learning for Early Detection of Autism (and Other Conditions) Using a Parental Questionnaire and Home Video Screening." *2017 IEEE International Conference on Big Data (Big Data)*, 2017, doi:10.1109/bigdata.2017.8258346.

[45] Salisbury, Louisa A., et al. "Sensitivity and Specificity of 2 Autism Screeners among Referred Children Between 16 and 48 Months of Age." *Journal of Developmental & Behavioral Pediatrics*, vol. 39, no. 3, 2018, pp. 254–258, doi:10.1097/dbp.0000000000000537.

[46] Hine, Jeffrey F., et al. "Embedding Autism Spectrum Disorder Diagnosis within the Medical Home: Decreasing Wait Times through Streamlined Assessment." *Journal of Autism and Developmental Disorders*, vol. 48, no. 8, 2018, pp. 2846–2853, doi:10.1007/s10803-018-3548-3.

[47] Sharma, Anurag, et al. "Fast and Accurate Diagnosis of Autism (FADA): A Novel Hierarchical Fuzzy System Based Autism Detection Tool." *Australasian Physical & Engineering Sciences in Medicine*, vol. 41, no. 3, 2018, pp. 757–772, doi:10.1007/s13246-018-0666-3.

[48] Thabtah, Fadi, et al. "A New Computational Intelligence Approach to Detect Autistic Features for Autism Screening." *International Journal of Medical Informatics*, vol. 117, 2018, pp. 112–124, doi:10.1016/j.ijmedinf.2018.06.009.

[49] Dow, Deanna, et al. "Screening for Autism Spectrum Disorder in a Naturalistic Home Setting Using the Systematic Observation of Red Flags (SORF) at 18–24 Months." *Autism Research*, vol. 13, no. 1, 2019, pp. 122–133, doi:10.1002/aur.2226.

[50] Kamara, Dana, et al. "Socioemotional and Autism Spectrum Disorder Screening for Toddlers in Early Intervention: Agreement Among Measures." *Journal of Early Intervention*, 2019, p. 105381511988060, doi:10.1177/1053815119880607.

[51] Lebarton, Eve Sauer, and Rebecca J. Landa. "Infant Motor Skill Predicts Later Expressive Language and Autism Spectrum Disorder Diagnosis." *Infant Behavior and Development*, vol. 54, 2019, pp. 37–47, doi:10.1016/j.infbeh.2018.11.003.

[52] Cho, Sunghye, et al. "Automatic Detection of Autism Spectrum Disorder in Children Using Acoustic and Text Features from Brief Natural Conversations." *Interspeech 2019*, 2019, doi:10.21437/interspeech.2019-1452.

[53] Rahman, Rayees, et al. "Identification of Newborns at Risk for Autism Using Electronic Medical Records and Machine Learning." *European Psychiatry*, vol. 63, no. 1, 2019, doi:10.1101/19008367.

[54] Xu, Lingyu, et al. "Prediction in Autism by Deep Learning Short-Time Spontaneous Hemodynamic Fluctuations." *Frontiers in Neuroscience*, vol. 13, 2019, doi:10.3389/fnins.2019.01120.

[55] Khozaei, Aida, et al. "Early Screening of Autism Spectrum Disorder Using Cry Features." *PLoS ONE*, vol. 15, no. 12, 2020, doi:10.1101/2019.12.28.19016022.

[56] Yu, Qinlin, et al. "Differential White Matter Maturation from Birth to 8 Years of Age." *Cerebral Cortex*, 2019, doi:10.1093/cercor/bhz268.

[57] Drimalla, Hanna, et al. "Towards the Automatic Detection of Social Biomarkers in Autism Spectrum Disorder: Introducing the Simulated Interaction Task (SIT)." *NPJ Digital Medicine*, vol. 3, no. 1, 2020, doi:10.1038/s41746-020-0227-5.

[58] Baadel, Said, et al. "A Clustering Approach for Autistic Trait Classification." *Informatics for Health and Social Care*, 2020, pp. 1–18, doi:10.1080/17538157.2019.1687482.

[59] Xu, Lingyu, et al. "Classification of Autism Spectrum Disorder Based on Sample Entropy of Spontaneous Functional near Infra-Red Spectroscopy Signal." *Clinical Neurophysiology*, 2020, doi:10.1016/j.clinph.2019.12.400.

[60] Coben, Robert, et al. "EEG Power and Coherence in Autistic Spectrum Disorder." *Clinical Neurophysiology*, vol. 119, no. 5, 2008, pp. 1002–1009, doi:10.1016/j.clinph.2008.01.013.

[61] Yasuhara, Akihiro. "Correlation between EEG Abnormalities and Symptoms of Autism Spectrum Disorder (ASD)." *Brain and Development*, vol. 32, no. 10, 2010, pp. 791–798, doi:10.1016/j.braindev.2010.08.010.

[62] Ahmadlou, Mehran, et al. "Fractality and a Wavelet-Chaos-Neural Network Methodology for EEG-Based Diagnosis of Autistic Spectrum Disorder." *Journal of Clinical Neurophysiology*, vol. 27, no. 5, 2010, pp. 328–333, doi:10.1097/wnp.0b013e3181f40dc8.

[63] Bosl, William, et al. "EEG Complexity as a Biomarker for Autism Spectrum Disorder Risk." *BMC Medicine*, vol. 9, no. 1, 2011, doi:10.1186/1741-7015-9-18.

[64] M Cusenza, et al, "Analysis of awake and sleep EEG in autistic children." *International Journal of Biomagnetism*, vol. 14, no. 2, pp. 80–83, 2012.

[65] Kamel, Mahmoud I., et al. "EEG Based Autism Diagnosis Using Regularized Fisher Linear Discriminant Analysis." *International Journal of Image, Graphics and Signal Processing*, vol. 4, no. 3, 2012, pp. 35–41, doi:10.5815/ijigsp.2012.03.06.

[66] Ahmadlou, Mehran, et al. "Fuzzy Synchronization Likelihood-Wavelet Methodology for Diagnosis of Autism Spectrum Disorder." *Journal of Neuroscience Methods*, vol. 211, no. 2, 2012, pp. 203–209, doi:10.1016/j.jneumeth.2012.08.020.

[67] Diessen, Eric Van, et al. "Increased Power of Resting-State Gamma Oscillations in Autism Spectrum Disorder Detected by Routine Electroencephalography." *European Archives of Psychiatry and Clinical Neuroscience*, vol. 265, no. 6, 2014, pp. 537–540, doi:10.1007/s00406-014-0527-3.

[68] Galilee, Alena, et al. "Atypical Speech versus Non-Speech Detection and Discrimination in 4- to 6-Yr Old Children with Autism Spectrum Disorder: An ERP Study." *PLoS ONE*, vol. 12, no. 7, 2017, doi:10.1371/journal.pone.0181354.

[69] Djemal, Ridha, et al. "EEG-Based Computer Aided Diagnosis of Autism Spectrum Disorder Using Wavelet, Entropy, and ANN." *BioMed Research International*, vol. 2017, 2017, pp. 1–9, doi:10.1155/2017/9816591.

[70] Enzo Grossi, et al. "Diagnosis of Autism through EEG Processed by Advanced Computational Algorithms: A Pilot Study." *Computer Methods and Programs in Biomedicine*, vol. 142, 2017, pp. 73–79, doi:10.1016/j.cmpb.2017.02.002.

[71] Keehn, Brandon, et al. "Autism, Attention, and Alpha Oscillations: An Electrophysiological Study of Attentional Capture." *Biological Psychiatry: Cognitive Neuroscience and Neuroimaging*, vol. 2, no. 6, 2017, pp. 528–536, doi:10.1016/j.bpsc.2017.06.006.

[72] Bosl, William J., et al. "EEG Analytics for Early Detection of Autism Spectrum Disorder: A Data-Driven Approach." *Scientific Reports*, vol. 8, no. 1, 2018, doi:10.1038/s41598-018-24318-x.

[73] Dickinson, Abigail, et al. "Interhemispheric Alpha-Band Hypoconnectivity in Children with Autism Spectrum Disorder." *Behavioural Brain Research*, vol. 348, 2018, pp. 227–234, doi:10.1016/j.bbr.2018.04.026.

[74] Kang, Jiannan, et al. "EEG-Based Multi-Feature Fusion Assessment for Autism." *Journal of Clinical Neuroscience*, vol. 56, 2018, pp. 101–107, doi:10.1016/j.jocn.2018.06.049.

[75] Heunis, T., et al. "Recurrence Quantification Analysis of Resting State EEG Signals in Autism Spectrum Disorder—a Systematic Methodological Exploration of Technical and Demographic Confounders in the Search for Biomarkers." *BMC Medicine*, vol. 16, no. 1, 2018, doi:10.1186/s12916-018-1086-7.

[76] Abdulhay, Enas, et al. "Computer-Aided Autism Diagnosis via Second-Order Difference Plot Area Applied to EEG Empirical Mode Decomposition." *Neural Computing and Applications*, 2018, doi:10.1007/s00521-018-3738-0.

[77] Thapaliya, Sashi, et al. "Evaluating the EEG and Eye Movements for Autism Spectrum Disorder." *2018 IEEE International Conference on Big Data (Big Data)*, 2018, doi:10.1109/bigdata.2018.8622501.

[78] Ibrahim, Sutrisno, et al. "Electroencephalography (EEG) Signal Processing for Epilepsy and Autism Spectrum Disorder Diagnosis." *Biocybernetics and Biomedical Engineering*, vol. 38, no. 1, 2018, pp. 16–26, doi:10.1016/j.bbe.2017.08.006.

[79] Shou, Guofa, et al. "Resting-State Gamma-Band EEG Abnormalities in Autism." *2018 40th Annual International Conference of the IEEE Engineering in Medicine and Biology Society (EMBC)*, 2018, doi:10.1109/embc.2018.8512718.

[80] An, Kyung-Min, et al. "Altered Gamma Oscillations during Motor Control in Children with Autism Spectrum Disorder." *The Journal of Neuroscience*, vol. 38, no. 36, 2018, pp. 7878–7886, doi:10.1523/jneurosci.1229-18.2018.

[81] Lefebvre, Aline, et al. "Alpha Waves as a Neuromarker of Autism Spectrum Disorder: The Challenge of Reproducibility and Heterogeneity." *Frontiers in Neuroscience*, vol. 12, 2018, doi:10.3389/fnins.2018.00662.

[82] Bosl, William J., et al. "EEG Analytics for Early Detection of Autism Spectrum Disorder: A Data-Driven Approach." *Scientific Reports*, vol. 8, no. 1, 2018, doi:10.1038/s41598-018-24318-x.

[83] Wilkinson, Carol L., et al. "Reduced Frontal Gamma Power at 24 Months Is Associated with Better Expressive Language in Toddlers at Risk for Autism." *Autism Research*, vol. 12, no. 8, 2019, pp. 1211–1224, doi:10.1002/aur.2131.

[84] Hadoush, Hikmat, et al. "Brain Complexity in Children with Mild and Severe Autism Spectrum Disorders: Analysis of Multiscale Entropy in EEG." *Brain Topography*, vol. 32, no. 5, 2019, pp. 914–921, doi:10.1007/s10548-019-00711-1.

[85] Distefano, Charlotte, et al. "EEG Data Collection in Children with ASD: The Role of State in Data Quality and Spectral Power." *Research in Autism Spectrum Disorders*, vol. 57, 2019, pp. 132–144, doi:10.1016/j.rasd.2018.10.001.

[86] Nicotera, Antonio Gennaro, et al. "EEG Abnormalities as a Neurophysiological Biomarker of Severity in Autism Spectrum Disorder: A Pilot Cohort Study." *Journal of Autism and Developmental Disorders*, vol. 49, no. 6, 2019, pp. 2337–2347, doi:10.1007/s10803-019-03908-2.

[87] Jan, Reem K., et al. "Neural Processing of Dynamic Animated Social Interactions in Young Children with Autism Spectrum Disorder: A High-Density

Electroencephalography Study." *Frontiers in Psychiatry*, vol. 10, 2019, doi:10.3389/fpsyt.2019.00582.

[88] Hornung, Taylor, et al. "Dopaminergic Hypo-Activity and Reduced Theta-Band Power in Autism Spectrum Disorder: A Resting-State EEG Study." *International Journal of Psychophysiology*, vol. 146, 2019, pp. 101–106, doi:10.1016/j.ijpsycho.2019.08.012.

[89] Hadoush, Hikmat, et al. "Automated Identification for Autism Severity Level: EEG Analysis Using Empirical Mode Decomposition and Second Order Difference Plot." *Behavioural Brain Research*, vol. 362, 2019, pp. 240–248, doi:10.1016/j.bbr.2019.01.018.

[90] Haartsen, Rianne, et al. "Functional EEG Connectivity in Infants Associates with Later Restricted and Repetitive Behaviours in Autism; a Replication Study." *Translational Psychiatry*, vol. 9, no. 1, 2019, doi:10.1038/s41398-019-0380-2.

[91] Scheffler, Aaron W., et al. "Covariate-Adjusted Region-Referenced Generalized Functional Linear Model for EEG Data." *Statistics in Medicine*, vol. 38, no. 30, 2019, pp. 5587–5602, doi:10.1002/sim.8384.

[92] Lauttia, Jenni, et al. "Atypical Pattern of Frontal EEG Asymmetry for Direct Gaze in Young Children with Autism Spectrum Disorder." *Journal of Autism and Developmental Disorders*, vol. 49, no. 9, 2019, pp. 3592–3601, doi:10.1007/s10803-019-04062-5.

[93] Sinha, Tulikapriya, et al. "An Efficient Approach for Detection of Autism Spectrum Disorder Using Electroencephalography Signal." *IETE Journal of Research*, 2019, pp. 1–9, doi:10.1080/03772063.2019.1622462.

[94] Jayawardana, Yasith, et al. "Analysis of Temporal Relationships between ASD and Brain Activity through EEG and Machine Learning." *2019 IEEE 20th International Conference on Information Reuse and Integration for Data Science (IRI)*, 2019, doi:10.1109/iri.2019.00035.

[95] Haputhanthri, Dilantha, et al. "An EEG Based Channel Optimized Classification Approach for Autism Spectrum Disorder." *2019 Moratuwa Engineering Research Conference (MERCon)*, 2019, doi:10.1109/mercon.2019.8818814.

[96] Kang, Jiannan, et al. "EEG Entropy Analysis in Autistic Children." *Journal of Clinical Neuroscience*, vol. 62, 2019, pp. 199–206, doi:10.1016/j.jocn.2018.11.027.

[97] Bajestani, Ghasem Sadeghi, et al. "Diagnosis of Autism Spectrum Disorder Based on Complex Network Features." *Computer Methods and Programs in Biomedicine*, vol. 177, 2019, pp. 277–283, doi:10.1016/j.cmpb.2019.06.006.

[98] D'Croz-Baron, David F., et al. "EEG Microstates Analysis in Young Adults with Autism Spectrum Disorder during Resting-State." *Frontiers in Human Neuroscience*, vol. 13, 2019, doi:10.3389/fnhum.2019.00173.

[99] Cook, Ian A., et al. "EEG Spectral Features in Sleep of Autism Spectrum Disorders in Children with Tuberous Sclerosis Complex." *Journal of Autism and Developmental Disorders*, vol. 50, no. 3, 2019, pp. 916–923, doi:10.1007/s10803-019-04326-0.

[100] Gabard-Durnam, Laurel J., et al. "Longitudinal EEG Power in the First Postnatal Year Differentiates Autism Outcomes." *Nature Communications*, vol. 10, no. 1, 2019, doi:10.1038/s41467-019-12202-9.

[101] Kang, Jiannan, et al. "The Identification of Children with Autism Spectrum Disorder by SVM Approach on EEG and Eye-Tracking Data." *Computers in Biology and Medicine*, vol. 120, 2020, p. 103722, doi:10.1016/j.compbiomed.2020.103722.

[102] Donck, Stephanie Van Der, et al. "Rapid Neural Categorization of Angry and Fearful Faces Is Specifically Impaired in Boys with Autism Spectrum Disorder." *Journal of Child Psychology and Psychiatry*, 2020, doi:10.1111/jcpp.13201.

[103] Abdolzadegan, Donya, et al. "A Robust Method for Early Diagnosis of Autism Spectrum Disorder from EEG Signals Based on Feature Selection and DBSCAN Method." *Biocybernetics and Biomedical Engineering*, vol. 40, no. 1, 2020, pp. 482–493, doi:10.1016/j.bbe.2020.01.008.
[104] Pham, The-Hanh, et al. "Autism Spectrum Disorder Diagnostic System Using HOS Bispectrum with EEG Signals." *International Journal of Environmental Research and Public Health*, vol. 17, no. 3, 2020, p. 971, doi:10.3390/ijerph17030971.

Index

For Product Safety Concerns and Information please contact our EU
representative GPSR@taylorandfrancis.com
Taylor & Francis Verlag GmbH, Kaufingerstraße 24, 80331 München, Germany

www.ingramcontent.com/pod-product-compliance
Lightning Source LLC
Chambersburg PA
CBHW060341220326
41598CB00023B/2778

* 9 7 8 1 0 3 2 0 7 5 9 8 3 *